Complementary Therapies for LYMPHEDEMA

Jean LaMantia, RD

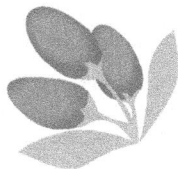

To all those with lymphedema,
I hope you find the ideal combination of conventional and complementary therapies to help you feel your best with lymphedema.

To lymphedema professionals,
I hope this book helps you find the ideal services to offer and enables you to expand your network so that you can cultivate a circle of providers working toward a common mission of helping people with lymphedema.

To the researchers,
thank you for all you do to improve our understanding of lymphedema and how to care for it. I hope this book inspires you to keep going!

Contents

Part One
Traditional Therapies

Part Two
Body Work

Part Three
Natural Health Products

Part Four
High-Tech Devices

Part Five
Final Thoughts

About the Author

I joined the lymphedema community in late 2016, when I started seeing clients for nutrition consultations at a lymphedema clinic near my city. As far as I knew, I was the only registered dietitian in this space, and my nerdy little self tingled at the idea of exploring a completely new area. It felt right to dedicate myself to lymphedema, because I had my own experience with the lymphatic system: Mine tried to kill me when I was diagnosed with lymphoma—cancer originating in the lymphatic system—at the age of twenty-seven.

Since I began helping to support individuals with lymphedema and the professionals that care for them, I've co-written *The Complete Lymphedema Management and Nutrition Guide*, now in its second edition, and I've spoken at the Canadian Lymphedema Framework Conference, the National Lymphedema Network Conference, the American Vein and Lymphatic Society Conference, the Food and Nutrition Conference and Expo, Power Lymphatics, and several provincial and state conferences to spread the word that nutrition matters for people with lymphedema. I am also the recipient of the Distinguished Practice Award from the Oncology Dietetics Practice Group, largely due to my contributions related to lymphedema risk reduction and management in the cancer community.

For professionals, I created the course Lymphedema Nutrition for Health Professionals, which is available on my website: www.jeanlamantia.com. I also offer a digital seminar on Nutrition Strategies for Lymphedema: Practical Solutions to Improve Patient Outcomes at PESI.com, where you can earn CEUs. If you want to become a certified lymphedema therapist in a program that includes my nutrition content, that option is available from the American Academy of Lymphatic and Wound Management certification program at aalwm.us. In addition, I'm working on publishing academic papers on lymphedema nutrition. In short, I think nutrition plays a huge role in lymphedema management, and I'm on a mission to share that message.

For individuals living with lymphedema, I've created Lymphedema Nutrition

School, which is available as a small-group, live, ten-week program over Zoom, as well as a self-study version. I've also produced several lymphedema and lipedema journals to help clients track their lymphedema, self-care and nutrition, as well as teaching tools for health professionals. I've even started my own creative little Etsy shop, called LymphedemaCollection, where I sell products to help spread awareness of lymphedema in a cute or clever way.

I'm grateful that my lymphatic system is now working well and my treatment was successful. I feel driven to help others that have issues with their lymphatic system and lymphedema specifically. I hope you are able to learn and advance in your lymphedema care based on my work, as I will continue to learn from my clients, fellow professionals and researchers in this space and to be an advocate for lymphedema.

Jean LaMantia
    Registered Dietitian
    www.jeanlamantia.com

SCAN ME

Preface

When you are dealing with lymphedema, you might sometimes find yourself wondering if there is something missing from your treatment or if you are really doing everything you can to improve your condition. Or, as a health care provider, you might ask yourself, "Is there is anything else I can do to help my patients?" You might do an online search or go on social media and see someone talking about a supplement they are taking or a device they are using, and wonder whether it would work for you. If you identify with this experience, then this book is for you!

My Motivation

I'm a self-professed nutrition nerd. That means I love to get lost in the PubMed database, the US National Institutes of Health's National Library of Medicine, developed and maintained by the National Center for Biotechnology Information. This library of published medical research is where scientists and medical practitioners look for research to answer our pertinent questions.

In March 2015, I was able to visit the location in person and peer into the glass-enclosed room that houses the servers when I traveled to Maryland as the recipient of the John Milner Nutrition and Cancer Prevention Research Practicum. On the tour, our guides told us that during a snowstorm, the folks that keep the servers working stay in that room until their replacements can make it to the site. That's how seriously they take their responsibility to keep the information accessible, and I appreciate them for it!

Although I'm a nutrition nerd, I am also open-minded. I don't dismiss new ideas out of hand simply because I'm not familiar with them. But I do approach each new idea with a healthy dose of skepticism. As I like to say, "I'm open-minded, but not so open-minded that my brain falls out." With this book, I try to strike the right balance between getting caught up in "shiny new object syndrome" and dismissing every new idea.

My Purpose

I created this resource to help you answer the question "What else can I do?" For many people in the cancer community, complementary therapies are part of the journey, but credible information about them is often lacking. I see the same need in the lymphedema community. I want to offer patients and practitioners an unbiased source of information on the complementary therapies you may see online so that you know your options, their pros and cons, and where you can learn more about them.

But I had to draw the line somewhere, or this book would never be finished. For that reason, I will not cover therapies involving medications, surgery or nutrition. And, of course, I will not discuss complete decongestive therapy (CDT) —that is not a complementary therapy, it is *the* mainstream therapy.

I do strongly believe that your diet affects your lymphedema, and I encourage you to access the many resources I created to get more information on nutrition for lymphedema. Spoiler: There isn't one "lymphedema diet," but there are many tested strategies that I have seen make a significant difference for my clients and students.

For lymphedema patients, I hope the information provided here enables you to believe you are doing everything possible for your lymphedema and have found the ideal self-care routine to help you feel your best. There are many new (and old) strategies you can try so that your lymphedema doesn't get too comfortable with the same routine. I also want to give you hope, as there is active research going on in this area.

For health professionals, my goal is to give you an excellent reference to help you address your patients' questions, determine which complementary therapies to incorporate into your practice and decide what new referral sources to bring into the circle of care you offer your patients.

For researchers, I hope this book inspires you to design the high-quality clinical trials that are so badly needed in this community. I've got 101 ideas for you!

Although I did have lymphoma—lymph node cancer—which has made me appreciate my lymphatic system, I do not personally live with lymphedema. But I hear every day from my clients and students the impact that this condition has on their lives; this book is one more way for me to be helpful and supportive.

Whether you choose to try any of these complementary therapies is up to you. You must decide for yourself, along with your lymphedema therapist and support team. A mention in this book is not a recommendation or endorsement for any particular therapy.

My Methodology

My methodology in writing this book involved three steps. First, figure out what people are talking about and promoting for lymphedema care. Second, track down the latest evidence on these therapies and review references to find other research. And third, provide an unbiased, easy-to-read analysis and summary of the research, stating both the findings and the side effects and risks. I did not use AI; I did it all the old-fashioned way—by reading every research article and highlighting the key points.

My goal is a balanced approach that shares both the potential benefits and the potential drawbacks of each therapy. I've included all my references, and I encourage you to use them as jumping-off points for your own research.

Considerations for Choosing a Therapy

How do you know what therapy to try? Here's where I take off my science hat and encourage you to notice what you are drawn to. With 101 different complementary therapies on offer, you need to have a starting place. You certainly don't want to do too much all at once, as you'll need to systemically evaluate what works and what doesn't work for your ideal lymphedema management and your ideal lymphedema management team. If all this book offers you is confirmation that you're already following the exact right protocol for your lymphedema, there is value in that peace too.

Building a team of trusted professionals around you is a good way to care for yourself. Nowadays, health professionals are highly specialized, and most are cautious to practice only within their scope, so it's not likely that one person can be a one-stop shop for all your needs. For example, your team may include a certified lymphedema therapist, a registered dietitian, an acupuncturist and a yoga instructor. Building a trusted team can take time, but referrals from health professionals or others with lymphedema can help. If you decide to try any of the complementary therapies discussed in this book, please do so with the full knowledge of your certified lymphedema therapist.

Limitations

I was educated in English, and while I have a working knowledge of other languages, I restricted this work to include research (or at least abstracts) published in English only. Also, because I am registered to practice in Canada and the United States, this work is written from that perspective, which will inevitably introduce some unintended bias.

Another limitation of this work is the focus of researchers on breast cancer survivors with arm lymphedema. There are only a few studies of gynecological cancer survivors with leg lymphedema, a few on filarial lymphedema in the legs and one on breast lymphedema. These gaps in the research will likely be discouraging for those with less studied types of lymphedema, and I sincerely hope they are filled in soon.

I may be missing some therapies or some studies; although I did my best to find them all, it's inevitable that I missed some. My goal is to continually update this book as new research is published and new complementary therapies are introduced. I chose to self-publish this book to make updates fast and easy. If I've missed something, please reach out.

These are summaries of the research, and although not every detail is included, I've been diligent about providing accurate references so you can read the studies yourself. In the end, you may not agree with my "bottom line"—it is not intended to be universally accepted, but simply a synopsis of the information. I encourage you to use your own personal and professional experience to come to your own conclusions.

Finally, I was educated in allopathic, evidence-based Western medicine, and that is the framework for my analysis. Not all complementary therapies evolve from this structure.

My Hope

I hope you find answers here that will support you as you live with this chronic disease. Know that this book comes to you along with my best wishes.

Chapter 1
Introduction to the Lymphatic System and Lymphedema

Everybody has a lymphatic system, although some admittedly work better than others. The lymphatic system is a collection of lymphatic vessels, capillaries and nodes that transport fluid, are a key part of the immune system and allow the body to absorb fats and fat-soluble vitamins from the diet.

Lymphedema is a chronic swelling condition in which the body pools lymphatic fluid. The first line of treatment, and the gold standard of lymphedema management, is complete decongestive therapy (CDT), also referred to as "conservative treatment" in the research. CDT has four components: exercise, skin care, compression and manual lymphatic drainage (MLD).

The professionals who treat lymphedema are called certified lymphedema therapists. They are health professionals such as massage therapists, physical therapists, occupational therapists and nurses who have completed additional training in lymphedema management. If you don't already have a therapist, finding one should be your first step. Check out my blog *Lymphedema Resources*, which has links to lymphedema associations and training schools to help you find a therapist near you, see About the Author, page x, for a QR code to my website, or go to www.jeanlamantia.com.

Detailed information on the lymphatic system, lymphedema and complete decongestive therapy, including lots of photos and diagrams, can be found in the book *The Complete Lymphedema Management and Nutrition Guide*, by Jean LaMantia and Ann DiMenna, available wherever books are sold.

This book will not cover conventional CDT. Instead, it covers all of the *other* therapies, which I call complementary therapies. I can't emphasize enough that complementary therapies are meant to *complement*, not replace, CDT. If you are brand-new to learning about lymphedema, then be sure to read *The Complete Lymphedema Management and Nutrition Guide* as well as this book so that you understand both CDT and complementary therapies, and be sure to keep an open communication with your lymphedema therapist if you are considering any changes to your care.

Chapter 2
Complementary, Alternative and Integrative Care

I've worked in the cancer community for a few decades, and complementary and alternative care is big. I remember a book that came out about twenty years ago that detailed the basics of each therapy and how to find more information; it was such a relief for me, as a practitioner, to have all the information in one place. That resource was my inspiration for this book. Before we jump in, let's begin with two important definitions:

- **Alternative therapy** is done *in place of*, or as an alternative to, the standard therapy.
- **Complementary therapy** is done *in addition to*, or as a complement to, the standard therapy.

This is an important distinction; complementary and alternative therapies are not the same thing, even though people often use these terms synonymously. For definitions of other important terms, see the glossary on page 289.

Classifying Complementary Therapies

Complementary approaches are generally classified into one of four categories: Nutritional, such as special diets or supplements, psychological, such as mindfulness, cognitive behavior therapy, physical, such as tai chi or dry brushing and combinations, such as yoga, which combines physical and psychological aspects, or mindful eating, which combines nutritional and psychological aspects.

I've divided this book into four parts: 1) Traditional Therapies; 2) Body Work; 3) Natural Health Products; and 4) High-Tech Devices. Within each category, I've provided the following information:

- **What Is It?**
- **History of** (in the Traditional Therapies section only)
- **Lymphedema-Specific Research** (human research)
- **Side Effects/Risks**
- **Bottom Line**
- **References**

Where there isn't any, or enough, lymphedema-specific human research, I've provided animal research on lymphedema labelled under **"Lymphedema Research in Animals"** or human research on a related condition, labeled as **"Related Research"**. I've designed the book so you can either read it cover to cover or use it as a reference guide to quickly get the information you need on a particular modality.

As much as I would like to think of myself as innovative for bringing complementary therapies for lymphedema to light, authors Michael Bernas and Marlys Witte from the University of Arizona wrote about them over two decades ago in their editorial entitled "Alternative/Complementary Treatment in Lymphology: Trying the Untried and Testing the Untested," where they stated:

> *"Because there is no ideal, simple clinical answer or cure for most patients with lymphedema and treatment commitment is life-long, we need to be open to new ideas and creative, low-cost, low-maintenance approaches while at the same time demanding evidence of efficacy and assurance of safety and protection for our patients. In this light, alternative/complementary therapies may in the future be important adjuncts in the developing as well as the more developed world"* (Bernas 2004).

I think their statement is still true today, and I hope my efforts help advance this goal.

Evaluating Complementary Therapies

As a patient or practitioner, how do you evaluate complementary therapies? When I was training to become a registered dietitian, the concept of "evidence-based practice" was drilled into us, with "evidence" meaning published scientific evidence, which was valued over anecdotal evidence (the experience of the practitioner when helping their patients). But any health care provider will need to balance these two sources of information, and patients may rely more heavily on one type of evidence over another.

When it comes to scientific evidence, there is a hierarchy, known simply as the "hierarchy of evidence." It is usually represented as a pyramid. The types of research at the top are the most valued, and those at the bottom are given the least amount of weight when it comes to evidence-informed decision-making. For example, an evidence-informed practitioner would not change their practice based on the results of an animal study or a case study, which are in the bottom tiers. A case study is essentially the experience of an individual patient, or a group of patients in a case series. The patient and the practitioner know what intervention was used, and the case study simply describes what happened as a result.

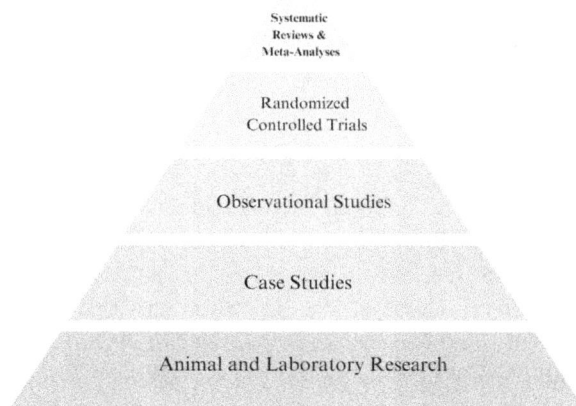

Hierarchy of Evidence. Image adapted from Wallace 2022

In the next tier up, observational studies are designed to find associations between two different factors. An example would be a finding that women who consume more soy foods have lower rates of breast cancer. In an observational study, you can't know that the soy foods were the *cause* of the lower rates, only that they were *associated* (correlated) with them. An expression used to emphasize this point is "correlation is not causation."

Next up are randomized controlled trials, clinical studies in which subjects are randomly assigned to receive either the intervention or a control. When the study is double-blinded, neither the patient nor the assessor know what intervention they received. For example, if fifty people with lymphedema are enrolled in a study, and twenty-five are randomly assigned to receive low-level laser treatment by a certified practitioner while the other half receive a fake laser treatment, the practitioner would know who gets the real treatment, but they wouldn't tell the patient or the assessor who measures the lymphedema. Double-blinding helps to reduce the risk of bias.

Finally, in the top tier, a systematic review is a detailed search of databases for research on a specific topic. First, researchers look in one or more databases for a defined set of search terms; for example, in a systematic review and meta-analysis of acupuncture, moxibustion and lymphedema, the researchers described their search terms as "breast cancer," "breast cancer–related lymphedema," "lymphedema," "acupuncture" and "moxibustion," as well as their relevant derivatives (Xu 2024). Researchers cast a wide net so they don't miss any research on a specific topic. In this case, they found 886 published articles. Then a team reviews the articles to make sure they fit any other criteria of the search, such as only randomized controlled trials, only trials published during certain years, or only leg lymphedema or arm lymphedema. Once only the studies that meet the criteria remain, then the detailed reading and analysis of the work begins. This meta-analysis is essentially a study of studies; by increasing the total number of participants studied, researchers can get a better understanding of true outcomes.

When deciding what research to include in this book, I chose from the top of the pyramid first. Unfortunately, both lymphedema and complementary therapies are under-researched, so I was often happy to find any type of research at all. When research from the top of the pyramid wasn't available, I shared with you whatever studies I found. My "Bottom Line" summary at the end of each treatment review bears this in mind. For example, I won't recommend a complementary therapy when the only research available is an animal study. (To be clear, I do not recommend any treatment discussed in this book as an alternative to complete decongestive therapy with a certified lymphedema therapist.)

In addition to sharing the evidence I uncovered, I conducted surveys of patients and professionals with first-hand experience of particular therapies, and I've included the results under the heading "Survey Says." Their comments, whether positive or negative, appear as "User Experiences" (reviews from patients) and "Anecdotal Reports" (reviews from lymphedema therapists). I offered my respondents the option of using their names (and their clinic names) or of being anonymous. Where explanations of technical or research lingo are needed, I provide them in "Technical Breakdown" boxes, and I offer my notes to other lymphedema professionals in boxes called "Between Professionals." For the professionals reading this book, you'll find the source citations listed at the end of each treatment review so you can do more research and decide what is right for your practice and your clients.

There are two factors to consider when deciding whether to try a complementary therapy for your lymphedema:

1. Cost versus benefit
2. Risk versus benefit

Lymphedema is an expensive condition to treat. When you spend money on a therapy, you want to see results. Granted, some of the therapies are quite inexpensive (for example, you can buy a head of cabbage for under five dollars), but the higher-tech options can cost hundreds or even thousands of dollars. Any money spent on a complementary therapy could be money spent on a proven therapy, so choose carefully. As a tip, before you invest, be sure you know the return policy and find out if you can try the product to evaluate whether you will tolerate it.

A risk-benefit analysis considers how you might respond to a treatment. A low-risk therapy like deep breathing is easy to say yes to, as it has an excellent risk-benefit profile. With coumarin, on the other hand, there is a risk of liver toxicity, so you would need to consider very carefully whether this risk is worth the potential benefits. I've reported the documented side effects, but do your own research before you begin. Some therapies also have a long list of contraindications, so be sure to check the manufacturer's website or ask your lymphedema therapist to avoid potential adverse reactions.

Direct Versus Indirect Risk

When it comes to complementary care, it's important to recognize two areas of risk: direct and indirect. Direct risk, often called a side effect or adverse reaction, comes from using a treatment, while an indirect risk occurs when a patient is harmed by a delay in getting effective treatment because they were using an ineffective one. Indirect risk is lessened by choosing to use a therapy as complementary rather than alternative (Stub 2018).

Anecdotal Report

"I have integrated complementary therapies into my clinic care for many years. I find that my patients improve and heal deeper with the combination of CDT, mindfulness practices and yoga interventions."

—**Barbara, lymphedema therapist, Balance With Babz Lymph Flow Yoga, Massachusetts**

Surveys of Complementary Therapy Use in Lymphedema

In an Australian study from 2011, researchers sent out surveys to members of the Lymphoedema Association of Queensland (Finnane 2011). They received ninety-five completed responses addressing questions about the members' use of complementary therapies for their lymphedema in the past twelve months. Of the women in the sample who had lymphedema due to breast or gynecological cancers, 45% reported using a complementary therapy, and half of those had used more than one. The most common complementary treatments at that time were Chi Machine, tai chi, vitamin E or selenium supplements, meditation and yoga. The study considered mainstream therapies to be compression, exercise, skin care, manual lymphatic drainage, laser therapy and ultrasound (I include laser and ultrasound as complementary therapies in this book). Interestingly, the perceived effectiveness of the complementary therapies and mainstream therapies were almost the same.

I couldn't find any similar surveys published more recently, but I suspect the use of complementary therapies for lymphedema has grown since this research was published. While I was writing this book, I prepared a survey about complementary therapy use, and I've included the results and relevant comments in the appropriate sections. Forty people responded to my survey, of whom twenty-six had lymphedema, three had lymphedema themselves and were also lymphedema therapists, seven were certified lymphedema therapists and two were the parent of a child with lymphedema; two didn't respond to that question. Of my forty respondents, thirty-four (85%) had used a complementary therapy.

Integrative Therapy

An integrative therapy is one that considers mind, body and spirit and combines conventional and complementary therapies. Examples of integrated therapies are beginning to appear in the lymphedema research, as the examples below demonstrate.

REVIEW #1: LEAL 2009

Physiotherapists in Brazil published this review paper supporting complementary therapies. Specifically, they concluded that "combined techniques of complete decongestive therapy plus complementary therapies produce the most beneficial effects and depending on the physiopathology of the lymphedema, the physiotherapist should select the best combination, based on a detailed assessment of individual cases."

REVIEW #2: DENG 2024

In this systematic review and meta-analysis of medical interventions (such as ultrasound, shock wave therapy or laser therapy) as a complement to CDT for breast cancer–related lymphedema, the authors recognized that CDT is the first line of treatment but set out to analyze additional treatments patients might seek out. Their meta-analysis included sixteen randomized controlled trials, with a total of 690 participants, on the following complementary therapies: laser, extracorporeal shock wave therapy, electrotherapy, ultrasound, diet, diet + symbiotic supplements, traditional Chinese medicine (TCM), continuous passive motion, and negative pressure massage (cupping). The analysis revealed that the complementary therapies improved lymphedema volume, with laser and electrotherapy being especially effective.

The authors concluded that it is meaningful to discover and promote complementary therapies in clinical practice, to better help patients. But they emphasized that more research is needed to determine who will benefit, the best treatment options and when to begin treatment.

CLINICAL TRIAL: CAVEZZI 2020

The authors described this study as "an intensive CDT and holistic protocol." In a six-day experiment, forty-one patients with stage 2 or 3 leg lymphedema completed an intensive daily program with twenty minutes of manual lymphatic drainage, forty minutes of electro-sound lymphatic drainage, multilayer short stretch bandaging, a low-carbohydrate diet, anti-inflammatory supplements and exercise. The result was a progressive and statistically significant improvement in limb volume and reduced extracellular fluids.

Although the study was focused on testing a bioimpedance tool to accurately measure lymphedema volume, the authors concluded that their intensive holistic protocol was beneficial in the short term. Obviously, to evaluate whether it is a good integrative health plan for lymphedema, research on this particular protocol would need to be longer-term.

Case Study: Hamlett 2013

In this case study, a woman in her mid-fifties with severe primary lymphedema and painful neuropathy in her lower extremities, obesity and mental stress was treated with a holistic plan designed to address mind, body and spirit. The four-month treatment protocol consisted of resistance training twice a week, cardiovascular training at 70% of perceived exertion, whole-body vibration using the I-Shape vibrating platform, daily meditation and reflection, chair yoga and healthy eating with the guidance of a registered dietitian, using the WeightWatchers Points program. At her final evaluation, the client had lost 20 kilograms (45 pounds) and reduced her cholesterol. Her overall health, stress, quality of life and general outlook on life greatly improved. Her legs had improved fluid movement and less swelling.

Holistic Care Teamwork

A team that thinks holistically can address not just physical issues but other aspects of health as well. You may not have access to a holistic care team, as the woman in the Hamlett case study did, but you can be the center of your own care team by pulling in and coordinating all the team members you need to support you. This type of holistic care plan can also provide culturally sensitive treatment that conforms to your values or those of your patients (Stub 2018).

As the above research indicates, it may be time to start practicing more holistic medicine, building multidisciplinary teams and incorporating more complementary therapies. This book will help you start thinking about your next steps.

Bottom Line on Complementary Therapies

Individuals living with lymphedema and their therapists vary widely in their experience with complementary therapies and willingness to use them. The right balance of conventional and complementary care will evolve as all parties become more familiar and comfortable with the different options. Carefully consider the risk and cost of each treatment versus its potential benefit before making any decisions. The tables on pages 276–77 will help you identify which complementary therapies may be best suited to your particular symptoms.

References for Complementary, Alternative & Integrative Care

Bernas M, Witte M. 2004. Alternative/Complementary Treatment in Lymphology: Trying the Untried and Testing the Untested. *Lymphology* 37 (2): 43–44.

Cavezzi A, Urso SU, Paccasassi S, et al. 2020. Bioimpedance Spectroscopy and Volumetry in the Immediate/Short-Term Monitoring of Intensive Complex Decongestive Treatment of Lymphedema. *Phlebology* 35 (9): 715–23.

Deng C, Wu Z, Cai Z, et al. 2024. Conservative Medical Intervention as a Complement to CDT for BCRL Therapy: A Systematic Review and Meta-Analysis of Randomized Controlled Trials. *Front Oncol* 26 (14): 1361128.

Finnane A, Liu Y, Battistutta D, et al. 2011. Lymphedema After Breast or Gynecological Cancer: Use and Effectiveness of Mainstream and Complementary Therapies. *J Altern Complement Med* 17 (9): 867–69.

Hamlett P. 2013. "A Holistic Approach to Lymphedema Treatment and Case Study." Accessed July 12, 2025. https://www.researchgate.net/publication/273772739_A_HOLISTIC_APPROACH_TO_LYMPHEDEMA_TREATMENT_1_A_Holistic_Approach_to_Lymphedema_Treatment.

Leal NF, Carrara HH, Vieira KF, Ferreira CH. 2009. Physiotherapy Treatments for Breast Cancer-Related Lymphedema: A Literature Review. *Rev Lat Am Enfermagem* 17 (5): 730–36.

Stub T, Quandt SA, Arcury TA, et al. 2018. Attitudes and Knowledge About Direct and Indirect Risks Among Conventional and Complementary Health Care Providers in Cancer Care. *BMC Complement Altern Med* 18 (1): 44.

Wallace SS, Barak G, Truong G, Parker MW. 2022. Hierarchy of Evidence Within the Medical Literature. *Hosp Pediatr* 12 (8): 745–50.

Xu Y, Yu J, Shen R, et al. 2024. Comparison Efficacy and Safety of Acupuncture and Moxibustion Therapies in Breast Cancer-Related Lymphedema: A Systematic Review and Network Meta-analysis. *PLoS One* 19 (5): e0303513.

Part One
Traditional Therapies

Introduction to Traditional Therapies

These therapies are low-tech approaches—no power outlets needed. Many of them also lack robust scientific evidence; they are more like folk medicine or home remedies, though some have been used for hundreds or even thousands of years. I reveal and discuss their origins and share what I found in the research to help you decide if one of these treatments is right for you.

SURVEY SAYS

In my survey of complementary therapy use, the most popular traditional therapies were yoga (eighteen respondents, 45%), castor oil (fourteen respondents, 35%), meditation (thirteen respondents, 33%) and cupping (ten respondents, 25%). All of the therapies discussed in this section had been tried by at least one of my respondents, with the exceptions of moxibustion, tuina and Wenyang Huoxue compress.

Acupressure

What Is It?

Acupressure, sometimes called acupoint massage, involves applying pressure to specific points on the body using hands, fingers, thumbs, elbows, feet or various noninvasive devices. It is typically painless and does not include needles; you can think of it as needle-free acupuncture. The goal is to stimulate acupressure points, or trigger points, to clear blockages in qi (energy).

"Acupressure" can also be used as a general term for any therapy that stimulates acupoints on the meridians. Others include acupuncture (page 15), tuina (page 56), moxibustion (page 46), Lidong needling therapy (page 89) and transcutaneous electrical acupoint stimulation (page 262). Using the term "acupoint massage" can help avoid confusion.

History of Acupressure

Acupressure is part of traditional Chinese and Indian medicine practice and is based on the belief that the body contains energy that flows through meridians throughout the body. By applying pressure to certain points, the practitioner can remove blockages and bring harmony back to the body. Acupressure may have originated in China, or may have been brought from India to China along with Buddhism.

Lymphedema-Specific Research

A meta-analysis reported on sixteen studies that focused on stimulating acupressure points to either prevent or treat lymphedema (Shen 2025). Nine of the studies used acupoint massage for breast cancer–related lymphedema. One used tuina and one used transcutaneous electrical acupoint stimulation.

A study that compared acupressure plus Chinese medicine poultices and medium-frequency pulse therapy to CDT found that the combined complementary therapies achieved superior results (Bi 2017). Another study demonstrated lowered blood levels of inflammation with acupoint massage (Li 2022).

In their summary, the authors of the meta-analysis stated that the studies had consistently shown acupressure to be effective for lymphedema prevention and treatment, and for improving limb function and quality of life. They concluded that acupressure is an accessible and cost-effective complementary therapy for lymphedema, to alleviate swelling, pain and discomfort.

However, due to the small sample sizes of the studies, further research is needed and could help to define the ideal acupoints to use and the frequency and duration of treatments.

Side Effects/Risks

None reported.

Bottom Line on Acupressure

Acupressure—or, more specifically, acupoint massage—is a needle-free method of stimulating acupressure points to improve the flow of energy in the body. One meta-analysis described sixteen studies of acupressure, including nine specifically on acupoint massage, and found it to be effective at reducing lymphedema volume, discomfort and pain. Acupoint massage seems like an excellent candidate for further exploration: The risk is low, as is the cost, because it can be self-administered. It can alleviate concerns about needles. While Western medicine can't explain how this ancient treatment works, it does appear to have benefits that may make it worth exploring.

References for Acupressure

Bi J, Wang F, Feng J. 2017. Clinical Observation of Acupoint Massage Nursing Intervention on Postoperative Limb Lymphatic Edema of Breast Cancer Patients. [In Chinese.] *Guangm J Chin Med* 32: 136–37.

Li R, Wang Y, Fan Y. 2022. Effect of Acupoint Massage Combined with Early Rehabilitation Training on Short-Term and Midterm Prognosis of Patients after Breast Cancer Surgery. [In Chinese.] *J Clin Nurs Prac* 8 (9): 6–14.

Shen A, Li M, Ning H, et al. 2025. The Promising Application of Acupressure for Management of Cancer-Related Lymphedema: A Scoping Review. *Asia Pac J Oncol Nurs* 12 (February): 100669.

Acupuncture

What Is It?

Acupuncture is an important part of traditional Chinese medicine that has been brought into more mainstream Western medicine by physiotherapists, chiropractors and other health care workers. It is based on activating points along meridians using fine needles that move energy (qi) throughout the body. It can also include moxibustion (see page 46)—heating of the acupressure points, usually by burning dried and ground mugwort plant (*Artemisia vulgaris*).

History of Acupuncture

Acupuncture is believed to have originated in China thousands of years ago. Knowledge of it spread along Arab trade routes toward the west. In 1972, President Nixon visited China along with *New York Times* reporter James Reston, who received acupuncture after an emergency appendectomy and then wrote about it in the newspaper. In 1997, the US National Institutes of Health (NIH) formally recognized acupuncture as a mainstream medicine and healing option (Hao 2014).

> **User Experience**
> "I have lymphedema in my right leg due to removal of lymph nodes during a hysterectomy for uterine cancer. I used acupuncture every two weeks for a year. I just began drinking Traditional Medicinals ginger tea once daily. The tea seems to be helping. It's difficult to know whether the acupuncture helps, since I also wear compression stockings, which definitely do make a huge difference."
>
> **—Anonymous, Massachusetts (uterine cancer–related lymphedema)**

Lymphedema-Specific Research

There have been many studies and at least three systematic reviews of using acupuncture to treat lymphedema (Chien 2019; Gao 2021; Xu 2024). The most recent systematic review (Xu 2024) analyzed eighteen studies conducted between 2014 and 2023 that included 1,217 patients who had acupuncture or related therapies for breast cancer–related lymphedema. The treatments studied were simple acupuncture and/or moxibustion; bloodletting cupping (also called wet cupping; see page 35); electroacupuncture; gentle moxibustion; and needle-warming moxibustion. Here are the results:

CLINICAL EFFECTIVENESS

- Gentle moxibustion, bloodletting cupping and simple acupuncture had a significantly higher clinical effectiveness rate than functional exercise.
- The treatments with the highest clinical effectiveness rate were needle-warming moxibustion (83%), gentle moxibustion (72%), bloodletting cupping (65%) and simple acupuncture (61%).

REDUCTION IN ARM CIRCUMFERENCE

Six studies including 291 participants revealed that:

- Needle-warming moxibustion was more effective than oral medication.

- There was no significant difference between gentle moxibustion and pneumatic injection.
- Bloodletting cupping performed no better than functional exercise.

REDUCING SWELLING AT THE ELBOW

None of the treatments were shown to reduce swelling at the elbow when the data was analyzed in a network meta-analysis (comparing multiple treatments); however, a pairwise meta-analysis (comparing two treatments) found that:

- Needle-warming moxibustion and bloodletting cupping were both better than usual care (defined in the review as "life care, health education, skin care and so on").
- Bloodletting cupping performed better than oral medication.

A statistical plotting of the results revealed that needle-warming moxibustion was the most effective treatment for elbow swelling, followed by gentle moxibustion and bloodletting cupping.

PAIN REDUCTION

In an analysis of three studies:

- Bloodletting cupping reduced pain significantly more than usual care.
- Simple acupuncture reduced pain better than functional exercise.
- Bloodletting cupping performed no better than functional exercise.

Side Effects/Risks

Five studies reported on a total of ten patients who experienced an adverse event (Xu 2024). In seven of these cases, acupuncture and moxibustion treatments caused local skin discomfort, mild scalding from positional changes, flushing, itching, xerostomia (dry mouth) or swelling. None of the patients withdrew from the research as a result. The treatment with the most reported adverse events was gentle moxibustion.

Many people in the lymphedema community are concerned about needles, especially in a limb with lymphedema, as a possible trigger. Research on the use of acupuncture in over 35,000 Korean cancer survivors found no increased risk of lymphedema for the 5.8% who received acupuncture in the three to six months after cancer surgery (Lee 2024). That said, if you want to experience the benefits of pressure point stimulation without needles, you may wish to try acupressure instead of acupuncture.

Bottom Line on Acupuncture

Unlike many complementary therapies, the effectiveness of acupuncture and related treatments for lymphedema has been evaluated in many trials and at least three meta-analyses. There have been mixed results from the various acupuncture therapies. But looking at simple acupuncture only, the Xu (2024) study found that it had a 61% clinical effectiveness rate and reduced pain better than functional exercise. I've included the other meta-analyses in the references below so you can do additional research if you wish.

Without research comparing the various acupuncture and moxibustion techniques against each other, it's difficult to say which one is most useful, safest and most cost-effective. For the time being, given the multiple parameters, it is difficult to make a blanket statement about the efficacy of acupuncture for lymphedema.

References for Acupuncture

Chien TJ, Liu CY, Fang CJ. 2019. The Effect of Acupuncture in Breast Cancer-Related Lymphoedema (BCRL): A Systematic Review and Meta-analysis. *Integr Cancer Ther* 18 (January–December): 1534735419866910.

Gao Y, Ma T, Han M, et al. 2021. Effects of Acupuncture and Moxibustion on Breast Cancer-Related Lymphedema: A Systematic Review and Meta-Analysis of Randomized Controlled Trials. *Integr Cancer Ther* 20 (January–December): 15347354211044107.

Hao JJ, Mittelman M. 2014. Acupuncture: Past, Present, and Future. *Glob Adv Health Med* 3 (4): 6–8.

Lee Y-S, Lim Y, Yeo J. 2024. Acupuncture Needles and the Risk of Lymphedema After Breast Cancer Surgery: A Retrospective National Cohort Study. *Perspect Integr Med* 3 (1): 29–36.

Xu Y, Yu J, Shen R, et al. 2024. Comparison Efficacy and Safety of Acupuncture and Moxibustion Therapies in Breast Cancer-Related Lymphedema: A Systematic Review and Network Meta-analysis. *PLoS One* 19 (5): e0303513.

Apple Cider Vinegar

What Is It?

Apple cider vinegar (often known simply as ACV) is the fermented juice of crushed apples. It contains pectin, vitamins, minerals and acetic acid or citric acid (NatMed 2024), as well as amino acids and polyphenols—specifically flavonoids, which are believed to have health benefits (Abou-Khalil 2024).

Like other vinegars, ACV goes through two fermentations. In the first, yeast converts the natural sugars in the apples to ethanol alcohol; in the second, acetic acid bacteria convert the ethanol to acetic acid.

ACV is found in most grocery stores, and most brands contain 5% acetic acid. Check the label for other considerations that may be important to you, such as whether the product is filtered, pasteurized, raw, and/or organic, and whether it includes the "mother." Here's a rundown of what these terms mean:

- **Filtered:** The vinegar is passed through a filter that captures the solid particles. Filtered apple cider vinegar will be less cloudy, and there will be less sediment in the bottle.
- **Pasteurized:** The vinegar is heated to destroy bacteria; people who are immunocompromised should choose pasteurized vinegar to avoid exposure to potentially harmful bacteria.
- **Raw:** The product is unpasteurized; its bacteria have not been destroyed by heat.
- **Organic:** The apples are produced according to organic agricultural practices.
- **Mother:** The mother is the biofilm made up of the bacteria and yeast that participated in the fermentation process, along with cellulose. Vinegar with the mother is cloudier and has more sediment. The mother is harmless if consumed.

Be careful not to buy apple cider–flavored vinegar—white vinegar with apple flavoring and caramel color added—instead of ACV. The research cited below used authentic apple cider vinegar made from fermented crushed apples.

ACV can be eaten in food, is often used as a salad dressing, can be taken in larger amounts for therapeutic benefit and can be applied to the skin. My summary of the related research is divided into oral and topical uses.

Lymphedema-Specific Research

I was unable to find any published studies specifically covering the oral or topical use of ACV for lymphedema.

Related Research

Because there are many online claims that ACV can be used (mostly topically) to treat lymphedema, I will discuss the research on using ACV for weight loss and skin ailments, which may be relevant to assisting with lymphedema.

WEIGHT LOSS

In a double-blinded, placebo-controlled study, 120 overweight and obese adolescents and young adults aged twelve to twenty-five years old living in Lebanon were divided into four groups (Abou-Khalil 2024). Each received one of the following drinks every morning for twelve weeks and were told to drink it on an empty stomach:

- 5 milliliters (1 teaspoon) of ACV + 250 milliliters (8 ounces) of water
- 10 milliliters (2 teaspoons) of ACV + 250 milliliters (8 ounces) of water
- 15 milliliters (1 tablespoon) of ACV + 250 milliliters (8 ounces) of water
- Placebo (water that tasted and looked like ACV had been added, but that in fact contained lactic acid)

Neither the participants nor the researchers knew which participant had received which solution. Importantly, the subjects were instructed to continue with their usual diet and activities.

The addition of ACV to the diet resulted in significant decreases in body weight at weeks four, eight and twelve as compared to starting weight. The greatest weight reduction came from the group drinking 15 milliliters (1 tablespoon) of ACV in 250 milliliters (8 ounces) of water. In addition to weight loss, there were reductions in waist and hip circumference and body fat ratio.

Those who drank the look-alike placebo experienced no significant changes in their weight, circumference measurements or body fat ratio. Because the participants had not altered their food intake or exercise, the ACV was the only new variable.

BLOOD LIPIDS

A systematic review and meta-analysis examining the role of ACV and blood lipid levels found that ACV had a favorable effect on lowering blood cholesterol and triglycerides, as well as blood sugar levels (Hadi 2021). This finding may have some relevance to lymphedema, as preliminary evidence has found a correlation between an elevated atherogenic index (a calculation of total cholesterol minus HDL cholesterol, divided by HDL cholesterol) and lymphedema risk (Ryu 2016).

SKIN CONDITIONS

Several skin issues are common in lymphedema, including bacterial infections (cellulitis); lymphorrhea (leakage of lymph fluid through cracks in the skin); ulceration (wounds, bed sores, pressure injuries or skin fissures); hyperkeratosis (thickening of the skin, specifically an excess of keratin, which is the fibrous protein that forms our skin); papillomas (benign wart-like growths) and fibromas (benign growths of fibrous or connective tissue); mossy lesions (a large number of small papillomas); frog spawn (multiple larger papillomas); and fungal infections. A well-written paper by Fife et al. (2017) includes plenty of photos if you're interested in seeing what these conditions look like. That study does not mention vinegar as a treatment. Instead, it recommends:

- Carefully washing the skin daily with non-drying cleansers
- Avoiding skin damage by, for example, wearing well-fitting shoes that don't rub, using electric razors to shave and protecting the skin from sunburns
- Moisturizing with bath oils or ceramide-containing emollients
- Using antifungal or antimicrobial dermatological treatments or topical steroids

A review on home remedies reported on the use of different types of vinegar (including ACV) as an antibacterial and antifungal to promote wound healing and treat seborrheic keratosis, among other skin issues (Gaurav 2023). As an antibacterial, daily wound baths or compresses with 1% to 5% vinegar were used for several days to treat chronic non-healing wounds. As an antifungal, vinegar was used in combination with ketoconazole shampoo or as a soak. One study even used vinegar-soaked cotton socks. Unfortunately, this review provided insufficient detail to warrant a recommendation for using any of the treatments for lymphedema.

Outside of the published research, on social media some certified lymphedema therapists report excellent results from treating hyperkeratosis, a common skin issue in lymphedema, with diluted ACV applied topically.

Side Effects/Risks for Oral Use

In the studies where apple cider vinegar was taken by mouth, stomach burning and a vague mention of "apple cider vinegar intolerance" (Hadi 2021) were reported. Another possible side effect is heartburn, also known as gastroesophageal reflux (GER). The Abou-Khalil study excluded those subjects who reported GER in the initial stages of the research; the remaining 120 participants reported no side effects over the twelve weeks.

There is one case report of hypokalemia (low blood potassium levels), hyper-reninemia (an elevated renin response linked to kidney decline) and osteoporosis when 250 milliliters (1 cup) of ACV was taken daily for six years (NatMed 2024). However, this is an extreme amount, sixteen times more than is used in most studies.

Side Effects/Risks for Topical Use

Irritation of the skin and chemical burns are the main risks of topical application (NatMed 2024). Seek the guidance of a health care professional before using ACV topically.

If you have cellulitis, a bacterial infection of the skin common in lymphedema, don't fool around with home remedies; go to your doctor or emergency room immediately and get medical treatment. Cellulitis can become a serious medical issue if not treated properly at the first signs.

Bottom Line on Apple Cider Vinegar

Although there is currently no published research on the oral use of apple cider vinegar for lymphedema, one double-blinded trial found benefits for reducing body weight, cholesterol and blood sugar—outcomes that may benefit lymphedema. Four out of five studies to date have found that weight loss reduces lymphedema (Schmitz 2019; Shaw 2007a; Shaw 2007b; Keith 2017; Vafa 2020). Given all the unknowns, it is hard to state emphatically that ACV can directly affect lymphedema, but it may provide an indirect benefit through weight loss and/or improvements in blood lipid levels.

When it comes to topical use, the only available evidence comes from home remedies and anecdotal reports. I look forward to research in this area. In the meantime, if you have skin issues related to your lymphedema, your dermatologist, certified lymphedema therapist or other health care professional may be able to share their anecdotal experience with apple cider vinegar.

References for Apple Cider Vinegar

Abou-Khalil R, Andary J, El-Hayek E. 2024. Apple Cider Vinegar for Weight Management in Lebanese Adolescents and Young Adults with Overweight and Obesity: A Randomised, Double-Blind, Placebo-Controlled Study. *BMJ Nutr Prev Health* 7 (1): 61–67.

Fife CE, Farrow W, Hebert AA, et al. 2017. Skin and Wound Care in Lymphedema Patients: A Taxonomy, Primer, and Literature Review. *Adv Skin Wound Care* 30 (7); 305–18.

Gaurav V, Bhoi AK, Mehta N. 2023. Home Remedies in Dermatology. *Indian Dermatol Online J* 14 (6): 864–70.

Hadi A, Pourmasoumi M, Najafgholizadeh A, et al. 2021. The Effect of Apple Cider Vinegar on Lipid Profiles and Glycemic Parameters: A Systematic Review and Meta-Analysis of Randomized Clinical Trials. *BMC Complement Med Ther* 21 (1): 179.

Keith L, Rowsemitt C, Richards L. 2017. Lifestyle Modification Group for Lymphedema and Obesity Results in Significant Health Outcomes. *Am J Lifestyle Med* 14 (4): 420–28.

NatMed. 2024. "Apple Cider Vinegar." Accessed July 29, 2024. https://naturalmedicines.therapeuticresearch.com/Home/ND.

Ryu E, Yim SY, Do HJ, et al. 2016. Risk of Secondary Lymphedema in Breast Cancer Survivors Is Related to Serum Phospholipid Fatty Acid Desaturation. *Support Care Cancer* 24 (9): 3767–74.

Schmitz KH, Troxel AB, Dean LT, et al. 2019. Effect of Home-Based Exercise and Weight Loss Program and Breast Cancer-Related Lymphedema Outcomes Among Overweight Breast Cancer Survivors: The WISER Survivor Randomized Clinical Trial. *JAMA Oncol* 5 (11): 1605–13.

Shaw C, Mortimer P, Judd, PA. 2007a. Randomized Controlled Trial Comparing a Low-Fat Diet with a Weight-Reduction Diet in Breast Cancer-Related Lymphedema. *Cancer* 109 (10): 1949–56.

Shaw C, Mortimer P, Judd PA. 2007b. A Randomized Controlled Trial of Weight Reduction as a Treatment for Breast Cancer-Related Lymphedema. *Cancer* 110 (8): 1868–74.

Vafa S, Haghighat S, Janani L, et al. 2020. The Effects of Synbiotic Supplementation on Serum Inflammatory Markers and Edema Volume in Breast Cancer Survivors with Lymphedema. *EXCLI J* 19 (January): 1–15.

Ayurveda

What Is It?

Ayurveda is a system of medicine that originated in the Indian subcontinent, which includes India, Pakistan, Bangladesh, Bhutan, Maldives, Nepal and Sri Lanka. It is considered an alternative medicine system, separate from allopathic medicine (also called science-based medicine or Western medicine). Its written history documents an origin in which wisdom was passed from gods to sages and then to human physicians. One of Ayurveda's key principles is that everything in the world, including our own bodies, is made up of five key components: earth, water, fire, air and space (ether). Ayurvedic treatments include herbal products, diets, meditation, yoga, massage, laxatives, enemas and medicinal oils. The focus of Ayurveda is on restoring balance.

Lymphedema-Specific Research

India is located between 8 and 37 degrees latitude, which is similar to the latitude of Mexico. As a tropical country, it is home to many mosquitos, including those that carry filarial parasites, so India has a high incidence of filarial lymphedemas (see "Technical

Breakdown," page 133). A 2007 study set out to test an Ayurvedic-based lymphedema protocol on 240 people with filarial lymphedema (Narahari 2007). The researchers chose to test Ayurvedic treatments because they were affordable and culturally accepted by the rural people included in the study. Their particular protocol was adapted based on Ayurvedic concepts from European practice that were available locally at a low cost.

The patients were first assessed by an Ayurvedic doctor on 100 clinical parameters, which were used to select the specific herbal medicines each patient would ingest. The protocol began with a two-week hospitalization, during which the foot of the bed was elevated 20 to 30 centimeters (8 to 12 inches). The patients had daily treatments, lasting one and a half to two hours, that included:

- Skin care with low-pH soap
- Wound care
- Immersion in a phanta solution made up of manjistha, sariva, yestimadhu and triphala
- Yoga
- Indian manual lymphatic drainage consisting of Unmardhana—a dry massage—followed by Vimlapana with a massage oil called Nalpamaradi Thailam
- Limb elevation
- Cotton cloth wrapping + long stretch bandages
- More yoga with the bandages on

Those with more advanced lymphedema also received:

- Ekanga Swedana (a steam treatment) with the medicinal herb khadira (*Senegalia catechu*, previously known as *Acacia catechu*)
- More elevation
- More bandaging

All of the patients were sent home with instructions on how to self-administer these treatments at home, as well as oral Ayurvedic prescriptions called Kanchanar Guggulu and Mahamanjishtadi Kwatha and a strict vegetarian diet.

Results were assessed throughout the protocol and at the final session, six months after the patients' admission, and showed gradual and progressive reduction in limb volume. The Ekanga Swedana treatment did not appear to be helpful beyond the original protocol.

The authors concluded that their protocol was a cost-effective treatment (about one-quarter of the cost of complete decongestive therapy) that could be delivered by Ayurvedic practitioners in rural, filariasis-endemic areas.

Side Effects/Risks
None noted.

Bottom Line on Ayurveda

This research seems significant for Indian health authorities struggling to treat millions of poor and underserviced people, but it's impossible to say, based solely on this study, whether Ayurvedic practices should be adopted as complementary care for lymphedema in the Western world. The protocol was tested as a low-cost *alternative* to CDT in rural Indian areas, not as complementary care. In the Western world, Ayurvedic practitioners and herbs are less accessible and more expensive. In addition, this protocol was quite time-intensive in an era when most people are looking for time-saving strategies. An evidence-based systematic evaluation through an allopathic lens is needed to determine whether Ayurvedic treatments offer benefits as complementary care for lymphedema. (But see page 61 for further discussion of yoga, which was part of this protocol.)

References for Ayurveda

Narahari SR, Ryan TJ, Mahadevan PE, et al. 2007. Integrated Management of Filarial Lymphedema for Rural Communities. *Lymphology* 40 (1): 3–13.

Balneotherapy

What Is It?

Balneotherapy, which means "bath therapy," involves soaking in mineral water (usually from hot springs or thermal spas) or clay or mud baths. In addition to minerals, the baths can contain gases such as carbon dioxide or hydrogen sulfide. Balneotherapy may also be called health resort medicine, spa therapy or thermal mineral baths. The mineral-rich waters or muds are thought to have anti-inflammatory, relaxing and pain-relieving properties. Balneotherapy can take place in either natural or man-made formations. Some popular natural balneotherapy spas include Banff Upper Hot Springs in Banff National Park, Alberta; Hot Springs National Park in Arkansas; and Saratoga Springs in New York.

History of Balneotherapy

Many cultures have used hot springs, mineral waters or mud baths, depending on their local geographical formations. Balneotherapy is over 4,000 years old and was used in ancient Egyptian, Roman, Greek, Celtic and Hebrew civilizations (Moss 2010). Ancient Roman bathers would move from the warm bath (tepidarium) to the hot (caldarium) and then the cold (frigidarium). The baths were considered therapeutic, relaxing the muscles and joints and improving circulation, digestion and appetite (Moss 2010). Historically significant balneotherapy sites include Bath, England; the source of the Seine River in France; and the Dead Sea.

Lymphedema-Specific Research

One exploratory review argues in favor of mineral baths for lymphedema, citing as key benefits the buoyancy, hydrostatic pressure and viscosity of aqua therapy; the anti-inflammatory effect, relaxation and pain relief offered by the minerals; and the social atmosphere of the health resort environment, with its focus on overall well-being (Maccarone 2023).

Related Research

The same researchers also published a narrative review of both cell culture and human studies on the immune response to balneotherapy (Maccarone 2017). The ten human trials evaluated mud packs, mud baths, hot mineral baths, geothermal sea water baths and high-radon-concentration bathing. The treatments lasted from nine to twenty-eight days, and results were mixed, possibly due to the different mud and mineral water baths used.

Side Effects / Risks

Mineral baths present the same risks as aqua therapy when it comes to water temperature and the safety of surrounding surfaces. See page 78 for details on minimizing these risks.

Bottom Line on Balneotherapy

Mineral baths and mud packs have a long history of traditional use across many cultures, but although the 2023 Maccarone review provides a detailed position in favor of balneotherapy for lymphedema, as yet there are no clinical trials specific to this population. That said, the risks of water or mud bathing are minimal if safety measures are taken and the water temperature is appropriate. As with any complementary therapy, discuss it with your lymphedema therapist first.

References for Balneotherapy

Maccarone MC, Magro G, Solimene U, et al. 2017. From In Vitro Research to Real Life Studies: An Extensive Narrative Review of the Effects of Balneotherapy on Human Immune Response. *Sport Sci Health*. 17 (4): 817–35.

Maccarone MC, Venturini E, Masiero S. 2023. Exploring the Potential Role of Health Resort Medicine in the Management of Breast Cancer-Related Lymphedema: A Viable Alternative for Innovative Rehabilitation Opportunities? *Int J Biometeorol* 67 (9): 1505–7.

Moss GA. 2010. Water and Health: A Forgotten Connection? *Perspect Public Health* 130 (5): 227–32.

Cabbage Leaves

What Are They?

Cabbage is a head-forming brassica vegetable with the botanical name *Brassica oleracea L.* It is grown in many regions around the world and is popular in dishes such as coleslaw, cabbage rolls and okonomiyaki (Japanese cabbage pancakes). It may seem totally out of left field to consider cabbage leaves as a treatment for lymphedema, but they come up in internet searches for home remedies. They are used in the form of a cabbage leaf compress, which is made by rolling one of the thick outer leaves with a rolling pin or bottle and then applying it to the skin.

Lymphedema-Specific Research

I was unable to find any human studies specifically on using cabbage leaves to treat lymphedema.

User Experience
"Cabbage leaf therapy helped ease the pain of lymphatic swelling combined with arthritis on the shoulder of the lymphatic arm. I just started this therapy during the last six months."

—**Robin, Washington (left arm, hand and underarm lymphedema)**

Lymphedema Research in Animals

In a quest to explain how cabbage leaves worked on pain and inflammation, Polish researchers set out to isolate microRNAs in cabbage leaf juice (Kasarello 2022). They discovered over 280 microRNAs, with one in particular—miR172—present in large quantities.

The researchers chemically synthesized miR172 and tested it on twenty male mice. Eight mice were injected with collagen to induce arthritis in their paws, then were injected with synthetic miR172a. Over the next fifty days, they received six more collagen injections, followed by synthetic miR172a injections. The mice were weighed and had their paw swelling measured weekly. Of the other twelve mice—the control group—four were injected with collagen but not with synthetic miR172a; four were injected with synthetic miR172a but not with collagen; and four received neither collagen nor synthetic miR172a.

After three weeks, the mice injected with collagen showed increased knuckle size in their front and back paws. Those who were treated with synthetic miR172a had less swelling than those who were not, demonstrating some anti-inflammatory effects.

Although this experiment was done on mice, used a synthetic version of the RNA found in cabbage, and injected it rather than applying it topically, the results give researchers some clues to explain what might be happening at a cellular level and why the use of cabbage leaves as a folk remedy has survived for so long.

Related Research

Researchers in Italy interviewed 137 residents of Caspoggio, a small village in the Bernina Alps, about their use of home remedies. They used cabbage leaves to relieve musculoskeletal pain and inflammation in conditions such as arthritis (Bottoni 2020). Similarly, in Polish folk medicine, cabbage leaf compresses are one of the most widely used anti-inflammatory remedies, mainly for rheumatic pain, vein and lymphatic vessel inflammation, bruises, sprains, mastitis and gastrointestinal problems (Kasarello 2022).

OSTEOARTHRITIS

In an open-label clinical trial that compared cabbage leaves with cooling gel pads or Diclofenac gel for knee pain from osteoarthritis (Chobpenthai 2022), patients with moderate to severe osteoarthritis were randomized as follows:

- Twenty people used a reusable cooling gel pad made by Nexcare for twenty minutes per day.
- Twenty people rubbed on 2 to 4 grams of diclofenac gel four times per day.
- Twenty people applied a cabbage leaf that was first bruised by a bottle, placing it on their knee for one hour per day, after dinner or before going to bed. (It's not clear if the bottle was rolled on the leaf like a rolling pin or used to hammer the leaf like a kitchen mallet; either way, breaking down some of the fibers appears to be an important stage in releasing the active ingredients.)

Each patient completed the Oxford Knee Score (OKS) questionnaire and recorded their pain scores before and after each application, and they attended weekly follow-ups and assessments for four weeks. None developed an allergic reaction to the cabbage leaves. Both the cabbage leaf group and the cooling gel pad group showed a significant improvement in their OKS and pain scores, superior to the results for the diclofenac gel group. The researchers concluded that "cabbage leaf application is an effective treatment in terms of relieving pain and reducing the severity of osteoarthritis much more effectively than topical pain medication."

It's important to point out, though, that this study was short-term and relied on the subjects to report their symptoms, which could potentially introduce bias or a placebo effect. But it's good to know that no side effects were reported. Knee arthritis can be a comorbidity of lymphedema; if arthritis pain can be improved, people with lymphedema may be able to tolerate more movement, more compression or a pneumatic pump. It is also possible that cabbage leaf compresses might have a similar pain-relieving and anti-inflammatory effect on lymphedema that they did for osteoarthritis.

Breast Pain and Hardness

A Cochrane review and meta-analysis examined the use of cabbage leaves to treat breast pain and hardness due to engorgement in breastfeeding moms (Zakarija-Grkovic 2020). After reviewing twenty-one randomized controlled trials including 152 women, the authors concluded that cold cabbage leaf compresses may be more effective than routine care or cold gel packs for breast pain; cold cabbage leaves may be better than routine care for breast hardness; and room temperature cabbage leaves may be better than a hot water bottle for breast engorgement. All of these conclusions were classified as low-certainty evidence.

It is unclear whether physiological commonalities exist between lymphedema and breast pain, hardness and engorgement, or if the same active ingredients that improved symptoms of breast engorgement would also improve painful or fibrotic lymphedema tissue.

Side Effects/Risks

There were no side effects noted in the published studies, but with lymphedema there is always a risk of cellulitis. After consulting with your lymphedema therapist, you may choose to try a cabbage leaf compress on non-lymphedema skin first to test your skin's sensitivity.

Bottom Line on Cabbage Leaves

I could not find any published evidence that cabbage leaves will help lymphedema, although it's theoretically possible that the results seen with breast engorgement and knee arthritis might be transferable to similar symptoms in lymphedema. But whether or not you should try a cabbage leaf compress depends on your skin's sensitivity level, as some people with very sensitive skin can develop cellulitis. As with any complementary therapy, consult your medical team first.

If you do decide to try this therapy, it's likely best to begin by testing your skin's tolerance to the cabbage by placing the compress on a non-lymphedema area. For added cooling relief, keep the cabbage in the fridge or a cold cellar. Pull off one leaf and rinse it under cold water, then place it on a clean surface and roll it with a rolling pin or a bottle to break up some of the cell membranes and release the active ingredients. Apply it to your skin, monitor your skin for sensitivity, and take note of any changes in your pain levels to assess whether you are experiencing relief. As with any new treatment, starting with a low dose—in this case, time exposure—would be sensible.

References for Cabbage Leaves

Bottoni M, Milani F, Colombo L, et al. 2020. Using Medicinal Plants in Valmalenco (Italian Alps): From Tradition to Scientific Approaches. *Molecules* 25 (18): 4144.

Chobpenthai T, Arunwatthanangkul P, Mahikul W. 2022. Efficacy of Cabbage Leaf Versus Cooling Gel Pad or Diclofenac Gel for Patients with Knee Osteoarthritis: A Randomized Open-Labeled Controlled Clinical Trial. *Pain Res Manag* (June): 3122153.

Kasarello K, Köhling I, Kosowska A, et al. 2022. The Anti-Inflammatory Effect of Cabbage Leaves Explained by the Influence of bol-miRNA172a on FAN Expression. *Front Pharmacol* 13 (March): 846830.

Zakarija-Grkovic I, Stewart F. 2020. Treatments for Breast Engorgement During Lactation. *Cochrane Database Syst Rev* 9 (9): CD006946.

Castor Oil

What Is It?

Castor oil is the oil pressed out of the castor bean (*Ricinus communis*). Like any vegetable oil, it can be extracted by cold-pressing or by methods involving heat and solvents. Castor oil contains 80% to 90% ricinoleic acid, not to be confused with ricin (see the box below). Some of its other constituents include oleic, linoleic and stearic fatty acids, as well as vitamin E

Technical Breakdown

Did you watch Breaking Bad? In one episode, the protagonist, a chemist named Walter White, suggests that he can make ricin from the lily of the valley plant. Ricin is one of the most potent and lethal substances known. It is considered an important bioweapon and is an attractive agent for bioterrorist activities (Franke 2019). Ricin is present in the hull of the castor bean, which is why you cannot eat the whole bean. Thankfully, when the oil is extracted from the bean, care is taken to exclude the hull. In addition, the oil is sampled and tested to be sure it meets safety standards.

History of Castor Oil

A 1982 article in the *Journal of Ethnopharmacology* is exhaustive in describing the historical and current uses of the castor plant, including the trunk, stem, wax, leaves and oil. A highlight is that castor oil has been found in 4,000-year-old Egyptian sarcophagi (Scarpa 1982). The Papyrus Ebers, 3,500-year-old scrolls detailing ancient Egyptian healing arts, state that it was used to treat rash (exanthem), with a ten-day application; the scrolls also extol castor oil's wound-healing properties, which led to it being called palma Cristi, or "palm of Christ" (Franke 2019). From Egypt, the castor plant was brought to Greece, India and China. In ancient Greece, it was used to treat constipation. It was introduced to London in 1764 (Scarpa 1982).

Components of the castor plant have been used in over twenty countries and by several indigenous tribes to treat conditions ranging from stomachaches, infections, jaundice and ascites to pneumonia, asthma and strokes. Sometimes the castor components were used on their own in simple preparations, and sometimes they were mixed with other ingredients or had elaborate preparation methods (Scarpa 1982).

User Experience
"I think that massaging castor oil on my breast daily has slowed down the thickening of the damaged tissues."

—Kathy, Ontario (breast and arm lymphedema)

CURRENT USES OF CASTOR OIL

In North America today, castor oil is mainly promoted for skin and hair care, for treating constipation and as a "liver detoxifier" (in quotation marks because many health professionals consider this term to be inappropriate as the liver is its own detoxifier). The oil can be taken by mouth or applied topically to the skin, belly button, eyes or scalp.

Various sources proclaim castor oil's efficacy in a broad range of medical uses, including as a laxative, to induce labor, to aid in the metabolization of lipids, as an antimicrobial, to assist in wound healing and to ease the pain of arthritis, headaches and menstrual cramps. However, the FDA has approved its use only as a stimulant laxative (Final Report 2007). Although evidence-based practitioners tend to use modern laxative and stool softening products in place of castor oil, some people do prefer traditional, natural medicines over the modern replacements.

A StatPearls article on castor oil offers this assurance: "With increased scientific research regarding castor oil and its longstanding historical use, clinicians can confidently consider prescribing this medication" (Alookaran 2024).

Lymphedema-Specific Research

I was unable to find any human research on using castor oil to improve lymphatic drainage. But people on social media certainly report that it works, and a quick web search yields results like: "by using castor packs, the flow of lymph is increased throughout the body"; "castor oil for lymphatic system support definitely works"; and "by using castor oil packs the flow of lymph is increased throughout the body." Unfortunately, these websites are limited in their credibility because they do not include links to any research.

Lymphedema Research in Animals

A 2000 study tested a castor oil component on mice and guinea pigs with induced inflammation and edema (Vieira 2000). The researchers induced inflammation in two ways: by injecting carrageenan into the inner layer of skin (the dermis) of a mouse paw and by injecting histamine into the eyelid of a guinea pig. Both injections led to an edema.

Each mouse's paw then received one of three topical applications: peanut oil alone; capsaicin diluted in peanut oil; or 99% ricinoleic acid diluted in peanut oil. (Castor oil is 80% to 90% ricinoleic acid, so this treatment is similar to but not identical to using castor oil.) On the first day, both the ricinoleic acid and the capsaicin treatments caused an increase in the paw edema, while the peanut oil by itself did not. The applications continued every day for eight days, and the ricinoleic acid and capsaicin treatments resulted in a "marked reduction in edema."

A similar result was seen for the guinea pigs: an increase in edema with the first application, then a reduction after eight days of application. The researchers noted that "the topical administration of capsaicin resulted in a local hyperemic response and activation of behavioral defensive responses including scratching of the eyelid" (as one might expect, given that capsaicin is the ingredient that provides the heat in chili peppers; if you've ever tried putting in contact lenses after touching jalapeño peppers, you can relate). They observed no such response with the ricinoleic acid treatment. Overall, the researchers concluded that:

- The anti-inflammatory effect of ricinoleic acid was more pronounced in the carrageenan-induced inflammation than the histamine-induced inflammation, as different mechanisms of action are responsible.
- Ricinoleic acid provided the same anti-inflammatory result as capsaicin without the pungent and painful effects.

Although this study is an interesting model of using ricinoleic acid as a topical treatment for lymphedema, we are not mice or guinea pigs, and castor oil is not the same thing as 99% ricinoleic acid in peanut oil. Still, as evidence supporting castor oil's traditional uses, we can see how it may have added momentum to recommendations to use castor oil to combat inflammation and edema.

User Experience

"I used castor oil to decrease localized areas of swelling when I had deep pitting. I soaked a boiled wool cloth with castor oil, put it on the area and wrapped it with plastic cling wrap and a bandage. This decreased swelling, left the skin soft and often eliminated pitting."

—Patti, Idaho (breast cancer–related lymphedema)

Related Research

Castor oil could potentially help address certain issues related to lymphedema, including relief from constipation, wound healing and scar treatment, as well as reducing inflammation and edema (discussed in "Lymphedema Research in Animals," above).

RELIEF FROM CONSTIPATION

My clients confirm that their lymphedema is often worse when they are constipated. Although constipation and lymphedema may seem like independent conditions, the intestines are rich in lymphatic capillaries called lacteals, and the mesentery—the lining that holds the intestines to the abdominal wall—has a large collection of lymph nodes. Castor oil can relieve constipation when taken orally in a dose of 15 to 60 milliliters (1 to 4 tablespoons) per day (Alookaran 2024), or when it is applied to the skin of the abdomen via a flannel cloth (known as a castor oil pack) or poured into the belly button.

WOUND HEALING

People with lymphedema can develop wounds for a variety of reasons, including ill-fitting garments, lymphorrhea and skin maceration, or poor blood circulation due to phlebolymphedema. Despite castor oil's lengthy history of use in wound healing, I could not find any modern research to support its efficacy. However, one review of various vegetable oils, including castor oil, describes their anti-inflammatory, antioxidant, antibacterial and anticancer properties and their potential use in the creation of biomaterials (Ribeiro 2022).

SCAR TREATMENT

People sometimes develop lymphedema after surgery or an injury. Most commonly, it develops after cancer treatment in which lymph nodes are surgically removed, creating scar tissue that can impair lymph flow. Breaking down scar tissue is another one of castor oil's traditional uses, and some lymphedema care professionals offer anecdotal evidence that it works; however, there is no published research available on this topic that I could find.

Anecdotal Report

"In my experience, consistent use of castor oil packs softens the scar tissue and fibrotic tissue, which then helps with my MLD treatment and drainage. Sometimes the results would show after just two applications, but it usually needs daily or overnight packs over a month."

—Biljana Bozic, RMT, Balanced Body by RMT, Kitchener, Ontario

Side Effects/Risks

Documented side effects of castor oil include abdominal cramping, vomiting, bloating, dizziness and premature contractions in pregnancy. There is a potential for reduced absorption of other drugs when castor oil is used as a laxative. Do not use castor oil if you have gastrointestinal obstruction, appendicitis, perforation or inflammatory bowel disease.

Bottom Line on Castor Oil

Castor oil has both oral and topical uses. Applying castor oil to your skin as part of a daily skin care routine appears to be safe and is a very common practice. Of course, as with any topical application, you may want to do a skin test first, especially if you tend to have sensitive skin. Animal research suggests that castor oil applied to the skin can reduce inflammation and edema, and anecdotal reports support this evidence.

The main reason for ingesting castor oil is to treat constipation. If you have never taken it for this purpose, consult your pharmacist or physician before trying it. It's best to start with a small dosage and gradually increase it, to avoid over-treating.

References for Castor Oil

Alookaran J, Tripp J. 2024. "Castor Oil." In StatPearls [Internet]. StatPearls Publishing. Accessed April 17, 2024. https://www.ncbi.nlm.nih.gov/books/NBK551626/.

Final Report on the Safety Assessment of Ricinus Communis (Castor) Seed Oil, Hydrogenated Castor Oil, Glyceryl Ricinoleate, Glyceryl Ricinoleate SE, Ricinoleic Acid, Potassium Ricinoleate, Sodium Ricinoleate, Zinc Ricinoleate, Cetyl Ricinoleate, Ethyl Ricinoleate, Glycol Ricinoleate, Isopropyl Ricinoleate, Methyl Ricinoleate, and Octyldodecyl Ricinoleate. 2007. *Int J Toxicol* 26 (Suppl 3): 31–77.

Franke H, Scholl R, Aigner A. 2019. Ricin and *Ricinus communis* in Pharmacology and Toxicology—From Ancient Use and "Papyrus Ebers" to Modern Perspectives and "Poisonous Plant of the Year 2018." *Naunyn Schmiedebergs Arch Pharmacol*. 392 (10): 1181–1208.

Ribeiro AR, Silva SS, Reis RL. 2022. Challenges and Opportunities on Vegetable Oils Derived Systems for Biomedical Applications. *Biomater Adv* 134 (March): 112720.

Scarpa A, Guerci A. 1982. Various Uses of the Castor Oil Plant (*Ricinus communis L.*): A Review. *J Ethnopharmacol* 5 (2): 117–37.

Vieira C, Evangelista S, Cirillo R, et al. 2000. Effect of Ricinoleic Acid in Acute and Subchronic Experimental Models of Inflammation. *Mediators Inflamm* 9 (5): 223–28

Cupping

What Is It?

Part of traditional Chinese medicine, cupping is widely used in Asia and the Middle East to enhance blood circulation and relieve swelling and pain (Wang 2018). It is also known as *hijama* in Arabic-speaking countries (Al-Reefy 2014) and *ventosa* in Native Latin American culture (Paz 2024). The cups create negative pressure via suction on the skin. Traditional cupping uses glass bowls that are heated with a flame, but these days we also have high-tech negative pressure machines (see LymphaTouch, page 246, and Vacumed, page 269).

There are three cupping methods: dry, wet and sliding. Dry cupping draws the skin and the underlying tissue into the cup via suction. Wet cupping adds a laceration to the skin, drawing blood out; it is sometimes called bloodletting cupping. Sliding cupping is dry cupping with light suction so that the cups can be moved along the skin.

History of Cupping

Cupping has been used in traditional Chinese medicine since 1550 BCE, was described in ancient Ayurvedic texts, was practiced in ancient Mesopotamia, Egypt and Greece, and is documented in Macedonian medical texts dating back to around 3300 BCE. Hippocrates (460–375 BCE), the father of medicine, recommended using cupping for menstrual cramps and cardiac angina (Al-Reefy 2014).

Lymphedema-Specific Research

I found three studies of cupping's use in treating lymphedema. One was only available in Chinese (Sun 2017), so I was unable to read it, but I've included it in the references in case you read Chinese. I have summarized the other two studies.

STUDY #1: WANG 2018

Seventy-five women with breast cancer–related upper arm lymphedema were given exercise training once a day for thirty minutes. Patients could choose to do the exercise on its own (the control group of twenty-five patients) or add a fifteen-minute bloodletting cupping treatment every five days (the cupping group of fifty patients). The study lasted for fifty days.

Cupping treatment points were selected for each patient based on areas of swelling. The skin was disinfected and a sterile needle was used to make a puncture in each swollen area. Sterilized cups were applied to absorb the draining fluid from the bleeding areas. The cups were left on for ten minutes, then removed and the skin was cleaned.

Arm circumference was measured before and after treatment. Circumference reductions were greater in the cupping group than in the control group from the tenth day of treatment onward, and arm circumference reduced progressively with each treatment. The authors concluded that bloodletting cupping safely and effectively reduced arm circumference and relieved upper limb pain in women with post–breast cancer lymphedema.

STUDY #2: XIONG 2019

Sixty patients with breast cancer–related lymphedema received multilayer compression bandaging, followed by exercise and deep breathing for thirty minutes. Prior to the bandaging and exercise, roughly half of the women were randomly allocated to receive manual lymphatic drainage and the other half to receive sliding cupping. The cupping was done along three yin meridians and three yang meridians on the hand and arm to the shoulder and back for twenty-five to thirty minutes, followed by wrapping in short stretch bandages. These treatments took place once a day for fourteen days.

All the women had improvements in circumference at each of six measuring points along the arm after their treatments. In the cupping group, seven cases were markedly effective, nineteen cases were effective and four cases were ineffective, for a total efficacy rate of 86.6%. In the MLD group, two cases were markedly effective, twenty-two cases were effective and six cases were ineffective, for a total efficacy rate of 80%. This difference between the two groups is not statistically significant.

The study also measured skin thickness. The sliding cupping group had reduced skin thickness at both the full skin layer and the subcutaneous tissue layer. The MLD group did not experience any change in skin thickness.

The authors concluded that sliding cupping + bandaging and exercise was more effective than MLD + bandaging and exercise.

Side Effects/Risks

No adverse events were reported in the wet cupping study (Wang 2018) or the sliding cupping study (Xiong 2019). But the authors did specify that the negative pressure of the cups should not be too high, to avoid pain and possibly skin damage. The amount of pressure should be based on the patient's tolerance, and treatment should stop when the skin is reddish and there are slight spots of rash (Xiong 2019).

In two published case studies, side effects including skin lesion, lipoma, anemia and skin pigmentation were reported (Kim 2012; Schumann 2012). Another case study described a forty-nine-year-old Bahraini woman who underwent breast cancer surgery and lymphonodectomy of nineteen nodes. Upon discharge from the hospital, she had wet cupping therapy, after which she noted swelling in her upper arm. The authors of the case study postulated that the wet cupping played a major role in the onset of her lymphedema (Al-Reefy 2014).

Other sources caution that you should not try cupping if you have a bleeding disorder, clotting problems, eczema or psoriasis (Cleveland Clinic 2023). The National Lymphedema Network advises avoiding trauma to the skin and recommends using soap and water to wash the skin after any breaks or punctures (NLN 2012).

Bottom Line on Cupping

Two studies demonstrated reduced lymphedema circumference after cupping treatment, with one study also showing improvement in skin thickness (Xiong 2019) and one reporting improvement in pain (Wang 2018). However, there are several potential side effects and precautions, not least of which is the NLN's advice to avoid skin trauma and needle punctures. Wet cupping (bloodletting cupping) may pose additional risks even though no side effects were noted in the Wang study. Caution is suggested with any cupping method to avoid causing skin trauma through excess pressure. Mechanically controlled suction pressure (see LymphaTouch, page 246, and Vacumed, page 269) may offer the practitioner more control over the amount of suction used.

References for Cupping

Al-Reefy S, Parsa-Nezhad M. 2014. Lymphedema Following Cupping Therapy Hijama Post Breast Cancer Surgery and Axillary Clearance. *Bahrain Medical Bulletin* 36 (1): 44–45.

Cleveland Clinic. 2023. "Cupping Therapy." Accessed December 30, 2024. https://my.clevelandclinic.org/health/treatments/16554-cupping.

Kim KH, Kim TH, Hwangbo M, Yang GY. 2012. Anemia and Skin Pigmentation After Excessive Cupping Therapy by an Unqualified Therapist in Korea: A Case Report. *Acupunct Med* 30 (3): 227–28.

NLN Medical Advisory Committee. 2012. "Lymphedema Risk Reduction Practices." Position Statement of the National Lymphedema Network. Accessed April 22, 2025. https://lymphnet.org/page/risk-reduction/.

Paz A, Yasin H, Mathis S. 2024. Parallels Between Cupping in Traditional Chinese Medicine and Ventosas in Native American Cultures. *Med Acupunct* 36 (6): 330–36.

Schumann S, Lauche R, Hohmann C, et al. 2012. Development of Lipoma Following a Single Cupping Massage: A Case Report. [In German.] *Forsch Komplementmed* 19 (4): 202–5.

Sun XH, Fu JR, Cao XC. 2017. The Clinical Observation on Bloodletting Puncture and Cupping and Moving Cupping to Treat Severe Lymphedema Related to Breast Cancer. [In Chinese.] *Chin J Surg Integr Tradit West Med* 23 (2): 167e170.

Wang C, Zhang Y, Yang M, et al. 2018. Bloodletting Puncture and Cupping as an Adjuvant Therapy for Breast Cancer-Related Lymphedema in Female Adults: A Non-Randomized Controlled Pragmatic Trial. *J Trad Chin Med Sci* 5 (3): 255–63.

Xiong Z, Wang T, Wang H, et al. 2019. Sliding-Cupping Along Meridian for Lymphedema After Breast Cancer Surgery: A Randomized Controlled Trial. *World J Acupunct -Moxibustion* 29 (3): 179–85.

Essential Oils

What Are They?

Essential oils, also known as volatile oils, are concentrated hydrophobic (water-avoidant) liquids containing volatile chemicals extracted from plants by either steam distillation or mechanical cold-pressing. The oils can be extracted from the stem, bark, flower, root, rhizome, seed, needles, rinds, fruits, woods, grasses or resins of the plant (Farrar 2020). Some are ingested orally or through other internal routes (such as suppository or douche), some are used topically (applied to the skin), and others are used for aromatherapy (breathing in the scent). Be careful not to ingest oils meant only for topical applications.

Aroma oil, or aromatherapy oil, is a blend of essential oil(s) with a carrier to reduce the concentration and provide a pleasant, not overpowering scent. Aromatherapy is based on an ancient healing art intended to promote harmony between body and mind (Krishbaum 1996). The oils are used to stimulate the olfactory receptors that connect to the limbic system in the brain, sometimes called the emotional center of the brain. The limbic center can affect heart rate, blood pressure, breathing, memory and stress response, among other roles (Kirshbaum 1996).

In the US, the regulation of aromatherapy varies depending on the intended use of a product as indicated on the labeling (FDA 2023). For example, if the essential oil is part of a cleanser or perfume, it's considered a cosmetic, and FDA approval is not required. If it is intended to treat or prevent disease or affect the function of the body, then it's considered a drug and must meet FDA requirements for safety and effectiveness before being sold to consumers. Essential oils that claim to treat colic, reduce pain, relax muscles, treat depression or anxiety, or help you sleep, for example, would all be subject to FDA approval. To learn whether a product you are considering is approved, visit https://www.fda.gov/drugs. You can also search on the FDA database to see if the manufacturer has had any warnings issued against them.

In Canada, under the Chemicals Management Plan, the government reviews and manages the potential risks that chemical substances can pose to people and the environment and maintains a list of essential oils and botanical extracts that may be associated with a range of health effects To check the list, visit https://www.canada.ca/en/health-canada/services/chemicals-product-safety/essential-oils-botanical-extracts.html.

User Experience
"I have tried essential oils, castor oil, meditation and yoga, and for me, nothing has really helped. I also have lipedema."

—Nicole, North Carolina (lipo-lymphedema)

Lymphedema-Specific Research

I found two studies that used essential oils to treat lymphedema. The first was a case series of eight patients who received at least six twenty- to thirty-minute therapeutic aromatherapy massages using lavender oil (Kirshbaum 1996). The massages were applied by nurses who had undergone specific training in aromatherapy massage for lymphedema.

Lavender was chosen for its calming, antiseptic and restorative properties, as well as its reputation as a safe agent. The patients were also educated on the use of compression sleeves, skin care and exercise. Arm volume measurements were taken, and functional assessments were made after each visit. The results revealed a slight reduction in the circumference of the affected arms. Common themes emerging from the interviews included pain reduction, less swelling and improvement in comfort, relaxation, self-esteem and well-being.

Although it sounds like aromatherapy massage provided great benefits for the cancer survivors, this study did not reveal much about the effects of lavender essential oil on lymphedema, as there was no control group for comparison and no attempt to standardize the other lymphedema tools, such as compression garment use.

The second study included seventy-nine adults who performed daily self-massage using lotion, randomly selected to include or exclude aromatherapy oil (Barclay 2006). The oil was a specially designed blend of wheat germ oil with fennel, sage, geranium, black pepper and juniper added to a base cream. The oil's components were selected by the cancer center's qualified complementary therapist as ones that could help stimulate the lymphatic system and relieve skin conditions. The patients were taught how to apply the cream using principles of lymphatic drainage. They were also instructed on exercise and skin care, and the use of compression garments was continued as prescribed for each individual. Measurements were taken monthly for three months via self-tensioning tape measurements every 4 centimeters (1.5 inches).

After about three months, twenty-one people dropped out of the study, noting that there was no improvement. The people who remained in the study had seen a slight improvement in limb volume. Importantly, there was no difference in results between the aromatherapy-infused lotion and the base lotion alone. The patients who remained in the study continued their daily self-massage for another three months. They did not have follow-up measurements taken, but were asked for their assessment of symptom improvement and reported that their symptoms and well-being continued to improve.

These are not positive results if you were hoping to read that essential oils are beneficial. This particular combination of essential oils, at least, did not outperform the base cream alone. And according to the Natural Medicines Database, although there is interest in using inhaled and topical aromatherapy for lymphedema, there is insufficient reliable information about the clinical effects of aromatherapy for this condition (NatMed 2025).

> **User Experience**
> "I use a mix of tamanu, sweet almond oil, vitamin E oil and sandalwood essential oil to keep the skin soft."
>
> **—Patti, Idaho (breast cancer–related lymphedema)**

Related Research

A comprehensive descriptive review of aromatherapy in the cancer population examined eighteen studies that, as a whole, showed a short-term benefit from aromatherapy that could last up to two weeks, with a reduction in anxiety and depression scores, improved sleep and an overall increase in well-being (Boehm 2012). However, some of the trials reported no significant difference between the group using essential oils and the control group. The quality of the publications was judged as low to mediocre, and the studies were usually done without blinding (which would be difficult to achieve, as participants can easily detect whether the product they are testing includes fragrant essential oils).

The authors of the review concluded that there is "weak evidence" that aromatherapy might have short-term effects on anxiety and depression, and possibly on pain relief, and that it is unclear whether any benefits come from expectation or from an actual pharmacological effect.

A systematic review of the use of complementary therapies for improving breast surgery outcomes included four studies that examined aromatherapy (Abushukur 2022). Overall, there were no adverse effects, but the evidence supporting the benefits was mixed.

Side Effects/Risks

Documented side effects of essential oils include dermal toxicity—usually from using undiluted essential oils or from being in the sun after applying an essential oil that is phototoxic (activated by the sun)—burning in the mouth, throat and stomach from excess oral intake of essential oil, poisoning, chemical burn and difficulty breathing (Farrar 2020). That said, the overall risk is considered minimal (Boehm 2012), although the use of lavender and tea tree oils present potential problems for estrogen-sensitive cancers, as these oils are thought to have weak estrogenic and antiandrogenic actions. It's best to work with an aromatherapist or another health practitioner trained in the use of essential oils.

To avoid side effects, the proper dosage is important. The effective dilution for most essential oils is 2.5% for adults, which is two drops of essential oils in 100 drops of carrier oil (Boehm 2012). For a full-body bath, it is usually five to ten drops per bath.

Bottom Line on Essential Oils

To date there have been only one small clinical trial and one older case series on essential oil aromatherapy for lymphedema. The clinical trial showed that self-massage improved lymphedema, but no additional benefit was seen from adding essential oils to the carrier cream over a three-month period. The case series revealed that cancer survivors enjoyed aromatherapy massage and reported benefits, but it is unknown what effect the lavender oil contributed to these outcomes. Overall, the evidence in support of aromatherapy for lymphedema is weak.

As you can imagine, there are countless essential oils and combinations of oils that could be used. If you are considering using essential oils to treat your lymphedema, consult an aromatherapist or another experienced complementary care practitioner, and monitor your skin for signs of reactions.

If you are hoping for an actual clinical benefit, not just a pleasant, nice-smelling massage, be diligent about recording your observations in an objective way, to help you evaluate whether there is any measurable benefit. So far, the available research would caution you to temper your expectations.

References for Essential Oils

Abushukur Y, Cascardo C, Ibrahim Y, et al. 2022. Improving Breast Surgery Outcomes Through Alternative Therapy: A Systematic Review. *Cureus* 14 (3): e23443.

Barclay J, Vestey J, Lambert A, Balmer C. 2006. Reducing the Symptoms of Lymphoedema: Is There a Role for Aromatherapy? *Eur J Oncol Nurs* 10 (2): 140–49.

Boehm K, Büssing A, Ostermann T. 2012. Aromatherapy as an Adjuvant Treatment in Cancer Care—A Descriptive Systematic Review. *Afr J Tradit Complement Altern Med* 9 (4): 503–18.

Farrar AJ, Farrar FC. 2020. Clinical Aromatherapy. *Nurs Clin North Am* 55 (4): 489–504.

Food and Drug Administration (FDA). 2023. "Aromatherapy." Accessed August 7, 2024. https://www.fda.gov/cosmetics/cosmetic-products/aromatherapy.

Kirshbaum M. 1996. Using Massage in the Relief of Lymphoedema. *Prof Nurse* 11 (4): 230–32.

NatMed. 2025. "Aromatherapy." Accessed August 4, 2025. https://naturalmedicines.therapeuticresearch.com/Tools/EffectivenessByCondition?id=1361&title=Lymphedema&type=Condition

Hypnosis

What Is It?

Hypnosis involves a two-step process in which a trained hypnotherapist guides the patient into a deep relaxation or trance-like state, then makes verbal suggestions to facilitate an outcome, such as quitting smoking or reducing anxiety. It can also be self-induced using technology such as smart phone apps or recorded sessions. Virtual reality can also be used for self-hypnosis, and could be a powerful tool due to the enhanced immersion experience. Hypnosis is similar to guided visualization (see page 57).

History of Hypnosis

The use of hypnosis dates back 6,000 years to Egyptian "sleep temples," but modern hypnotherapy began in eighteenth-century Paris with Franz Anton Mesmer, who used it for pain management. In 1842, James Braid published the first book on hypnotherapy, *Neurypnology*, in the United Kingdom (Zhao 2024).

Lymphedema-Specific Research

I was unable to locate any research on hypnosis used for lymphedema.

Related Research

An extensive review of over 1,500 publications describes the growing popularity of hypnosis over the past thirty years, especially in the US (Zhao 2024). In particular, it has been researched for pain, irritable bowel syndrome (IBS) and anxiety. Many of the studies include MRI or EEG testing to examine the body's response to the hypnotic process.

> **Between Professionals**
> I took a class called "Self-Hypnosis for Childbirth," during which we would practice pain management techniques. It was important to listen to the tapes each night before bed and really practice getting into a deep relaxation state. I was able to have a drug-free delivery, which was very different from the birth of my first child. Learning self-hypnosis let me experience how powerful my mind is.

Side Effects/Risks

General side effects of hypnosis include dizziness, headache, nausea, drowsiness and the creation of false memories (Mayo Clinic 2022).

Bottom Line on Hypnosis

Although no research exists on using hypnosis or self-hypnosis specifically for lymphedema, thousands of articles have been published on its successful use in managing pain, IBS and anxiety. Self-hypnosis has a low cost, is accessible in underserviced areas and has the potential to expand into the high-tech realm by integrating virtual reality. If you decide to pursue this complementary therapy, seek out a trained practitioner who understands lymphedema and can guide you on the best verbal suggestions to use.

References for Hypnosis

Mayo Clinic. 2022. "Hypnosis." Accessed January 26, 2025. https://www.mayoclinic.org/tests-procedures/hypnosis/about/pac-20394405.

Zhao FY, Li L, Xu P, et al. 2024. Mapping Knowledge Landscapes and Evolving Trends of Clinical Hypnotherapy Practice: A Bibliometrics-Based Visualization Analysis. *Int J Gen Med* 17 (December): 5773–92.

Meditation

What Is It?

Meditation is a general term for training in mental presence, which, through the quieting of the mind and a deeper level of awareness, acts on the physical, energetic, mental and spiritual levels (Pagliaro 2019). It is described as focused awareness on the body or the breath. The basic practice involves sitting quietly with your feet on the floor and your palms open on your lap while you focus your attention on your breath. Like any skill, meditation requires practice, and it can deepen with a regular routine. There are various forms of meditation, but they all fall under the category of contemplative practice.

History of Meditation

Meditation has a long history across many cultures. There is no surviving record of its creation, but it is thought to have evolved from the natural human capacity for introspection. The oldest mention of meditation is from the Indian Vedic period, in 1500 BCE. There is also evidence of ancient Greek, pagan and Christian practices (Nash 2019).

> **Between Professionals**
> I like to recommend meditation to my clients because I have personal experience with it and can provide guidance. Many clients say, "I tried it, but I can't do it." People often give up on meditation because, when they first try it, their mind remains busy with thoughts. I reassure my clients that this is normal; like anything, it just takes practice, and a few minutes a day is enough.

Lymphedema-Specific Research

In a survey of ninety-five Australian women living with lymphedema as a result of breast or gynecological cancer, 45% reported using a complementary therapy, and meditation was among the most common (Finnane 2011). The study was not designed to measure the effectiveness of the individual therapies, though, only the uses of the therapies and the perceived effectiveness—which was high, equal to that of conventional therapies.

In a similar study, 148 breast cancer survivors in Vermont were asked about their use of complementary therapies that they thought were helpful in managing their treatment and recovery (Ashikaga 2022). Their use of such therapies was high, with 72% reporting that they used at least one and 32% using at least two. Among the most frequently used were vitamins and non-food supplements (63%), herbal products (21%) and meditation (21%). Of the women interviewed, 36% reported swelling (lymphedema) in either the arm or the chest, and these woman were more likely to use a complementary therapy.

One possible interpretation of this finding is that when few options are presented by a cancer center, patients are more likely to seek out other types of treatments to help them cope with their symptoms. But this is only speculation, as we have no information on the types of lymphedema care provided to the women in this study.

One popular protocol that features meditation is mindfulness-based stress reduction, a program created by Jon Kabat-Zinn that combines Hatha yoga, breathing exercises, body scans and meditations. The research on this protocol has shown it to improve anxiety, depression, stress and pain (Srour 2024).

Side Effects/Risks

There was no mention in the studies cited of any side effects or risks of meditation.

Bottom Line on Meditation

The only available lymphedema-specific research examines whether people with lymphedema choose to include meditation as a complementary therapy, but that alone says little about the effectiveness of meditation for lymphedema—though presumably people wouldn't do it if they didn't find it helpful. Related research offers evidence that meditation combined with other introspective practices reduces anxiety, depression, stress and pain. Most health care practitioners would likely be comfortable recommending meditation despite a lack of lymphedema-specific evidence, as it has excellent risk-benefit and cost-benefit profiles.

References for Meditation

Ashikaga T, Bosompra K, O'Brien P, Nelson L. 2022. Use of Complementary and Alternative Medicine by Breast Cancer Patients: Prevalence, Patterns and Communication with Physicians. *Support Care Cancer* 10 (7): 542–48.

Finnane A, Liu Y, Battistutta D, et al. 2011. Lymphedema After Breast or Gynecological Cancer: Use and Effectiveness of Mainstream and Complementary Therapies. *J Altern Complement Med* 17 (9): 867–69.

Nash J. 2019. "The History of Meditation: Its Origins and Timeline." PositivePsychology.com. Accessed January 23, 2025. https://positivepsychology.com/history-of-meditation/.

Pagliaro G, Bernardini F. 2019. A Specific Type of Tibetan Medicine Meditation for Women with Breast Cancer: A Pilot Survey. *Oncology* 97 (2): 119–24.

Srour RA, Keyes D. 2024. "Lifestyle Mindfulness in Clinical Practice." In StatPearls [Internet]. StatPearls Publishing. Accessed January 23, 2025. https://www.ncbi.nlm.nih.gov/books/NBK599498/.

Moxibustion

What Is It?

Moxibustion is the heating of acupressure points. It is traditionally done using the dried extract of the mugwort plant (*Artemisia vulgaris*), also called moxa, moxa cone, moxa stick or moxa wool. The herb is burned, eliciting smoke, a very strong smell and heat. Moxibustion is part of traditional Chinese medicine, where it is used for tonification and purgation (Deng 2013).

There are three main types of moxibustion therapy in current use: traditional, drug and modern. Traditional therapy uses either direct contact—the moxa cone touches the skin as it burns—and indirect contact, where it is insulated from the skin by air or materials such as garlic, ginger or salt (Deng 2013). Drug moxibustion is applied to skin that has been first exposed to an irritant compound. Modern moxibustion uses microwave, laser or electrothermal technologies to provide heat to the chosen acupressure points (see electronic moxibustion, page 210); it has the advantages of less smoke and ash, a lower burning risk and greater efficiency, as it heats faster (Lu 2023).

The modern understanding of moxibustion is that it works via its thermal effects (the creation of heat), its radiation effects (the cellular penetration of that heat into the shallow and deep tissues of the skin) and its pharmacological effects from the smoke of the mugwort plant (Deng 2013).

History of Moxibustion

Moxibustion has been used to prevent and cure disease for more than 2,500 years, appearing in written text dating back to 581 BCE. From a traditional Chinese medicine perspective, it is used to dredge meridians and regulate qi (vital energy). It was used to treat many diseases throughout the reign of numerous Chinese emperors.

Lymphedema-Specific Research

The majority of studies on moxibustion for lymphedema combine it with acupuncture (see page 15).

CLINICAL TRIAL: WANG 2023

This randomized controlled trial studied the effects of two different combinations of treatments on forty patients with breast cancer–related lymphedema. One combination was tuina (see page 56) in this case, applying kneading manipulation to selected acupressure points for twenty minutes followed by moxibustion for twenty minutes; the other was pneumatic compression pump (see page 256) for thirty minutes followed by compression sleeve for eight hours. Each group received four weeks of one combination of treatments (two sessions per week), followed by a two-week break and then the other combination, for a total of eight treatments for each treatment type.

Both treatments (tuina + moxibustion and pneumatic pump + compression garment) reduced lymphedema volume. After the first treatment, when group A had started with tuina and group B had started with the compression pump, group A had significantly superior results for reduction in arm volume, as measured by water displacement. However, there was no significant difference in arm circumference between the two groups. The treatment effects were short-lived, with lymphedema returning to baseline by the end of the two-week break.

The authors concluded that adding traditional Chinese medicine therapies such as moxibustion and tuina to conventional CDT may become a new way to treat breast cancer–related lymphedema.

REVIEW: LU 2023

This review article examined the use of moxibustion to treat cancer side effects, including lymphedema. In summary, it concluded that moxibustion has been found to improve gastrointestinal toxicity, low white blood cell count, fatigue, pain and lymphedema. The lymphedema studies reviewed included the one discussed above plus one included in the section on electronic moxibustion (see page 210).

Side Effects/Risks

No adverse events occurred during moxibustion treatment in the Wang trial, but two patients quit because they couldn't tolerate the smell of the burning moxa. Risks of moxibustion include skin burns, coughing caused by the noxious smoke, inhalation of potentially harmful substances, headache and dry throat.

Bottom Line on Moxibustion

It's difficult to evaluate the effects of moxibustion on its own, as it is usually done in combination with acupuncture or tuina. While current lymphedema practice would caution against heat, some benefits have been noted from moxibustion, so you would need to weigh the risk-benefit profile before trying this treatment. Given the importance of skin integrity when you are living with lymphedema, the risk of skin burns should not be taken lightly. This therapy requires more controlled study and evaluation before safety-conscious practitioners can be enthusiastic about recommending it.

References for Moxibustion

Deng H, Shen X. 2013. The Mechanism of Moxibustion: Ancient Theory and Modern Research. *Evid Based Complement Alternat Med* 2013: 379291.

Lu S, Wang B, Wang J, et al. 2023. Moxibustion for the Treatment of Cancer and Its Complications: Efficacies and Mechanisms. *Integr Cancer Ther* 22 (January–December): 15347354231198089.

Wang C, Liu H, Shen J, et al. 2023. Effects of Tuina Combined with Moxibustion on Breast Cancer-Related Lymphedema: A Randomized Cross-Over Controlled Trial. *Integr Cancer Ther* 22 (January–December): 15347354231172735.

Qigong

What Is It?

Qigong (also known as dao yin, meaning "guiding the qi") is a mind-body exercise from traditional Chinese medicine (Fong 2014). It includes slow and controlled physical movements guided by mental exercises (internal qigong), deep breathing and relaxation. There are three main types of qigong—medical, martial arts and meditative—each with different styles. Examples include Baduanjin (meaning "eight brocades"), a gentle series of movements to improve circulation and balance; yin and yang qigong, which focuses on balancing opposing forces; and dragon and tiger qigong, which aims to improve agility and flexibility for martial arts.

History of Qigong

According to *Brittanica*, "qigong has its roots in Daoist traditions dating back to 2146 BCE" (Colón 2025). Practitioners believe that it has the power to direct the energy force of the body, which can promote longevity and revitalize people suffering from ill health.

Lymphedema-Specific Research

In a small single-blinded, non-randomized study on the use of qigong after breast cancer treatment, the twenty-three women enrolled had to have completed at least three training sessions a week in qigong for the past six months and be able to perform 18 Forms Tai Chi internal qigong independently (Fong 2014). This style of qigong, popular among cancer survivors, focuses on relaxation, deep breathing and slow, coordinated upper and lower body movements.

A physical therapist with no knowledge of how the patients were divided into groups took baseline lymphedema measurements, then eleven participants completed a six-minute qigong exercise while the twelve people in the control group sat still for six minutes. After qigong, remeasurements revealed a reduction of circumference of the upper arm (4.1%), elbow (3.1%), forearm (3.9%) and wrist (2.7%), while the control group had a slight increase in circumference of the upper arm (1.6%) and forearm (1.9%).

This study also used Doppler ultrasound to measure the participants' blood flow resistance index. In the qigong group, the radial arterial blood flow resistance reduced while the blood flow velocity increased compared with those of the control group. These results were consistent independent of age or duration of lymphedema.

It's important to note that when the participants arrived for each session, their lymphedema was similar, meaning that any benefits from the qigong did not last from one session to the next. On average, the women in the study had been doing qigong for about ten months, and their lymphedema circumference measurements at the beginning of the study were not significantly different from those of women who do not do qigong, which suggests that for sustained benefit, an even longer practice would be required (or that it's only effective in the short term).

Related Research

See the chapter on tai chi (page 52) for a study comparing tai chi and qigong in cancer patients.

Side Effects/Risks

There was no mention of side effects or risks in the Fong study.

Bottom Line on Qigong

One small short-term study demonstrated improvements in arm circumference measurements, reduction in radial arterial blood flow resistance and increased blood flow velocity after six minutes of 18 Forms Tai Chi internal qigong compared with a control group, but the benefits were not sustained over time. It is unclear how often or for how long qigong would need to be performed in order to see sustained improvements.

References for Qigong

Colón, Suzan. 2025. "Qigong: Exercise and Meditation Technique." Britannica. Accessed April 18, 2025. https://www.britannica.com/topic/qigong.

Fong SS, Ng SS, Luk WS, et al. 2014. Effects of Qigong Exercise on Upper Limb Lymphedema and Blood Flow in Survivors of Breast Cancer: A Pilot Study. *Integr Cancer Ther* 13 (1): 54–61.

Singing Bowls

What Are They?

Singing bowls, also called sound bowls, Tibetan singing bowls or Himalayan singing bowls, are round metal bowls designed to emit a pleasant resonating sound when they are struck or circled with a mallet. The frequency of the sound vibration varies depending on the thickness, height, radius, curvature and cone angle of the bowl. Different qualities of sound can also be produced based on the technique of striking the bowl, the force applied and the number of strikes. Single or multiple bowls can be used during a singing bowl session, and different sound frequencies can be targeted to different areas of the body (Seetharaman 2024). Research has explored the bowls' effects on blood pressure, heart rate, respiratory rate, brain waves, binaural beats, mood, tension, anxiety, depression and well-being.

History of Singing Bowls

Singing bowls sound meditation has been practiced for thousands of years in Tibetan and Buddhist societies to promote healing and relaxation. Specifically, the vibrations are thought to interact with the body's energy center, known as chakras (Seetharaman 2024). The singing bowls are placed on or near the body, allowing the sound vibrations to influence the body systems. In addition, the calming tones can induce relaxation and relieve stress and tension. Singing bowls sound meditation is considered a holistic treatment, impacting the body, mind and spirit. Breath work is generally done in conjunction with the sound emitting from the bowls.

Lymphedema-Specific Research

I was unable to find any lymphedema-specific studies, but I know of a couple of lymphedema clinics that use singing bowls. The use of vibration for lymphedema is fairly common; in addition to singing bowls, other vibration-based therapies include tuning forks (page 110) and vibration plates (page 270), among others.

Related Research

A randomized controlled trial explored the effects of singing bowls versus progressive muscle relaxation (see page 95) in a single session with a group of fifty people with non-clinical anxiety (Rio-Alamos 2023). Electroencephalographic activity (EEG), heart rate variability and self-reported anxiety were measured before and after treatment. Both the singing bowls and the progressive muscle relaxation induced a relaxation response, but the effect was more evident with the singing bowls.

A meta-analysis of singing bowl research examined four studies that measured various outcomes, including pain, tension, anger, fatigue, sleep duration, blood pressure and more (Stanhope 2020). The authors found that there was promising evidence for the health benefits of singing bowl therapy and acknowledged that it is a low-cost and low-risk option, but given that the research is in its infancy, they concluded that they cannot recommend it at this time.

Side Effects/Risks

There were no adverse events reported in the research, so singing bowl treatment appears to be very safe; however, potential side effects could include headaches, agitation, emotional distress and an impact on implanted medical devices. Caution is recommended for people with seizure disorders, pregnant women and those with mental health issues or non-healed postsurgical wounds (Hersh 2022).

Bottom Line on Singing Bowls

Singing bowls have a long traditional use, but there are few published studies on their therapeutic value, and none at all on their effectiveness for treating lymphedema. That said, they are known to induce relaxation, which may have an indirect benefit for lymphedema management. No side effects have been noted, the cost is low, and the treatment is relatively accessible, especially if patients purchase their own singing bowls and perform the therapy themselves. Some training may be required regarding the best type of bowl, where to place the bowl, and the intensity and frequency of striking or stroking the bowl, so people who are interested may wish to begin by working with a health practitioner familiar with this modality.

References for Singing Bowls

Hersh E, Lamoreux K. 2022. "Are There Health Benefits to Tibetan Singing Bowls?" Healthline. Accessed December 30, 2024. https://www.healthline.com/health/dangers-of-singing-bowls.

Rio-Alamos C, Montefusco-Siegmund R, Cañete T, et al. 2023. Acute Relaxation Response Induced by Tibetan Singing Bowl Sounds: A Randomized Controlled Trial. *Eur J Investig Health Psychol Educ* 13 (2): 317–30.

Seetharaman R, Avhad S, Rane J. 2024. Exploring the Healing Power of Singing Bowls: An Overview of Key Findings and Potential Benefits. *Explore* (New York) 20 (1): 39–43.

Stanhope J, Weinstein P. 2020. The Human Health Effects of Singing Bowls: A Systematic Review. *Complement Ther Med.* 51 (June): 102412.

Tai Chi

What Is It?

Tai chi is a Chinese martial art, initially developed for combat and self-defense, that has evolved into a gentle, low-impact exercise. It claims to balance the body's qi (vital energy). It can be done standing or seated, and there is a version performed in water called ai chi (see page 74).

History of Tai Chi

Tai chi and Qigong share a common history, which has evolved from Traditional Chinese medicine, martial arts and philosophy (Wayne 2018).

Lymphedema-Specific Research

I was unable to find any research specifically on tai chi for lymphedema. In their position paper on exercise, the National Lymphedema Network states: "There are many other types of exercise that have health benefits such as Pilates, yoga, tai chi, qigong, aquatic exercise, trampoline rebounding, breathing exercises and relaxation exercise that have not been adequately studied in people with lymphedema. However, the person with lymphedema can use the benefits of any system of exercise if he/she follows the general safety principles of exercise with lymphedema, seeks medical guidance, and uses caution in starting any new exercise program" (NLN 2011).

Related Research

A systematic review of exercise for cancer patients examined the effects of tai chi and qigong (see page 48) mind-body exercises on symptoms affecting quality of life, including fatigue, sleep difficulty, depression and pain (Wayne 2018). Over 1,500 patients participated in the exercises for between three and twelve weeks. A meta-analysis revealed that mind-body exercises were associated with a significant improvement in fatigue, sleep difficulty, depression and overall quality of life. There was a nonsignificant trend towards improvement in pain. There was no mention of lymphedema in any of the studies and therefore no evaluation of how the mind-body exercises might impact this cancer side effect.

Side Effects/Risks

None noted.

Bottom Line on Tai Chi

Tai chi is a set of gentle, slow movements that incorporate mind-body elements. To paraphrase the NLN's position statement, exercise is beneficial, and people with lymphedema should choose an exercise program that resonates with them. Finding a program that you enjoy and can participate in on a regular basis will provide countless benefits.

References for Tai Chi

NLN Medical Advisory Committee. 2011. "Exercise." Position Statement of the National Lymphedema Network. Accessed April 22, 2025. https://nlnmembership.com/wp-content/uploads/2022/02/Exercise.pdf.

Wayne PM, Lee MS, Novakowski J, et al. 2018. Tai Chi and Qigong for Cancer-Related Symptoms and Quality of Life: A Systematic Review and Meta-Analysis. *J Cancer Surviv* 12 (2): 256–67.

Traditional Chinese Medicine

What Is It?

Traditional Chinese medicine (TCM) is an integrative set of practices that include herbal treatments, acupuncture, acupressure, moxibustion, cupping, medicinal plants and dried animal parts (Britannica 2025). The goal of TCM is to balance the qi (life force), blood, yin (passive force) and yang (active force), promote self-healing and enhance quality of life.

History of Traditional Chinese Medicine

TCM originated during the Shang Dynasty at least twenty-three centuries ago from a shamanistic practice. It is one of the world's oldest medical systems. It acts to restore harmony between yin and yang because an imbalance can result in illness. Today, TCM has regulatory colleges in many jurisdictions outside of China. According to Britannica (2025), "Nearly 200 modern medicines have been developed either directly or indirectly from the 7,300 species of plants used as medicines in China." Although China has adopted a science-based approach to medicine, TCM is still commonly practiced, and China endorses a health system that incorporates the best of both worlds (Hong 2004).

> **Between Professionals**
>
> Over the years, clients have asked me about contradictions between what I am teaching them and what their TCM practitioner advises. For example, I might suggest that they eat more fruits and vegetables to improve their intake of fiber, while their TCM practitioner has told them to avoid certain vegetables that are hot/yang because their issue (for example, constipation) is also hot/yang. It can be very difficult for a patient to determine what to do when the information is contradictory. In some situations, they may have to choose one system to follow, as trying to do both when they don't integrate well may lead to frustration.

Lymphedema-Specific Research

There may be studies published in Chinese that evaluate TCM for lymphedema, but being limited to research published in English, I had access to only one trial, which combined TCM protocol with art therapy for arm lymphedema in breast cancer survivors (Liu 2024). Researchers recruited 120 patients, with half in the treatment group and half in the control group.

The control group received three phases of rehabilitation, beginning with deep breathing, shoulder mobility exercises and gentle, passive joint mobilization to prevent stiffness (weeks one and two post-surgery). The intermediate rehabilitation phase included gradually increasing active shoulder movements, arm elevation and manual lymphatic drainage (weeks two to six). The advanced rehabilitation phase added strength, flexibility, balance and coordination exercises (weeks six to eight).

The treatment group received TCM from a trained practitioner, which included acupuncture, herbal therapy (*Panax ginseng*, *Angelica sinesis* and astragalus), tuina and massage. In addition, they met with a psychological counselor. For the art therapy portion, participants did mandala painting.

Both groups reported improved pain, ability to perform activities of daily living, range of motion and muscle strength, but the improvement scores were greater for the TCM + art therapy protocol than for the control group. Fewer people in the TCM group developed lymphedema (nineteen cases versus nine cases), and there was a lower incidence of fatigue in the TCM group (fifty-six cases versus forty-four cases).

Side Effects/Risks

There was no mention of side effects or risks in the Liu study.

Bottom Line on Traditional Chinese Medicine

Traditional Chinese medicine combines healing practices designed to balance qi and restore life force. The only lymphedema study published in English included an entire TCM protocol, as opposed to testing the individual elements, which would be challenging since TCM is a holistic protocol. The study found that breast cancer survivors experienced improved outcomes over conventional rehabilitation when TCM was combined with psychological counseling and art therapy. This study took place in China, where the participants' belief system and comfort with TCM might have played a role in its acceptance and effectiveness—a factor that may be relevant when testing TCM protocols in other cultures.

References for Traditional Chinese Medicine

Britannica. 2025. "Traditional Chinese Medicine." Accessed April 18, 2025. https://www.britannica.com/science/traditional-Chinese-medicine.

Hong, FF. 2004. History of Medicine in China: When Medicine Took an Alternative Path. *McGill J Med* 8 (1): 79–84.

Liu J, Shi Y, Wu L, Feng X. 2024. Effects of Chinese Medicine Comprehensive Care Combined with Art Painting Therapy in Upper Limb Lymphedema and Shoulder Joint Mobility After Breast Cancer Surgery. *Eur J Gynaecol Oncol* 45 (3): 130–37.

Tuina

What Is It?

Tuina (also spelled tui na) is a massage technique similar to shiatsu. Part of traditional Chinese medicine (see page 54), it is often used in conjunction with acupuncture (page 15), moxibustion (page 46), cupping (page 35), herbalism, tai chi (page 52) or qigong (page 48). It is a hands-on treatment designed to bring the body into balance. The name comes from the Chinese words *tui*, meaning "to push," and *na*, meaning "to lift and squeeze"—two of the techniques used to move qi. The Korean approach to tuina is known as *chu na*; Japanese-style tuina is called *anma*.

Tuina techniques include brushing, kneading, rolling, pressing and rubbing the area between the joints to open the body's defenses and get the energy moving in the meridians and muscles by applying pressure to certain acupoints. Tuina treats the muscular tension surrounding the bony structures in a way that minimizes rebound effects and the short-term return of symptoms (Kim, n.d.).

History of Tuina

Like other TCM-based practices, tuina has been used for centuries in China. Chinese texts that are 2,000 years old document the use of manual therapies (Kim, n.d.).

Lymphedema-Specific Research

A randomized controlled trial studied the effects of two different combinations of treatments on forty patients with breast cancer–related lymphedema (Wang 2023). One combination was tuina for twenty minutes followed by moxibustion for twenty minutes; the other was pneumatic compression pump (see page 256) for thirty minutes followed by compression sleeve for eight hours. Each group received four weeks of one combination of treatments (two sessions per week), followed by a two-week break and then the other combination, for a total of eight treatments for each treatment type.

The tuina was modified for lymphedema, treating from distal to proximal for both the three yin meridians and the three yang meridians; it was designed to warm yang and activate blood circulation while purging yin and reducing swelling. Only gentle manipulations were used, to focus on the skin and lymphatic structures and avoid stimulating deep muscle tissue.

Both treatments (tuina + moxibustion and pneumatic pump + compression garment) reduced lymphedema volume. After the first treatment, when group A had started with tuina and group B had started with compression pump, group A had significantly superior results for reduction in arm volume, as measured by water displacement. However, there was no significant difference in arm circumference between the two groups. The treatment effects were short-lived, with lymphedema returning to baseline by the end of the two-week break.

Side Effects/Risks

No side effects were noted in this study, but importantly, the tuina was modified from the usual pattern to include distal to proximal movement and a light touch.

Bottom Line on Tuina

This gentle manual technique based on principles of traditional Chinese medicine may prove to be a relaxing addition to complete decongestive therapy. If you pursue tuina, be sure to work with a practitioner who understands lymphedema and is willing to modify their technique to provide the best decongestive results. Although tuina is a manual technique, the research to date does not demonstrate that it can replace manual lymphatic drainage by a certified lymphedema therapist.

References for Tuina

Kim JM, Cheng SM, Yu D-F. n.d. "Orthodox Tui-Na Treatment." The World Tui-Na Association. Accessed January 25, 2024. https://www.tui-na.com/tuina.html.

Wang C, Liu H, Shen J, et al. 2023. Effects of Tuina Combined with Moxibustion on Breast Cancer-Related Lymphedema: A Randomized Cross-Over Controlled Trial. *Integr Cancer Ther* 22 (January–December): 15347354231172735.

Visualization

What Is It?

Visualization—also called guided visualization, guided meditation, guided imagery or mental rehearsal—is similar to hypnosis (see page 42). It involves becoming very relaxed and then listening to suggestive messages that invoke a multisensory conscious experience. A participant may feel like they are actually experiencing an event through their mind's eye (Giacobbi 2017).

Visualization has a traditional use in many cultures, including Tibetan Buddhism, Indian Tantra and Chinese medicine (Pagliaro 2019). It can be used to increase physical activity, modify food intake, reduce cravings and cope with stress, among other applications. Many mental health and complementary care practitioners, such as psychologists and hypnotherapists, use guided visualization as part of their treatment. For example, guided visualization is a common practice in sports psychology, especially for elite athletes.

Lymphedema-Specific Research

I was unable to locate research on guided visualization being used to treat lymphedema.

Related Research

A review of 320 randomized controlled trials with 17,979 adults published in 216 peer-reviewed journals found that visualization improved coping skills, pain, stroke recovery, anxiety, stress management and sports skills (Giacobbi 2017). In 77% of the studies, visualization resulted in significant improvement in a variety of outcomes. The authors of the review concluded that:

- Guided imagery offers great potential for future research and application.
- Deep breathing and visualization are low-risk complementary therapies.
- Deep breathing, visualization and yoga can be done individually or combined into one practice and are excellent protocols to consider when finances are limited.

Another review of ten studies on breast cancer survivors who used complementary therapies concluded that visualization did not provide any additional pain control when used in combination with pain medication, but that hypnosis and meditation both independently demonstrated significant pain reduction and psychological benefit (Abushukur 2022).

A study of sixty-two female breast cancer survivors used visualization in the form of Tibetan medicine meditation (Pagliaro 2019). Participants were asked to quiet their mind, have a deep level of awareness, picture a sphere of white light on a precise point of their chest and then see it start to border the area around the wound, leaving a luminous trail of light. They were told to imagine the light as a beneficial energy acting around the wound, increasing the effectiveness of their treatments and evoking a feeling of joy and happiness. After five sessions, the researchers noted a significant reduction in follow-up scores for anxiety-tension, depression-dejection, anger-hostility, fatigue and confusion, as well as a nonsignificant increase in vigor. No side effects were noted, but there was no control group for comparison. This study is just one example of visualization being used to treat not only psychological issues, such as depression and anxiety, but also somatic issues like fatigue.

Side Effects/Risks

None noted.

User Experience

"I have had lymphedema in my arm following breast cancer treatment more than twenty years ago. As part of manual lymph drainage massage from one practitioner, I was asked to visualize the movement of lymph fluid. I didn't notice any particular benefit."

—Anonymous, Ontario (post–breast cancer arm lymphedema)

Bottom Line on Visualization

Visualization is a low-cost, low-risk complementary therapy. Although there is no published research on using visualization for lymphedema, there is plenty of evidence on its benefits for other medical conditions. If you would like to try it, look for a practitioner who understands both visualization and your lymphedema-specific goals. Alternatively, you can purchase prerecorded visualizations to listen to on your own, and the use of virtual reality may soon become an option. You may choose to pair visualization with practices such as yoga, deep breathing and/or self-MLD. The mind can be a powerful healing tool, and we often fail to use it to its full potential.

References for Visualization

Abushukur Y, Cascardo C, Ibrahim Y, et al. 2022. Improving Breast Surgery Outcomes Through Alternative Therapy: A Systematic Review. *Cureus* 14 (3): e23443.

Giacobbi PR Jr, Stewart J, Chaffee K, et al. 2017. A Scoping Review of Health Outcomes Examined in Randomized Controlled Trials Using Guided Imagery. *Prog Prev Med* (New York) 2 (7): e0010.

Pagliaro G, Bernardini F. 2019. A Specific Type of Tibetan Medicine Meditation for Women with Breast Cancer: A Pilot Survey. *Oncology* 97 (2): 119–24.

Wenyang Huoxue Compress

What Is It?

The Wenyang Huoxue (WYHX) washing prescription is a bandage soak and compress based on principles from traditional Chinese medicine. It was created by Professor Hu Kaiwen of the oncology department of Donggang Hospital in China. It includes 300 grams each of dried ginger (*Zingiber officinale Rosc.*), cassia (*Cinnamomum cassia Presl.*), Chinese prickly ash (*Zanthoxylum bungeanum Maxim.*) and dong quai

(*Angelica sinensis*). The warm herbal poultice is thought to alleviate symptoms of yang deficiency and blood stasis.

A study published in 2018 offers instructions on making the herbal solution (Chen 2018), though some important details are missing that would make it challenging to prepare at home. For example, the recipe says to combine eight parts water and one part herbs, then cook them twice, for forty-five minutes each time, but it is unclear what cooking method to use (though I would guess boiling). After several other steps, including filtering the decoction, letting it stand overnight and then concentrating it, the solution is packed into bags. Before use, a bag is added to hot water in an insulated bowl and allowed to stand for three minutes.

There are two ways to apply the liquid solution. For the first, you wrap the affected arm in gauze extending 2 centimeters (¾ inch) beyond the lymphedema in each direction, then drench the gauze with the solution; spray the gauze with more solution every five to ten minutes to keep it warm and moist for forty to sixty minutes. For the second, you soak the gauze in the solution, wring it out using tweezers to get the proper dampness, then apply the soaked gauze to the arm and keep it warm. This is done daily for fourteen days. The study also specifies using the compress between 9:00 and 11:00 a.m., as part of the spleen meridian.

History of the Wenyang Huoxue Compress

Like other traditional Chinese medicines, the Wenyang Huoxue compress has been around for centuries. It is similar to acupuncture and moxibustion in that the goal is to warm yang and activate blood circulation.

> **Technical Breakdown**
> Botanical names are formal scientific names assigned to plant species by the International Code of Nomenclature. It's important for each plant to have a single universal name, as a plant may grow in many different countries and have different names and nicknames throughout the world; the use of the formal name ensures that everyone is confident they are referring to the same plant. One of the ingredients in Wenyang Huoxue is dried ginger, known as gan jiang in Chinese. Its scientific name is Zingiber officinale Roscoe.

Lymphedema-Specific Research

The trial that used the recipe described briefly above involved seventy-eight patients with arm lymphedema (Chen 2018). After fourteen days, the functional scores in twenty-three patients improved by ten points. A further forty-one cases improved by five to ten points, while six patients had improvements that were less than five points. Eight cases experienced a worsening of their functional scores. The functional scores ranked factors such as the ability to put on a sweater, the ability to cut vegetables, shoulder discomfort, numbness, stiffness and range of movement.

It's unclear whether the researchers were observing the functional changes or the patients were reporting them; either way, there was some opportunity for bias since there was no mention of blinding in the study. That said, the compress does appear to have had a positive impact on seventy out of seventy-eight patients.

Side Effects/Risks

No adverse reactions were noted in the Chen study.

Bottom Line on Wenyang Huoxue Compress

In the Chen study, the Wenyang Huoxue compress was applied by nurses in a hospital. If you were to try it at home, you would have to give some thought to how to set everything up or you might end up with a big mess, especially if you are trying to do everything one-handed. The recipe is quite involved, and monitoring the temperature as you work through the instructions seems challenging. On the positive side, your arm would smell nice—like cinnamon and ginger.

Ultimately, traditional Chinese medicine is an entirely different approach to health, and it may be best to work with a TCM practitioner. Like most research on traditional medicines, the Chen study was small, follow-up was not done, and the study quality was limited, so Western-trained evidence-based practitioners are unlikely to enthusiastically recommend this therapy until more research is done. If it proves to be helpful, a convenient, ready-to-use version of the herbal solution would make it more practical.

References for Wenyang Huoxue Compress

Chen H, Wang X-Y, Zhao, B-Y, et al. 2018. Clinical Experience in Treating 78 Cases of Upper Limb Edema After Breast Cancer Operation by WenYang HuoZue Washing Prescription. *TMR Modern Herb Med* 1 (4): 198–202.

Yoga

What Is It?

Yoga is a combination of meditation, relaxation, breathing, stretching, and posture control exercises; for some practitioners, it is also a spiritual practice. It originated in India and was designed to balance physical, mental, psychological and emotional needs (Wei 2019).

There are various types of yoga, usually named after their creator, emphasizing different meditative or physical aspects of the practice. Examples include:

- **Hatha:** A generic term for any type of yoga that teaches physical postures.
- **Jivamukti:** A vigorous and physically challenging style with lively music.
- **Satyananda:** A form of yoga with the goal of increasing inner awareness.
- **Vinyasa:** A dynamic style with smooth transitions from one pose to the next, creating a continuous, synchronized flow. Also called "flow yoga."

History of Yoga

Yoga dates to 2700 BCE. The word derives from the Sanskrit *yuj*, which means "to unite." According to ancient spiritual texts, yoga leads to the union of individual consciousness with universal consciousness. When you experience this oneness, you are in yoga or are being a yogi. The aim of yoga, as it was traditionally practiced, was self-realization, to overcome suffering and live in a state of liberation (Basavaraddi 2015).

User Experience

"Lymphatic yoga has been very beneficial, combining breathing, manual lymphatic drainage, muscle/yoga poses and mindfulness with meditation to help maintain swelling. I have been using lymphatic yoga for approximately two years."

—Robin, Washington (left arm, hand and underarm lymphedema)

Lymphedema-Specific Research

Several studies have been done on yoga for lymphedema. I'll share two systematic reviews of randomized controlled trials on breast cancer–related lymphedema and yoga, and one clinical trial that involved the creation of a lymphedema-specific yoga sequence.

REVIEW #1: WEI 2019

This systematic review included five studies, totaling eighty-five participants: three randomized controlled trials comparing yoga with usual care (Douglass 2012; Loudon 2014; Loudon 2016), and two quasi-experimental studies measuring lymphedema before and after yoga (Fisher 2014; Lai 2017). All of the studies used similar therapies, namely breathing exercises, physical postures (asanas), meditation and relaxation. One study also included education on avoiding static postures of the affected arm. Three of the studies lasted four weeks (and one, Douglass 2012, had a six-month follow-up), and two were for eight weeks. The set-up was also similar: ninety-minute yoga classes with a professional trainer one to three days a week, and a forty-five-minute CD or DVD for home use six days a week. Three of the studies used Satyananda yoga, one used Hatha yoga, and one used aerobic yoga training.

The results were mixed: Two studies found no significant difference in lymphedema (Douglass 2012; Lai 2017), one found a significant improvement (Fisher 2014), one found an increase in lymphedema volume (Loudon 2014) and one did not measure lymphedema volume but did see an improvement in posture and shoulder strength (Loudon 2016).

The write-up of this review confounded me. After reading the results, my impression was that the impact of yoga on lymphedema was lukewarm. But the authors of the review concluded that despite no standardization for yoga practice, there was "significant improvement of lymphedema." While that was true for one study, another two that measured lymphedema volume found no significant improvements and a fourth found an increase, so it's unclear to me how the authors came to this conclusion.

User Experience

"Yoga is a regular activity for me (three times per week) that helps significantly with the heaviness and aches."

—Christina, Ontario (secondary lymphedema in the arm, stomach and leg)

REVIEW #2: FREGUIA 2024

This review comparing routine care to yoga included three randomized controlled trials with a total of ninety-six patients. Those in the yoga group participated in ninety-minute sessions with an

instructor, as well as a forty-five-minute home practice watching a recording. One study included twenty asanas and five breathing exercises chosen to expand the chest, maximize range of motion of the neck, shoulder and elbows, and stretch the skin by activating muscles around the armpits and lymph nodes (Pasyar 2019). The other two studies designed their Satyananda protocols to mimic manual lymphatic drainage, with gentle range of motion of the shoulder and spine, core and shoulder stabilization, and stress reduction (Loudon 2014 and 2016).

The results included improvements in physical and emotional functioning and reduced fatigue, pain and insomnia. The Loudon studies reported reductions in tissue induration (an indication of how hard and thick the skin is, measured using a tool called a tonometer) and increased shoulder strength and spinal mobility, but none of the studies found a significant improvement in lymphedema volume.

The authors of the review concluded that yoga showed promise in improving quality of life, musculoskeletal function and some aspects of lymphedema management, but that further research is needed to clarify yoga's role in reducing lymphedema swelling.

CLINICAL TRIAL: NARAHARI 2016

The researchers for this study analyzed past protocols for lymphedema and designed their own unique yoga sequence for upper limb lymphedema (referred to as "Narahari et al. yoga"). They observed the action of anatomical areas on lymph node and skin stretch with the goal of developing a yoga and breathing sequence that would improve range of motion, reduce fibrosis and drain lymph. They decided that the protocol should begin with massage of the contralateral axillary nodes (the armpit on the healthy side) and inguinal nodes (the lymph nodes in the groin) on the same side and then incorporate:

- A proximal to distal sequence
- Posture progression from head to toe
- Joint movements to help drain lymph nodes
- Coordinated breathing to maximize lymph drainage
- Slow, methodical joint movements for pain management and range of motion
- Abdominal contractions to create a pressure difference between the abdomen and the thoracic regions and maximize lymph drainage

The protocol was pilot-tested on eight patients with stage 3 lymphedema. They were given in-person training for two weeks, then advised to continue their forty-five-minute yoga protocol at home for the next three months. The yoga was part of a holistic care plan that also included counseling to explain the treatment, Ayurvedic oil massage in the lymphedema arm and Indian manual lymphatic drainage (which is different from North American MLD) followed by long stretch bandaging (rather than the North American standard of short stretch bandaging).

At their three-month follow-up, the patients' limb volume had reduced from 2.5 to 1.2 liters (84 to 41 ounces). The protocol also improved limb heaviness, fibrosis, pain and range of motion. The authors concluded that their protocol was comparable to the effects seen with a combination of MLD and two previously described lymphedema yoga sequences. But given that there was no control group, and that the patients also received Indian MLD and compression, it's unclear what effects were due to the yoga itself.

Side Effects/Risks

In the Wei review, no adverse events were reported. The Freguia review reported on one study that saw an increase in lymphedema volume (Louden 2014). Yoga's risks vary depending on the poses and your joint restrictions; some poses may need to be modified. Poses that require holding a position for a long time may put pressure on a joint such as the wrist or shoulder that could aggravate the joint or have a negative impact on the lymphedema, especially if the yoga class is not specifically designed for cancer survivors or those living with lymphedema.

If you are a yoga teacher and want to offer a yoga protocol specific to lymphedema, I highly suggest reading the Narahari clinical trial, which describes their protocol in detail. If you have upper arm lymphedema, share the article with a qualified yoga instructor so they can evaluate it and teach you the sequence or one of the alternative postures included, as appropriate for your needs. If you have lymphedema in other parts of your body, work with a professional who understands lymphedema and can advise you on the best yoga protocol for your needs to complement complete decongestive therapy. Caution may be needed with Bikram yoga, which is also called "hot yoga" and is performed in a heated room.

User Experience
"Vinyasa or Jivamukti yoga paired with ujjayi breathing and a lot of stretching works very well for me."

—Anonymous, Germany (secondary lymphedema in the legs after cervical cancer)

Bottom Line on Yoga

There are several studies and meta-analyses specifically of yoga for lymphedema. The results show benefits in quality of life, strength, range of motion and tissue induration, and reduced scarring, pain, fatigue and insomnia. But there have been no consistent results in terms of lymphedema volume reduction.

One important consideration is that yoga is not one modality; there are several different types, as well as variations depending on the teacher. To limit injury and maximize benefit, clients should seek out instructors who can interpret and teach yoga sequences that have been designed specifically for lymphedema. In cases of financial limitation, patients may be able to perform the yoga sequences independently after instruction from a qualified instructor. Yoga should be done in a progressive manner, to build up tolerance. Deep breathing, visualization and yoga can be done individually or combined into one practice.

If yoga is something you already enjoy and find benefit in, by all means continue with your current practice. But if you are looking to begin a body movement or exercise practice that has consistent published results for lymphedema volume reduction, yoga may not be the best option based on research to date. On the other hand, if your goals are improvement in quality of life, insomnia, pain and other side effects of living with lymphedema, then yoga may be a good addition to your care plan.

References for Yoga

Basavaraddi IV. 2015. "Yoga: Its Origin, History and Development." High Commission of India, Ottawa, Canada. Accessed April 18, 2025. https://hciottawa.gov.in/newsevent?id=16.

Douglass J, Immink M, Piller N, Ullah S. 2012. Yoga for Women with Breast Cancer-Related Lymphoedema: A Preliminary 6-Month Study. *J Lymphoedema* 7 (2): 30–38.

Fisher MI, Donahoe-Fillmore B, Leach L, et al. 2014. Effects of Yoga on Arm Volume Among Women with Breast Cancer Related Lymphedema: A Pilot Study. *J Bodyw Mov Ther* 18 (4): 559–65.

Freguia S, Platano D, Donati D, et al. 2024. Closing the Gaps: An Integrative Review of Yoga's Benefits for Lymphedema in Breast Cancer Survivors. *Life* (Basel) 14 (8): 999.

Lai Y, Hsieh C, Huang L, et al. 2017. The Effects of Upper Limb Exercise Through Yoga on Limb Swelling in Chinese Breast Cancer Survivors—A Pilot Study. *Rehabil Nurs* 42 (1): 46–54.

Loudon A, Barnett T, Piller N, et al. 2014. Yoga Management of Breast Cancer-Related Lymphoedema: A Randomised Controlled Pilot-Trial. *BMC Complement Altern Med* 14 (July): 214.

Loudon A, Barnett T, Piller N, et al. 2016. The Effects of Yoga on Shoulder and Spinal Actions for Women with Breast Cancer-Related Lymphoedema of the Arm: A Randomised Controlled Pilot Study. *BMC Complement Altern Med* 16 (1): 343.

Narahari SR, Aggithaya MG, Thernoe L, et al. 2016. Yoga Protocol for Treatment of Breast Cancer-Related Lymphedema. *Int J Yoga* 9 (2): 145–55.

Pasyar N, Barshan Tashnizi N, Mansouri P, Tahmasebi S. 2019. Effect of Yoga Exercise on the Quality of Life and Upper Extremity Volume Among Women with Breast Cancer Related Lymphedema: A Pilot Study. *Eur J Oncol Nurs* 42 (October): 103–9.

Wei CW, Wu YC, Chen PY, et al. 2019. Effectiveness of Yoga Interventions in Breast Cancer-Related Lymphedema: A Systematic Review. *Complement Ther Clin Pract* 36 (August): 49–55.

Traditional Therapies Summary

Traditional therapies have been used for generations and have emerged from a verbal legacy rather than a written one. There tend to be few published studies on traditional therapies, but they generate strong opinions and have a loyal following. They are often low-risk and low-cost, which makes them very appealing. Some, such as acupuncture and yoga, have become very popular and have more supporting evidence.

The following pages provide a summary of the findings in this section. Be sure to consult the specific book chapters for more details.

Therapy	What It Is	Claims	Lymphedema Research	Results	Side Effects/Risks
Acupressure	Pressure applied to points on the meridians	Clears blockages in qi and restores harmony	Meta-analysis of nine acupoint massage studies (most published in Chinese)	Improved swelling, limb function and QoL, lower levels of blood inflammatory markers	None noted
Acupuncture	Fine needles inserted into meridians to align qi	Rebalances qi	Multiple studies and at least three systematic reviews	Reduced arm swelling and pain, especially with needle warming	Skin discomfort, scalding, flushing, itching, swelling and dry mouth
Apple cider vinegar	Fermented juice of crushed apples with 5% acetic acid	Promotes weight loss, reduces blood lipids, anti-inflammatory, repairs skin	None	n/a	Tooth enamel loss, stomach burning, heartburn, skin reactions
Ayurveda	Traditional Indian medicine	Restores balance	One study of 240 patients with filarial lymphedema	Gradual reduction in limb volume	None noted
Balneotherapy	Mineral water or mud bathing	Anti-inflammatory, relaxing, pain-relieving	One exploratory review	n/a	Hot water may increase edema, infection
Cabbage leaves	Rolled leaves of *Brassica oleracea L.*	Anti-inflammatory, pain relieving	One animal study using a synthetic version of a cabbage extract	Reduced swelling in mice	Skin reactions
Castor oil	Oil from the castor bean (*Ricinus communis*)	Laxative, anti-inflammatory, wound healing	One animal study using a topical application	Reduced swelling in mice and guinea pigs	Abdominal cramping, vomiting, bloating, dizziness, reduced drug absorption; contraindicated with GI obstruction, IBD

n/a = not applicable; QoL = quality of life, GI = gastrointestinal, IBD = inflammatory bowel disease

Therapy	What It Is	Claims	Lymphedema Research	Results	Side Effects/Risks
Cupping	Negative pressure via suction	Enhances blood circulation and relieves swelling and pain	Two studies in English with a total of 135 participants	Improved circumferences, pain and skin thickness	Skin trauma; contraindicated with clotting problems, eczema, psoriasis
Essential oils	Concentrated hydrophobic liquids extracted from plants	Multiple health claims, including stress reduction and improved sleep	One case series of 8 patients; one clinical trial with 79 participants	Essential oils were ineffective	Skin or allergic reactions
Hypnosis	Suggestions given while the patient is in a trance state	Reduces pain, anxiety and IBS symptoms	None	n/a	Dizziness, headache, nausea, drowsiness, the creation of false memories
Meditation	Focused awareness on the body or breath	Helps achieve a deeper level of awareness	Two surveys of complementary therapy use	Meditation is commonly used by cancer survivors	None noted
Moxibustion	Warming of acupressure points, usually by burning dried mugwort	Tonifies and purges meridians	Studies are on moxibustion combined with acupuncture or tuina, not on its own	Improved fatigue, pain, lymphedema, white blood cell count and GI toxicity	Skin burns, coughing due to noxious smoke, headache, dry throat
Qigong	Mind-body exercise from traditional Chinese medicine	Directs qi to promote healing and longevity	One human study with 23 patients on sitting still versus qigong	Improved arm circumference, reduction in radial arterial blood flow resistance and increased blood flow velocity	None noted
Singing bowls	Round metal bowls that emit a frequency when struck	Sound vibrations can be directed toward healing	None	n/a	Headaches, agitation, emotional distress, impact on implanted medical devices

n/a = not applicable, IBS = irritable bowel syndrome, GI = gastrointestinal

Therapy	What It Is	Claims	Lymphedema Research	Results	Side Effects/ Risks
Tai chi	Gentle, low-impact exercise	Rebalances qi and promotes healing and longevity	None	n/a	None noted
Traditional Chinese medicine (TCM)	An integrative set of practices that include medicinals, acupuncture, acupressure, moxibustion, and cupping	Balances qi, blood, yin and yang, promotes self-healing and enhances QoL	One study of TCM + art therapy with 120 participants	Improved pain, ability to perform activities of daily living, RoM and muscle strength	None noted
Tuina	Traditional Chinese massage	Brings the body into balance	One study of 40 patients on tuina + moxibustion	Reduced volume better than pneumatic compression pump + sleeve	None noted
Visualization	Guided imagery	Harnesses the power of the mind to make physical changes	None	n/a	None noted
Wenyang Huoxue compress	Chinese herbal poultice	Warms yang and increases blood circulation	One study of 78 patients with arm lymphedema	70 patients had improved functional scores; 8 got worse	None noted
Yoga	A combination of meditation, relaxation, breathing, stretching, and posture control exercises	Promotes mind-body harmony	Multiple studies and two systematic reviews with a total of 181 participants	Improved QoL, fatigue, RoM, pain and insomnia	Increased lymphedema volume, joint pain or injury

n/a = not applicable, QoL = quality of life; RoM = range of motion

Part Two
Body Work

Introduction to Body Work Therapies

This section is a catch-all of treatments that are too modern to be traditional therapies, aren't natural health products and are lower-tech in that they don't need to be plugged into an electrical outlet or use a battery. It includes therapies involving body movement, contact with the body by a practitioner, or bioresonance.

Survey Says

Of my forty survey respondents, thirty-seven had used a body work therapy. The most popular was deep breathing (twenty-four respondents, 60%), followed by dry brushing (twenty-three respondents, 58%) and taping (seventeen respondents, 43%). Several body work therapies, including ai chi, circle of healing and dry needling, had not been used by any of my respondents. The remaining therapies had been tried by at least one. You will see comments from the survey throughout this section in the form of "Anecdotal Reports" (from professionals) and "User Experience" (from people with lymphedema).

Ai Chi

What Is It?

Ai chi is a water-based exercise program that combines tai chi (see page 52), qigong (page 48) and aquatic exercise. It was developed in 1993 by Jun Konno of the Aqua Dynamics Institute in Yokohama, Japan. One of its purposes was to balance and stretch the meridians. It uses breathing techniques and slow, progressive resistance movements in shoulder-level water to relax and strengthen the body. Movement is slow and continuous, with an attention to body alignment and a calm, meditative state of mind focused on flowing movement. There are nineteen different katas (movements), done while the practitioner is breathing at about fourteen to sixteen breaths per minute (Lambeck 2011).

There are different versions of ai chi. Wall ai chi is done while holding a bar or wall. When ai chi is done with a partner, using pair work, it is called ai chi ne. When an individual is unable to stand, ai chi can be adapted so that they are sitting in a chair in shallow water. When it is used for specific therapeutic healing, such as stroke rehabilitation, it is called clinical ai chi (Lambeck 2011).

The main difference between ai chi and conventional aqua therapy (page 76) is that ai chi is performed at a slower pace.

> **Anecdotal Report**
> "Aqua therapy for cancer–related lymphedema and severe obesity provides great opportunities for deep breathing and exercise with the compression benefits of the water."
>
> —**Annie, lymphedema therapist, Minnesota**

Lymphedema-Specific Research

In a study that compared ai chi to conventional aqua therapy in an attempt to learn which is more effective at reducing arm lymphedema, eighteen women participated in both types of class, one week apart (Deacon 2019). Each class lasted for fifty minutes in the same pool at 34°C (93°F) and 1 to 1.5 meters (3 feet 3 inches to 4 feet 11 inches) of water depth. Most of the class was done in the deeper end, allowing the water level to be neck-high when knees were slightly flexed.

The conventional aqua therapy class started with a warm-up and stretching, followed by aerobic activity and then a cooldown. In comparison, the ai chi was slow and relaxing, with gentle exercise performed in time with the breath. Both classes included similar amounts of self-MLD and diaphragmatic breathing throughout, in an effort to compare only the slow movements of ai chi to the faster movements of aqua therapy.

Measurements were taken before, immediately after and one hour after each class, and included water displacement and bioimpedance. The participants also answered a twelve-question survey. The results showed that 72% of the women had a volume reduction immediately after ai chi, compared with 28% after conventional aqua therapy. The average reduction was 140 milliliters (4.7 ounces), with a range of 17 to 263 milliliters (0.6 to 8.9 ounces), but it was not sustained after one hour. There was no difference in bioimpedance immediately after the classes or an hour later.

One explanation for these results might be that, in the ai chi class, participants remained immersed in the water, while in the conventional aqua therapy class, some movements required participants to raise their arms above the water level. In addition, the aerobic aspects of the aqua therapy class, such as walking, punching, cycling and jumping, increased blood flow, which may have increased fluid volume, negating some of the benefits of the deep breathing and hydrostatic pressure.

The participants' satisfaction level was high for both classes. When questioned about their experience, 73% agreed or strongly agreed they would prefer to attend a full class of ai chi or a class with an ai chi cooldown, while 66% agreed or strongly agreed that they enjoyed the conventional aqua therapy class.

Side Effects/Risks

Some participants in the Deacon study reported that they got cold in the slower-moving ai chi class or that they preferred a more active class. No actual side effects were reported. Similar risks exist for ai chi as for any pool-related activity, such as falling on a slippery deck surface or toenail fungus from contact with wet surfaces in the pool or change rooms.

Bottom Line on Ai Chi

Women with arm lymphedema who participated in an ai chi class that was modified to include more diaphragmatic breathing and self-MLD showed a greater reduction in lymphedema volume, measured by water displacement, then they did after a conventional aqua therapy class. The improvements in lymphedema volume lasted for less than an hour, but most of the participants enjoyed the class. Ai chi may be a good option for individuals with lymphedema who would enjoy slow, mindful movements performed in neck-high water.

References for Ai Chi

Deacon R, de Noronha M, Shanley L, Young K. 2019. Does the Speed of Aquatic Therapy Exercise Alter Arm Volume in Women with Breast Cancer Related Lymphoedema? A Cross-Over Randomized Controlled Trial. *Braz J Phys Ther* 23 (2): 140–47.

Lambeck J, Bommer A. 2011. "Ai Chi: Applications in Clinical Practice." Chap. 7 in *Comprehensive Aquatic Therapy*, 3rd ed., edited by Bruce E. Becker and Andrew J Cole. Washington State University Publishing. Available at https://www.ewacmedical.com/wp-content/uploads/2017/08/Clinical-Ai-Chi-Lambeck-and-Bommer-2009-1.pdf.

Aqua Therapy

What Is It?

Aqua therapy is a series of exercises done in the water (usually a pool). The sequence and specific exercises may vary depending on your instructor. Aqua Lymphatic Therapy (ALT), also known as the Tidhar Method, is designed specifically for lymphedema; for more information, visit https://www.aqua-lymphatic-therapy.org/. Ai chi (see page 74) is another form of aqua-based therapy.

One of the benefits of being under the water is the hydrostatic pressure. Each inch below the surface adds an additional 1.85 mmHg. So if your feet are under 1 meter (3 feet 3 inches) of water, they are experiencing 73 mmHg of pressure. Compression garments provide much less (Medi, n.d.):

- Class 1—mild compression: 18 to 21 mmHg
- Class 2—moderate compression: 23 to 32 mmHg
- Class 3—strong compression: 34 to 46 mmHg
- Class 4—extra-strong compression: at least 49 mmHg

Moreover, underwater the compression is provided from all angles and on all body parts, not just the arms and legs. If you need compression on breasts or genitals, fingers or toes—which are sometimes difficult or awkward to compress with garments—you can achieve it with hydrostatic pressure.

In addition, movement in the water can help to direct lymph fluid and provide additional decongestion. The buoyancy of the water is beneficial for those who have joint pain or challenges with land-based exercise.

After an aqua therapy session, bandaging or applying compression garments can help preserve volume reductions.

User Experience

"Aqua therapy was amazing!! Deep breathing, stress reduction and progressive relaxation are helpful in almost any situation, especially after flying. I like to use a pool when I land at my destination."

—Patti, Idaho (breast cancer–related lymphedema)

Between Professionals

I encourage my clients and students to get in the water if they can. Thanks to what I learned in a webinar by Dorit Tidhar, I suggest walking in the water rather than swimming, so that more of the body is underwater. I also encourage them to do deep breathing and self-MLD while in the water. Most of my students who spend time in the water really love it. They are the water babies of the group.

Lymphedema-Specific Research

ALT was developed specifically with lymphedema in mind and has been studied in at least five randomized controlled trials and one systematic review and meta-analysis.

REVIEW AND META-ANALYSIS: YEUNG 2018

This study included four trials in the review, and two of the four in the meta-analysis. The four trials included 134 participants before dropout, all women with breast cancer–related lymphedema. They performed ALT for twenty to sixty minutes, one to four times a week, for eight to twelve weeks. In one study, participants had to keep their shoulders underwater (Johansson 2013), while two studies specified water at chest level (Letellier 2014; Tidhar 2010). The fourth study did not specify a water depth (Hayes 2009).

The authors of the review and meta-analysis concluded that ALT resulted in similar volume reductions to land-based treatments, and there was no additional benefit from water-based therapy. However, one ALT group experienced significant improvement in flexion range of motion compared to usual physical activity (Johansson 2013).

CLINICAL TRIAL: ALI 2021

In a randomized controlled trial published after the review and meta-analysis above, fifty women with breast cancer–related lymphedema were randomly assigned to either aquatic resistance exercise therapy or land-based exercise. Both therapies were done three times a week for eight weeks, and consisted of a ten-minute warm-up, forty minutes of strengthening and ten minutes of cooldown. Both included diaphragmatic breathing.

When designing the water-based protocol, the researchers took into account previous aquatic therapy studies and modified the exercises to target all of the upper limb muscles and movements that can be affected by arm lymphedema. The exercises were done in neck-deep water at 30°C to 32°C (86°F to 90°F).

The water-based group saw a significant reduction in limb volume by the end of the study, with an average loss of 344 milliliters (11.6 ounces), compared to 184 milliliters (6.2 ounces) in the land-based group. In addition, the participants in the aqua therapy group had a significant improvement in shoulder flexion and abduction range of motion.

User Experience
"Water therapy five to six days per week has kept me stable."

—Carleen, Texas (leg lymphedema)

Side Effects/Risks

No adverse events were reported in any of the clinical trials. However, there are a few important considerations when it comes to aqua therapy. First, the temperature of the water is important. If it is too hot, the capillaries in your skin will dilate, which may make your lymphedema worse. Hot tubs, which are usually above 38°C (100°F), are not recommended (Tidhar 2011). Aim for a water temperature of 29°C to 33°C (84°F to 92°F), choosing the lower end of the range when you are exercising in the water as opposed to just walking in it.

Sanitation of the pool water and deck areas is also important. Don't swim if you have an open wound, and wear deck shoes to protect your feet from exposure to sharps, bacteria and fungi (such as athlete's foot) and give you better grip on slippery deck surfaces.

> **User Experience**
> "Aqua therapy is amazing, but I tend to only do it in the summer, as I often get sick from community pools in the winter."
>
> **—Christina, Ontario (secondary lymphedema in the arm, stomach and leg)**

Bottom Line on Aqua Therapy

Aqua therapy is a great way to help move your lymph and has the added bonus of giving you a break from your compression garment. Plus, it is generally performed in a group class, which can provide social support as well. Learning the proven sequence of movements, manual lymphatic drainage and breath work will provide a framework for positive results. The depth of the water is important, with various studies suggesting chest-deep, shoulder-deep or neck-deep. Water that is too shallow may compromise the results. Remember, too, that this is a *complementary* therapy; you still need to wear your compression garment between sessions.

References for Aqua Therapy

Ali KM, El Gammal ER, Eladl HM. 2021. Effect of Aqua Therapy Exercises on Postmastectomy Lymphedema: A Prospective Randomized Controlled Trial. *Ann Rehabil Med* 45 (2): 131–40.

Hayes SC, Ruel-Hirche H, Turner J. 2009. Exercise and Secondary Lymphedema: Safety, Potential Benefits, and Research Issues. *Med Sci Sports Exerc* 41 (3): 483–89.

Johansson K, Hayes S, Speck RM, Schmitz KH. 2013. Water-Based Exercise for Patients with Chronic Arm Lymphedema: A Randomized Controlled Pilot Trial. *Am J Phys Med Rehabil* 92 (4): 312–19.

Letellier ME, Towers A, Shimony A, Tidhar D. 2014. Breast Cancer-Related Lymphedema: A Randomized Controlled Pilot and Feasibility Study. *Am J Phys Med Rehabil* 93 (9): 751–59.

Medi. n.d. "RAL Compression Classes." Accessed October 27, 2024. https://www.mediuk.co.uk/service/medi-compression/compression-classes/.

Tidhar D. 2011. Water—Is It Good for Lymphedema? *Lymphedema Matters* 14 (2): 2.

Tidhar D, Katz-Leurer M. 2010. Aqua Lymphatic Therapy in Women Who Suffer from Breast Cancer Treatment-Related Lymphedema: A Randomized Controlled Study. *Support Care Cancer* 18 (3): 383–92.

Yeung W, Semciw AI. 2018. Aquatic Therapy for People with Lymphedema: A Systematic Review and Meta-analysis. *Lymphat Res Biol* 16 (1): 9–19.

Art Therapy

What Is It?

Art therapy uses creative expression through art to explore emotions and gain understanding. Any of the arts, such as theater, painting, poetry, music, writing, photography or composing, can be a medium for art therapy.

Within art therapy, collage is a creative process of first collecting, then assembling, words and images into a new piece of art. As part of the creative process, the artist is free to reflect on their feelings, hopes and aspirations. Collages can have a theme, such as the new year, recovery or transition. Like any type of art, collage can be a way to help you process your feelings to allow you to move forward.

> **Between Professionals**
> When I worked at a cancer support center, one of the classes offered was art therapy. It was a popular class, and I could see how art helped people cope with their diagnosis and express their feelings about it.

Lymphedema-Specific Research

I found two studies on using art therapy for lymphedema, one using collage and ethnodrama, and the other using collage and presentation. Both were conducted in Canada.

COLLAGE STUDY #1: QUINLAN 2014

The goal of this Saskatoon, Saskatchewan, study was to use the expressive arts of collage and everyday object installations with a group of breast cancer survivors to create an ethnodrama of their lived experience that would be presented to other survivors and health care providers.

The researchers stated that a "cultural impoverishment of healthcare" had evolved due to medical experts' knowledge becoming disconnected from patients' everyday lived experience. They therefore undertook this project to offer an expressive art as a vehicle to offset expert culture and revitalize patients' lifeworlds.

Seven women were invited to create an authentic representation of their lives with lymphedema. They were assured that their pieces would not be judged according to standards of "high art," and they should feel free to express their intimate knowledge of life with lymphedema. The women attended two workshops that included gentle yoga, breathing activities, free-writing and collage. At the second workshop, they presented their work to the group. The discussions that followed were transcribed and used to develop an ethnodrama script, with some of the collages and images integrated. The ethnodrama was recorded and is available on YouTube (https://www.youtube.com/chan nel/UCewEVF6CcTlEKYlLNcc8FWQ).

Four to six months later, the women were interviewed about their experiences. Some of the outcomes observed from this qualitative observational study were the development of group cohesion, mutual support and sustained shared interest in seeking out new ways to understand lymphedema. The women engaged in active listening and noted feeling courage, shared power, empathy for their fellow participants and reduced confusion and isolation. They felt like their contributions were valued, that their nonverbal communication abilities were expanded, that they could share private thoughts in a safe space, and that increased confidence in their own lay knowledge had replaced their previously overwhelming feelings of helplessness and resignation.

COLLAGE STUDY #2: THOMAS 2016

This study, which took place in Ottawa, Ontario, focused on harnessing hope after a cancer diagnosis. During acute cancer care, many patients are able to sustain hope thanks to the short-term objective of successfully completing treatment, but after a diagnosis of lymphedema, which is a chronic condition, their hope may need to be regenerated.

Nineteen participants (sixteen women and three men) attended three Saturday workshops and were given the option to create either a piece of reflective writing or a collage with the theme of reflecting on their cancer and lymphedema diagnoses and looking forward with hope. Eleven of the women chose to create and present collages.

The transcripts of the collage presentations were coded and analyzed. The researchers described the qualitative results as initial hesitation followed by positive outcomes from the creative process. The group sharing provided opportunities for the participants to discuss their experiences and reflections, and to realize that they are not alone. The presentations also enabled them to discuss coping strategies and reframe negative experiences.

Side Effects/Risks

None noted.

Bottom Line on Art Therapy

Two group programs that included making a collage and then presenting it and participating in a group discussion were found to be beneficial in that participants felt more hopeful after expressing their experiences with lymphedema through a creative medium. While the creation of the collage was important, so too was the group presentation, which helped participants feel less isolated. Clinics and patient-facilitators looking to offer more creative coping outlets for their patients with lymphedema may wish to consider using art therapy as a low-cost, low-risk option, which could also likely be delivered virtually. See page 54 for a study that combined traditional Chinese medicine with art therapy.

References for Art Therapy

Quinlan E, Thomas R, Ahmed S, et al. 2014. The Aesthetic Rationality of the Popular Expressive Arts: Lifeworld Communication Among Breast Cancer Survivors Living with Lymphedema. *Soc Theory Health* 12 (3): 291–312.

Thomas R, Hamilton R. 2016. Composing Hope Through Collage: A Community-Based Intervention for Cancer Survivors Living with Lymphedema. *Health Psychol Open* 3 (2): 2055102916657674.

Circle of Healing

What Is It?

Developed by Marjorie McClure for the Breast Cancer Recovery Program, the Circle of Healing is a synergistic strategy aimed at achieving physical and emotional outcomes based on the immune system's role in healing. In layman's terms, it is a structured small-group program that teaches coping techniques, relaxation, deep diaphragmatic breathing and gentle exercise through live support meetings and recorded audio and video instruction. The premise is that improvements in one area, such as exercise or emotional status, encourage immune health, which leads to progress in other areas, creating a "feed-forward loop."

> **Between Professionals**
> I facilitate a small-group program (Lymphedema Nutrition School), and I love watching the relationships that develop among the members. By the end of our ten-week program, the students are all on a first-name basis and are very supportive and encouraging of each other. It's a beautiful experience to be part of.

Lymphedema-Specific Research

In a randomized controlled trial, thirty-two participants were divided into eight groups of four women each (McClure 2010). Four groups were the control, and four did the Circle of Healing protocol. The control groups were told to continue with the lymphedema instructions from their medical team (specifics not provided). The treatment group performed exercises and relaxation techniques and wore compression sleeves. They also participated in biweekly one-hour group sessions for five weeks, followed by three months of self-monitoring at home.

During the live group sessions, patients watched the video *From Lymphedema Onto Wellness (FLOW)* and practiced deep diaphragmatic breathing, relaxation, facial massage and gentle guided exercise while viewing images of natural scenery with flowing water and listening to relaxing background music. They also discussed how they were coping. The exercises were similar to tai chi or qigong, and were done to verbal instructions and relaxation imagery cues.

Compared to the control groups, the Circle of Healing groups experienced greater weight loss and improvements in range of motion, mood, quality of life, vitality, bioimpedance and general health. The adherence to the treatment was high.

The authors speculated that the relaxation techniques, including deep diaphragmatic breathing, may have helped to lower stress, which in turn had positive effects on the immune system, which provided healing in the lymphedema limb. They considered the Circle of Healing protocol to be self-motivating, as success in one area encouraged the participants to continue, allowing for success in other areas.

Side Effects/Risks

None noted.

Bottom Line on Circle of Healing

The Circle of Healing protocol includes wearing a compression garment and exercising, which are also components of CDT, the current standard of care. The aspects of the

Circle of Healing that might be considered complementary care are the live group support sessions and the deep diaphragmatic breathing and relaxation practices.

The Circle of Healing seems like an easy yes to add as a complementary therapy for lymphedema care. It's gratifying to see that quality of life and other measures can be improved by enjoyable and relaxing self-care practices done within a supportive small-group structure.

References for Circle of Healing

McClure MK, McClure RJ, Day R, Brufsky AM. 2010. Randomized Controlled Trial of the Breast Cancer Recovery Program for Women with Breast Cancer-Related Lymphedema. *Am J Occup Ther* 64 (1): 59–72.

Deep Breathing

What Is It?

Deep breathing—also called diaphragmatic breathing, deep diaphragmatic breathing or belly breathing—is the intake of large breaths of air, causing an expansion of the diaphragm, the muscle the separates the chest from the abdomen. Deep breathing is credited with reducing stress and anxiety, lowering blood pressure and heart rate, and reducing muscle tension. Although we breath multiple times per minute, our breaths are mostly shallow, sometimes called chest breathing, and don't engage the diaphragm.

Deep breathing is so universally accepted and recommended within the lymphedema community that it is commonly used as part of CDT. That said, I will treat it like a complementary therapy and analyze the available research, as I have done for the other therapies.

Lymphedema-Specific Research

Deep breathing is often part of a holistic set of lymphedema treatments, so it's difficult to find research that isolates it to evaluate the effect it has on its own, but I was able to find one study that paired deep breathing with a very subtle exercise practice (Moseley 2005). In this protocol, thirty-eight women with post–breast cancer lymphedema were instructed to do deep breathing combined with a simple arm exercise.

The exercise was described as follows: "Begin with your hands pointing into the sternum, then, as you take a deep inhale, slowly open your arms outwards until they reach full extension. Once in full extension, hold the breath, then move the arms back toward the starting position as the breath is released." This breath and arm movement was repeated five times, followed by a one-minute break, then another five breath and arm cycles, then another one-minute break. In total, five cycles of five repetitions were completed. The entire set took ten minutes.

Measurements were taken immediately before and after the set, then twenty-four hours later and one week later. After the one-week follow-up, twenty-four of the women were asked to continue this practice every morning and evening for one month and track their commitment to the process in a logbook. The remaining fourteen women served as the control group.

Immediately after the ten-minute set, there was an average reduction in limb volume of 52 milliliters (1.8 ounces), or 5.8% of the lymphedema volume. This decrease was sustained for thirty minutes, after which the fluid gradually returned, so that by sixty minutes the lymphedema had returned to the baseline volume. When measured twenty-four hours later, volume was down an average of 46 milliliters (1.5 ounces). One week later, volume was down an average of 33 milliliters (1.1 ounces).

Truncal fluid was also measured and was down, on average, 32 milliliters (1.1 ounces) immediately after the set and 21 milliliters (0.7 ounces) thirty minutes later. There was no improvement in truncal fluid beyond sixty minutes.

Pain, burning and limb temperature changed little. Self-reports of arm heaviness and tightness decreased after the breath-arm routine, and that improvement continued for the entire week. Feelings of pins and needles also reduced significantly at twenty-four hours and one week.

In the group of women who performed the twice-daily practice for a month, the average volume reduction at the end of the month was 101 milliliters (3.4 ounces), which was a 9% decrease. By comparison, the women in the control group were only down 7 milliliters (0.2 ounces). The anterior thorax measurement also improved in those who continued the exercises, while it got worse in the control group. The exercise group also saw an improvement in fibrotic tissue in the thorax, self-reported arm heaviness and perceived limb size.

Anecdotal Report
"Deep breathing and dry brushing were done by my patient in addition to the MLD treatment. Breathing helped with her sleeping, relaxation and pain, and with the dry brushing I noticed improvement with her skin appearance."

—Biljana Bozic, RMT, Balanced Body by RMT, Kitchener, Ontario

Side Effects/Risks

The deep breathing protocol in the Moseley study was well tolerated, with no adverse effects reported.

Bottom Line on Deep Breathing

Because deep breathing is often part of other therapeutic practices, it is difficult to assess its individual impact on lymphedema. I could only find one study that isolated deep breathing, combining it with minimal arm movement in a ten-minute set, twice a day. Its results support including deep breathing in lymphedema treatment, and the study's protocol provides a blueprint for frequency, duration and technique that can be incorporated into lymphedema education.

Particularly exciting is that this protocol transcends financial, social and mobility barriers that can make some complementary therapies inaccessible. With just a twenty-minute-per-day time commitment, the protocol had a 90% compliance rate over a one-month span.

It will be interesting to see if future research can determine whether different techniques, frequency or timing can improve even further on the results from this successful trial.

References for Deep Breathing

Moseley AL, Piller NB, Carati CJ. 2005. The Effect of Gentle Arm Exercise and Deep Breathing on Secondary Arm Lymphedema. *Lymphology* 38 (3): 136–45.

Dry Brushing

What Is It?

Dry brushing involves using a bristle brush and a specific technique, pressure and sequence to stimulate the lymphatic system, with the goal of reducing lymphedema.

Lymphedema-Specific Research

Despite its popularity on social media and many unsubstantiated claims that it detoxifies the lymphatic system and breaks down cellulite (among other things), I could not locate any published research on dry brushing.

> **User Experience**
> "Sensory-wise, I didn't like the brushing. But rebounding, little bits throughout the day, helps my stress, energy and lymphedema. So does the deep breathing."
>
> **—Heather, Colorado (secondary lymphedema, left truncal, arm, hand and fingers)**

Side Effects/Risks

Using a dry brush when surgical scars are still healing could spread bacteria into the wound. Caution is recommended.

Bottom Line on Dry Brushing

There are plenty of claims about dry brushing's multiple benefits, but no research has yet been done to substantiate any of them. If you plan to use a dry brush as part of your lymphedema care, consult your lymphedema therapist for guidance.

References for Dry Brushing

No references available at the time of printing.

Dry Needling

What Is It?

Dry needling uses the same needles as acupuncture but does not follow the Eastern principles of stimulating meridians to enhance qi or balance yin and yang. Instead, it is a Western-based practice focused on pain patterns, faulty movement patterns and orthopedic testing (Cleveland Clinic 2023). In essence, the same needles are used, but with a different purpose, placement, technique and duration. The treatment is also known as trigger point dry needling, intramuscular stimulation or therapeutic dry needling.

When your muscle fibers have an insufficient blood supply, they don't return to their normal resting state, and the muscles can develop knots and become tender. These knots, known as trigger points, are highly sensitive and can be painful when touched. A trigger point can be the location of the pain or a source of referred pain. Therapists use dry needling through a trigger point to draw a normal blood supply back to the muscle and release the tension (Cleveland Clinic 2023).

Technical Breakdown
Trigger point therapy is similar to dry needling, but instead of needles, it uses massage, compression, stretching, foam rollers or other tools to stimulate trigger points.

Lymphedema-Specific Research

I could not find any research where lymphedema management was the primary reason for using dry needling, but there is one case study of a forty-six-year-old woman with pain in her chest wall after breast cancer treatment (Bell 2019). The patient also had lymphedema, restricted range of motion in her shoulder, weakness and scarring. To address these issues, a physiotherapist provided low-level laser treatment, myofascial release and stretching, which led to improvements, but the patient's chest wall tightness remained and was limiting her daily activities, including the ability to spend time in her garden.

The patient was treated with dry needling for three sessions, three weeks apart. The first treatment started with three needles, directed into the areas with the greatest tightness and pain. Because she had breast implants, care was taken to insert the tips of the needles away from the implants, to prevent rupture. The needles were connected to an electrical pulse stimulator and left in place for five minutes. She experienced a 70% improvement in pain after this treatment.

After a second treatment three weeks later, the patient reported an 80% improvement in pain. After the third treatment, three weeks after the second, she felt a 90% improvement and was very satisfied with the outcome. There was no increase in lymphedema.

Side Effects/Risks

No side effects occurred in the Bell case study, but risks do exist for this therapy, including potential implant punctures. People with an allergy to metals, skin lesions or an infection should exercise caution. Check with your health provider for a full list of precautions.

Bottom Line on Dry Needling

Dry needling has a long history of use by physical therapists for a variety of musculoskeletal issues, but to date, no research has been done on its effectiveness for treating lymphedema. In one case study of a woman with post–breast cancer lymphedema, the focus was on her postsurgical pain, tightness and limited range of motion, which the dry needling addressed with great success and without a detrimental effect on the lymphedema. This therapy may be of interest to patients dealing with musculoskeletal issues alongside lymphedema, but until there is more research on using dry needling specifically to treat lymphedema, it may be difficult for an evidence-based practitioner to recommend it for that issue alone.

References for Dry Needling

Bell L, Stout NL, Geiser MB. 2019. Dry Needling for Chronic Breast/Chest Wall Pain After Breast Cancer Treatment. *Rehabil Oncol* 37 (3): E14–16.

Cleveland Clinic. 2023. "Dry Needling." Accessed January 1, 2025. https://my.clevelandclinic.org/health/treatments/16542-dry-needling.

Foam Roller

What Is It?

A foam roller is a tube of dense foam that is strong enough to hold your body weight. They come in various sizes, textures and densities. To use one, you place it on the floor and roll part of your body back and forth over it. You can adjust the pressure by changing how much body weight you support yourself and how much you allow to press into the roller. Foam rollers are popular in gyms and athletic environments, where people use them to work out muscle tightness and other issues. This type of tissue mobilization can also help to break up adhesions or fibrosis. When used in this way, foam rolling can help soften tissues and improve lymphatic flow. Other health claims regarding foam rollers include indications for improving proprioceptive exercise, balance and stability; rolling out trigger points and knots; and increasing muscle density.

> **User Experience**
> "Using a soft foam roller and the MELT Method of exercises have helped me. MELT focuses on rehydrating body tissues; it seems to help with my general fluid management issues."
>
> **—Meg, New York (mild lymphedema in both legs and abdomen post–ovarian cancer surgery)**

Lymphedema-Specific Research

I located YouTube videos of lymphedema therapists teaching patients how to use a foam roller, and lots of Google search results on sites hosted by lymphedema therapists, but could not find any published medical research on using a foam roller to treat lymphedema.

Related Research

There are almost 200 results on the search term "foam roller" on PubMed (a US government database of published medical research). The majority of the studies appear to be on myofascial release, sports injury rehabilitation, pain, proprioception, balance, flexibility, range of motion, performance and recovery—many of which have a direct and indirect impact on lymphedema.

Side Effects/Risks

A consensus document on the risks and contraindications for foam rollers mentioned avoiding use with open wounds and bone fractures (Bartsch 2021). Cautions were given for those with tissue inflammation, myositis ossificans, deep vein thrombosis or osteomyelitis.

Bottom Line on Foam Rollers

Foam rolling may or may not benefit lymphedema. It certainly seems like some lymphedema therapists are already using this tool in their practice. Ask your therapist if foam rolling would be a suitable therapy for you and, if so, the best foam roller and technique for your needs. Hopefully researchers will investigate whether foam rolling has any direct effect on lymphedema volume, in addition to the indirect benefits from relief of related issues.

References for Foam Rollers

Bartsch KM, Baumgart C, Freiwald J, et al. 2021. Expert Consensus on the Contraindications and Cautions of Foam Rolling—An International Delphi Study. *J Clin Med* 10 (22): 5360.

Lidong Needling Therapy

What Is It?

Lidong needling therapy is an "acupuncture technique combined with therapeutic movement of the body" (Zhao 2023).

Lymphedema-Specific Research

In a study of seventy-three patients with breast cancer–related lymphedema, half were chosen randomly for the control group and half were placed in a treatment group (Zhao 2023). The original study was published in Chinese, but the abstract, which is in English, provides a lot of detail. The control group received routine nursing care and performed functional exercises twice a day for ten to fifteen minutes each time, lasting for eight weeks.

In the treatment group, Lidong needling therapy was applied to acupoints on the affected arm and the most obviously swollen areas (see the paper for the exact points used). The needles were left in for thirty minutes while the participants held their lymphedema arm in front of them at a right angle to their body. With the arm kept elevated and the needles in place, the participants were asked to repeatedly make a fist and open their hand on their lymphedema arm. This treatment was repeated three times a week for eight weeks.

Several measurements were taken before and after each treatment in both the control and treatment groups. After two, four, six and eight weeks of treatment, there was a reduction in swelling in both groups compared with their starting measurements (except for the area 10 centimeters/4 inches below the elbow crease in the control group). The researchers made the following observations:

- **After six weeks of treatment:** The treatment group had less swelling in the hand and wrist than the control group.
- **After eight weeks of treatment:** The treatment group had less swelling in the arm than the control group (except for the area 5 centimeters/2 inches above and below the elbow crease). The visual analog scale scores for swelling were improved in both groups compared to baseline and were lower in the treatment group than in the control group.

In the end, the authors calculated the total effectiveness score as 83% in the Lidong needling therapy group, compared to 35% in the routine nursing care and functional exercise group. They concluded that Lidong needling therapy combined with functional exercise resulted in a satisfactory clinical effect on arm lymphedema after breast cancer, improving both swelling and upper limb function.

Technical Breakdown

Visual analog scales are used regularly in research as a way to quantify a patient's subjective observations on parameters such as pain, mood or discomfort. The scale is usually a horizontal line about 10 centimeters (4 inches) long, with small vertical markings spaced evenly along it.

In the Zhao study, the visual analog scale was used to assess swelling in addition to the circumference measurements done by the researcher (an objective way to measure changes in swelling). The patients would have been asked to describe their perception of the changes in their swelling, and the visual analog scale likely included parameters such as "greatly improved," "somewhat improved," "neither improved nor worsened," "somewhat worsened" and "greatly worsened." Having more than one outcome measure to evaluate a treatment is usually a good idea when doing research. Keep this in mind as you evaluate your own experiences with different complementary therapies.

Side Effects/Risks

No side effects or risks were described in the abstract for the Zhao study (the article is written in Chinese, so I was unable to assess the full details). However, cellulitis is a risk for people with lymphedema, and any time the skin is broken (such as by a needle), there is a risk of infection, though that can be mitigated by proper sterilization techniques.

Bottom Line on Lidong Needling Therapy

Lidong needling therapy is an interesting technique that combines the effects of dry needling, acupuncture and physical movement. However, with only one English-language abstract currently available on this therapy, more research is needed to validate its efficacy for the English-speaking population.

References for Lidong Needling Therapy

Zhao W, Zhang HR, Lu P, et al. 2023. *Lidong* Needling Therapy Combined with Functional Exercise in Treatment of Upper Limb Lymphedema After Breast Cancer Surgery: A Randomized Controlled Trial. [In Chinese.] *Zhongguo Zhen Jiu* 43 (10): 1123–27.

Music Therapy

What Is It?

Music therapy is the use of music to improve overall well-being. As a clinical practice, it is about seventy-five years old. In a therapeutic session, trained music therapists use music—listening to recorded music, playing musical instruments, singing or writing music—to provide a healing outcome. Music therapy can be used for mental, emotional, physical, social or cognitive benefits, and the focus is on cognitive processing of the music. It relies on memory recall, cultural context and the release of neurotransmitters like dopamine as a response to the music to affect mood, emotion, relaxation and stress levels (Bartel 2021).

User Experience
"I tried music therapy, not specifically for lymphedema, but music does help me relax to sleep."

—Anonymous (secondary lymphedema of the leg)

Lymphedema-Specific Research

I was not able to locate any research specifically on music therapy for lymphedema.

Related Research

A review of integrative therapies for cancer treatment by the American Society of Clinical Oncology (ASCO) gave music therapy a grade B for the treatment of anxiety and stress reduction and for improving mood disturbance (Lyman 2018). As defined by the U.S. Preventive Services Task Force (USPSTF), grade B means "There is high certainty that the net benefit is moderate or there is moderate certainty that the net benefit is moderate to substantial," and it recommends that clinicians "offer or provide this service" (USPSTF 2018).

The stress, anxiety and mood disturbances of lymphedema are similar to those faced by cancer patients, and it seems reasonable that the same level of confidence in recommending music therapy for cancer patients may be applied to using it for lymphedema treatment.

> **Anecdotal Report**
> "I use music in all of my massage sessions. It is helpful for stress reduction and pace of treatment."
>
> —**Deanna Staniszewski, BCMT, C-MLD, Virginia**

Side Effects/Risks

Although music therapy is safe and low-risk, certain music may trigger uncomfortable or painful memories, which, depending on the level of trauma experienced, may be overwhelming. To safeguard against this, music therapists should gather detailed histories from their patients before beginning therapy (Cleveland Clinic 2023).

> **User Experience**
> "Listening to music helped reduce my stress. Using a roller brush on my arm helped alleviate any pain."
>
> —**Lisa, Ontario (arm lymphedema)**

Bottom Line on Music Therapy

Music therapy is a safe, cost-effective and recommended therapy for anxiety, stress and mood disorders, which are common concerns for people with lymphedema.

References for Music Therapy

Bartel L, Mosabbir A. 2021. Possible Mechanisms for the Effects of Sound Vibration on Human Health. *Healthcare* (Basel) 9 (5): 597.

Cleveland Clinic. 2023. "Music Therapy." Accessed January 2, 2025. https://my.clevelandclinic.org/health/treatments/8817-music-therapy.

Lyman GH, Greenlee H, Bohlke K, et al. 2018. Integrative Therapies During and After Breast Cancer Treatment: ASCO Endorsement of the SIO Clinical Practice Guideline. *J Clin Oncol* 36 (25): 2647–55.

U.S. Preventive Services Task Force (USPSTF). 2018. "What the Grades Mean and Suggestions for Practice." Accessed June 12, 2025. https://www.uspreventiveservicestaskforce.org/uspstf/about-uspstf/methods-and-processes/grade-definitions

Pilates

What Is It?

Pilates is a form of exercise that includes resistance training and stretching, synchronized with breathing. It involves control, precision, centering, fluid movements and concentration, and uses about fifty repetitive exercises flowing from the five essentials: breath, alignment of the cervical vertebrae (neck bones), rib and scapula (shoulder blade) stabilization, pelvic mobility and use of the transverse abdominis (the deepest abdominal muscle).

Pilates was developed in Germany by Joseph Pilates (1880–1967), whose father was a gymnast and whose mother was a naturopath. His inspiration is said to have been the rehabilitation of soldiers during the First World War. He also designed apparatuses called the reformer, Cadillac, Wunda Chair, electric chair, spine corrector, ladder barrel and pedi-pole.

User Experience

"I have practiced Pilates once a week for the past four years, and my lymphedema is stable."

—MJ, Ontario (breast cancer–related lymphedema)

Lymphedema-Specific Research

A clinical trial of sixty patients, half randomized to a Pilates group and half to a control group, examined the impact of Pilates on the severity of lymphedema that developed after breast cancer treatment, as well as grip strength, shoulder function, quality of life and social image concerns (Şener 2017). The Pilates group exercised three times a week for eight weeks (the precise details of their exercise routine are included in the published article). The control group was taught lumbopelvic stability and a home exercise program.

At the end of the eight weeks, there was no statistically significant difference in the timeline of lymphedema development. The patients in the Pilates group had significant improvements in pain, lymphedema severity, grip strength, shoulder range of motion, quality of life and social appearance anxiety; those in the control group had the same improvements, except for grip strength, shoulder flexion and external rotation angles.

The researchers concluded that clinical Pilates decreased lymphedema and improved upper limb function and quality of life more than standard exercise. When explaining the results, they hypothesized that the superior results of the Pilates program could be due to the attention paid to spinal stabilization and contraction of the trunk muscles and diaphragm, which stimulates the thoracic duct and abdominal lymph nodes, facilitating lymphatic flow.

The results of a study comparing Pilates and belly dancing for breast cancer survivors, which will include measurements of lymphedema in its analysis, have not yet been published, though the planned protocol has been (Boing 2020).

> **User Experience**
> "Pilates helps significantly, especially with my abdominal fluid issues. I think the combination of gravity (lying down) and muscle movement and breathing are very effective."
>
> —**Meg, New York (lymphedema in both legs, abdomen and pelvis post–ovarian cancer surgery)**

Side Effects/Risks

There was no mention of side effects in the Şener trial, but as with any exercise program, a proper warm-up is important.

Bottom Line on Pilates

When you're living with a chronic condition, pursuing a diverse range of activities may prove helpful over time. Pilates is a good exercise option for cancer survivors and others with lymphedema. It does not prevent lymphedema from developing, but for those who have lymphedema, Pilates offers superior results compared to a standard exercise program, likely thanks to its emphasis on the spine and core muscles. A Pilates class also provides opportunities for social interactions. Working with a Pilates teacher who understands lymphedema is recommended.

References for Pilates

Boing L, do Bem Fretta T, de Carvalho Souza Vieira M, et al. 2020. Pilates and Dance to Patients with Breast Cancer Undergoing Treatment: Study Protocol for a Randomized Clinical Trial—MoveMama Study. *Trials* 21 (1): 35.

Şener HÖ, Malkoç M, Ergin G, et al. 2017. Effects of Clinical Pilates Exercises on Patients Developing Lymphedema After Breast Cancer Treatment: A Randomized Clinical Trial. *J Breast Health* 13 (1): 16–22.

Progressive Muscle Relaxation

What Is It?

Relaxation is an emotional state in which the body is low in tension, the sympathetic nervous system is less active, and a person is not in fight-or-flight mode. It is associated with good health and longevity. Relaxation can be achieved in a number of ways, such as with meditation (see page 44), tai chi (page 52), guided visualization (page 57), listening to music (page 91) or deep breathing exercises (page 83). Progressive muscle relaxation is a technique of contracting and relaxing muscles to achieve relaxation. It was made famous in a 1929 book by Dr. Edmund Jacobson entitled *Progressive Relaxation*.

> **User Experience**
> "Deep breathing, rebounding and stress reduction have been related to overall relaxation, which contributes to a sense of well-being and acceptance. I do think relaxation, especially of my shoulders and neck, has a positive effect on my lymphedema."
>
> **—Anonymous, Ontario (breast cancer–related lymphedema)**

Lymphedema-Specific Research

In a clinical trial, thirty-one women with post-mastectomy lymphedema were divided into two groups: those who received CDT alone, and those who received CDT and practiced progressive muscle relaxation (Abbasi 2018). There were two phases. The first included sixty-minute sessions held six days a week for three consecutive weeks in which CDT was performed, including multilayer bandaging, exercise, skin and nail care, and patient education so they could perform the tasks themselves. In the second phase, which lasted for six weeks, the patients continued the therapy on their own, following a CD recording of self-MLD and exercise, and wearing a compression sleeve during the day and multilayer compression bandaging at night.

Relaxation was induced via progressive muscle relaxation before the session with the lymphedema therapist. Patients were told to contract a muscle for five to seven seconds, then relax it for ten seconds. This was done in a progressive sequence guided by the therapist that lasted for fifteen minutes. In phase two, the progressive muscle relaxation was performed by the patients on their own.

The researchers measured and compared depression, anxiety and edema across the two groups, and the results from the two phases combined are summarized in the table that follows.

	CDT Only	CDT + Relaxation
Mean reduction in lymphedema volume	62.4%	64.3%
Mean reduction in anxiety score	27.3%	60.0%*
Mean reduction in depression score	33.3%	71.0%*

* Statistically significant

The researchers concluded that progressive muscle relaxation added to CDT was more effective at significantly reducing anxiety and depression than CDT alone. Progressive relaxation also led to a greater reduction in lymph volume, but the difference was not statistically significant compared to CDT alone.

Side Effects/Risks

None noted.

Bottom Line on Progressive Muscle Relaxation

A small study showed significant improvement in anxiety and depression, along with a slight improvement in lymphedema volume, when progressive muscle relaxation was added to CDT. Progressive muscle relaxation is a cost-effective complementary therapy that is easily taught to patients. While it will add time to their self-care routine, the investment would be worthwhile for those who need additional support with anxiety and depression. The study did not specify whether the particular sequence was important, which muscle groups were included in their sequence or how many cycles per muscle group were done within the fifteen-minute practice.

References for Progressive Muscle Relaxation

Abbasi B, Mirzakhany N, Angooti Oshnari L, et al. 2018. The Effect of Relaxation Techniques on Edema, Anxiety and Depression in Post-Mastectomy Lymphedema Patients Undergoing Comprehensive Decongestive Therapy: A Clinical Trial. *PLoS One* 13 (1): e0190231.

Pyro-Drive Jet Injector

What Is It?

A pyro-drive jet injector is a needle-free injection device that uses gun powder (yes, gun powder) to deliver a liquid pharmaceutical at high speed through the skin. The "pyro" in the name refers to pyrotechnics. Also called the Actranza Lab jet injector, it is made by the Daicel Corporation of Osaka, Japan. It delivers a single dose and is disposable after use (Miyazaki 2019). The components include a gas generator, piston, plunger and container. When activated, the ignition powder triggers the piston with combustion pressure, pushing the plunger into the container and releasing the high-pressure pharmaceutical through a nozzle into the skin (Nishiyama 2024).

> **Technical Breakdown**
> I feel like I've seen a similar needle-free injection device in every sci-fi TV show and movie, starting with Star Trek. Despite the jet injector's futuristic appearance, its first documented use to deliver water or medicine into the body was in France in 1866 (Béclard 1866).

Lymphedema-Specific Research

This novel device hasn't been tested in humans with lymphedema.

Lymphedema Research in Animals

Lymphedema was induced in the tail of eighteen rats after venous and lymphatic cauterization (Nishiyama 2024). The jet injector was prepared with 10 microliters of lactated Ringer's solution and 40 microliters of air. (Lactated Ringer's is a sterile solution of water and electrolytes, commonly used in hospitals to provide IV hydration to patients.)

The researchers had decided to test this technology on lymphedema because of previous observations that when medications were injected using the device, clefts formed between bundles of collagen fibers in the skin. They hypothesized that these clefts could be used as channels for the removal of lymph fluid.

The control group of rats did not receive any injections; the test group received either three or five injections, starting two weeks after lymphedema was induced. After the injections, the researchers performed sophisticated scanning and visualization tests of the lymphedema area. The rats that received the jet injections had a peak in their lymphedema two to four days after the first injection, after which it began to reduce. They also had fibrous granulation tissue, rather than the inflammatory granulation tissue in the control group. In the test group, the collagen fibers were thick and showed increased density; in the control group, they were thin and edematous. The smallest lymphatic vessels had a significantly greater density in the test group than in the control group. In the study paper, images of the tails clearly show a reduction of swelling in the rats that received the treatment.

The exact mechanism of action is unclear, but the formation of clefts caused by the jet injector appears to allow lymph to flow into the clefts, promoting lymphatic regeneration.

The authors of this unique study concluded that they had confirmed the therapeutic benefit of jet injectors in rats with induced lymphedema, but before using this therapy in humans, they need to be meticulous about the volume of injection, precise site of administration and configuration of the jet injector. Importantly, they noted that the lymphatic channels formed as a result of jet injection will not have anti-reflux valves, which means that compression bandages will be an important aspect of a successful long-term outcome.

Jet injection also has potential as a preventative treatment that can be used in the early stages following lymph node dissection. The study authors describe it as a "potential groundbreaking treatment" based on their results, as well as practical features such as low cost and the fact that no specialized skills are needed to deploy the device.

Side Effects/Risks

In the Nishiyama study, the jet injectors inflicted minimal tissue damage.

Bottom Line on Pyro-Drive Jet Injectors

Someone was certainly thinking outside the box, not only to come up with the pyro-drive jet injector, but to use it for its cleft-making ability instead of to deliver medication. It's what the pharmaceutical industry calls an off-label use. The Nishiyama study is recent, and its authors seem enthusiastic and are extremely detailed and analytical in their evaluation of using the device to treat lymphedema. I hope these exceptional researchers are able to overcome the challenges they have identified when it comes to studying the device for lymphedema in humans.

References for Pyro-Drive Jet Injectors

Béclard, F. 1866. Presentation of the Jet Injector of Galante, Meeting of 18 December 1866, Monsieur Bouchardat Presiding. [In French.] *B Acad Imp Méd* 32: 321–327.

Miyazaki H, Atobe S, Suzuki T, et al. 2019. Development of Pyro-Drive Jet Injector with Controllable Jet Pressure. *J Pharm Sci* 108 (7): 2415–20.

Nishiyama M, Sakaguchi Y, Morito S, et al. 2024. A New Lymphedema Treatment Using Pyro-Drive Jet Injection. *Hum Cell* 37 (2): 465–77.

Rebounding

What Is It?

Rebounding, also known as mini trampoline, is a low-tech device with an elastic surface stretched across a circular metal frame, supported by springs. It provides a cushioned landing, which may reduce trauma on the joints. The word "trampoline" was coined in 1936, and the device was called a "dynamic feedback mechanism" for exercise (Rathi 2024).

Lymphedema-Specific Research

Despite rebounding's huge popularity in the lymphedema community, I was unable to find any published research to substantiate lymphedema-specific claims.

User Experience

"I found rebounding really good for getting the lymph flow going. It was very energizing, especially if done with music. Five to ten minutes got me puffing. Even bouncing without jumping was beneficial. For safety, I would recommend a rebounder with a handrail."

—Kerry, New Zealand (secondary lymphedema of the leg)

Related Research

There are multiple studies on rebounding's use for physical health and rehabilitation. A recent meta-analysis that included eleven studies found that rebounding has applications for musculoskeletal rehabilitation, cardiovascular conditioning, balance training and neurological rehabilitation (Rathi 2024). Improvements were seen in body composition, insulin resistance, blood sugar, blood lipids, waist circumference, lung function, anaerobic performance, bone density, blood pressure, running speed, joint extension, balance, muscle strength, vertical jump, quality of life, mental health and pain. Many of these outcomes are relevant to lymphedema and its associated conditions.

User Experience

"Gentle rebounding has helped to stimulate the lymphatic flow in my whole body, and after ten minutes, my arm does not feel so heavy. I do it first thing in the morning, and I have done this for two years."

—Robin, Washington (left arm, hand and underarm lymphedema)

Side Effects/Risks

There is a risk of falling and injury, especially if you have balance issues or are attempting advanced maneuvers.

Bottom Line on Rebounding

There are many health advantages to using a rebounder, and it is a relatively safe and effective piece of exercise equipment. There are currently no studies published on its use for lymphedema, however, so the multiple online claims cannot be substantiated. To guard against injury, users should seek qualified instruction, make sure the rebounder is placed in an area with sufficient space, implement a gradual program and maintain their equipment. Some models have handles, making them a prudent choice for new users or when balance is a challenge. Adapted exercises may be required to accommodate physical limitations.

User Experience
"I haven't been consistent with rebounding, but I feel it helps when I do it."

—**Christina, Ontario (secondary lymphedema in the arm, stomach and leg)**

References for Rebounding

Rathi MA, Joshi R, Munot P, et al. 2024. Rebound Exercises in Rehabilitation: A Scoping Review. *Cureus* 16 (7): e63711.

Reflexology

What Is It?

Reflexology is the application of pressure to the feet or hands to stimulate a corresponding body part. It is often confused with acupressure, but they are distinct practices. Reflexology uses only pressure points on the feet and hands; acupressure uses the same meridians and pressure points as acupuncture, but without needles. Reflexology Lymph Drainage (RLD) is a protocol designed by reflexologist Sally Kay that mimics the pattern used for manual lymphatic drainage using pressure points on the feet only. For more information, visit reflexologylymphdrainage.co.uk.

User Experience
"Reflexology Lymph Drainage has been a life-changing therapy. There is much to feel good about with this therapy. I always feel so calm, cared for and even pampered after a session. Not only is this a relaxing, noninvasive therapy, but it has also been very successful in moving my lymph fluid. The positive effects have lasted for several days after the therapy session."

—**Kerry, New Zealand (secondary lymphedema of the leg)**

Lymphedema-Specific Research

There have been three studies of RLD for lymphedema by the same research team, which included the creator of RLD.

Study #1: Whatley 2016

In this non-blinded, non-randomized study, twenty-six women with arm lymphedema secondary to breast cancer received RLD lasting thirty to forty minutes weekly for four consecutive weeks. Results included significantly reduced volume of the swollen arm, which was maintained for over six months. In addition, there were improvements in pain, stress, self-confidence, body image, mobility and well-being. But the research design did not permit inferences about cause and effect, as there was no control group and no monitoring of weight or use of compression garments. The authors concluded that the data gained from this study was sufficient to warrant a randomized controlled trial.

User Experience
"Reflexology Lymph Drainage is a godsend therapy that stimulates lymphatic circulation. I can feel the lymph flow up my legs and arms, and it has helped reduce and maintain the swelling. I have done this for two years."

—Robin, Washington (left arm, hand and underarm lymphedema)

Study #2: Whatley 2018

The same group of women as in study #1 participated in a semi-structured interview for this qualitative study. The reflexology appeared to have empowered them to reconnect with the person they had once been, re-engaging with work life and hobbies.

Study #3: Whatley 2020

This case study included two patients with breast cancer–related lymphedema who had thermal imaging while they were receiving RLD. Heat patterns from the thermal imaging camera demonstrated changes in the lymphedema arm as reflexology was applied to the feet. Patient One's excess arm volume was reduced by 12% immediately after the reflexology, and by 13% twenty-four hours later. Patient Two experienced a 6% excess volume reduction immediately after the therapy, and 8% twenty-four hours later.

Side Effects/Risks

There were reports of some minor and transient discomforts in the 2016 Whatley study.

Bottom Line on Reflexology

Reflexologists are now being trained on the Reflexology Lymph Drainage protocol. Three small studies have shown changes in the heat pattern in the affected arm, as well as volume reductions. There were also improvements in pain, stress, self-confidence, body image, mobility and well-being. RLD appears to be a promising, safe, noninvasive complementary therapy, making reflexologists promising members of the multi-disciplinary care team. Ongoing research to strengthen the evidence would be welcome.

References for Reflexology

Whatley J, Kay S. 2020. Using Thermal Imaging to Measure Changes in Breast Cancer-Related Lymphoedema During Reflexology. *Br J Community Nurs* 25 (Sup10): S6–11.

Whatley J, Street R, Kay S. 2018. Experiences of Breast Cancer Related Lymphoedema and the Use of Reflexology for Managing Swelling: A Qualitative Study. *Complement Ther Clin Pract* 32 (August): 123–29.

Whatley J, Street R, Kay S, Harris PE. 2016. Use of Reflexology in Managing Secondary Lymphoedema for Patients Affected by Treatments for Breast Cancer: A Feasibility Study. *Complement Ther Clin Pract* 23 (May): 1–8.

Scar Therapy

What Is It?

There are several products available to treat scars, including silicone gel, onion extract, vitamin E, trolamine and microporous tape. Proponents claim that these products improve the healing of new scars, prevent the development of scar-related problems and, if successful, could play an important complementary role in lymphedema therapy.

Scars are left behind after wound healing when the skin has been opened due to either surgery or trauma. Although scar formation is a part of the normal, healthy healing and reconnection of the torn tissue, it sometimes goes wrong. Some of the issues that can occur are:

- **Hypertrophic scars:** These raised, red, often itchy and sometimes painful thick scars remain within the boundary of the original wound. They can restrict your movement, as they feel tight or pull, and tend to occur when there is a lot of tension on the wound while it is healing. They are quite common and sometimes improve on their own (Yoong 2022).
- **Keloids:** These firm, smooth, hard growths are a result of excessive scar formation. They extend beyond the border of the original injury and are most common on the chest, shoulders, ears and neck. They occur most commonly on people with darker-white to light-brown skin, known as the Fitzpatrick skin types III to IV (Yoong 2022).
- **Pathological scars:** These are hypertrophic scars or keloids that affect physical or psychological health and quality of life—for example, a scar that impairs lymphatic drainage by creating a barrier that lymph fluid cannot cross. Scars that negatively affect lymphatic flow tend to be the ones that run side to side (laterally) and intersect the normal lymphatic flow.

Lymphedema-Specific Research

Many lymphedema therapists have first-hand experience with the negative impact scars can have on lymphatic flow, but I was unable to locate any research published on this subject.

Related Research

A systematic review of topical scar treatment products analyzed thirty-four randomized controlled trials and prospective clinical trials that included silicone gel, onion extract, trolamine, vitamin E and microporous tape (Tran 2020). Although the studies did not address the impact of scar treatment on lymphedema, one can presumably expect a positive result for lymphedema if pathological scar formation can be prevented or treated.

Silicone Gel

Silicone gel is available as a sheet, gel or spray. The systematic review noted mixed results from the sixteen trials that investigated silicone gel, with some showing no evidence or weak evidence of clinical benefit. Numerous others, however, found that silicone gel prevented hypertrophic scars from forming and improved scar appearance. Sheets, gels and sprays were equally effective at improving appearance, but a combination of sheets and gel led to faster decreases in scar redness and height than gel sheets on their own.

Onion Extract

The active ingredient *Allium cepa*, extracted from onions, can be made into a topical gel, with or without heparin (an anticoagulant to prevent blood from clotting) and allantoin (a plant extract that promotes healing). The Tran review found that:

- Onion extract applied topically significantly improved scar texture, redness and appearance.
- Onion extract and petroleum jelly led to similar improvements in scar appearance.
- Onion extract and silicone gel sheets offered similar results for improving scar redness, height and texture.
- Onion extract was significantly less effective than silicone gel products in improving scar appearance after a burn injury.

The review authors suggested that a follow-up of twelve weeks or more was needed to see clinical evidence of scar improvement.

Trolamine

Trolamine, a topical analgesic, is said to improve the healing of superficial wounds by promoting new tissue formation. Although there were only three studies on trolamine included in the systematic review, they demonstrated efficacy in decreasing wound healing time. Trolamine was less effective than petroleum jelly at improving redness, texture, edema and crusting in the first seven days, but was equally effective by day fourteen.

Vitamin E

A fat-soluble vitamin found in many foods, such as almonds, avocados and wheat germ oil, vitamin E is one of the most popular and best-known scar therapies. The Tran review analyzed the results of three studies and found only weak evidence to support vitamin E's efficacy in scar management. One trial of vitamin E versus a placebo cream found no significant difference in outcome; however, another found that vitamin E was more effective than petroleum jelly at improving Vancouver Scar Scale scores and preventing keloid formation. The review authors noted that allergic reactions to vitamin E can cause contact dermatitis.

Microporous Paper Tape

A study of seventy women who applied microporous tape to their scars for twelve weeks after a Caesarean section found that they had reduced scar formation and fewer hypertrophic scars. Once the tape was removed, however, they developed hypertrophic scars.

Technical Breakdown

People with Noonan syndrome (also known as familial Turner syndrome) are more likely to form keloids. One of the hallmarks of this syndrome is lymphedema (Chan 2017). The formation of a keloid can impair lymphatic drainage, adding another challenge to lymphedema management.

CONCLUSIONS OF REVIEW

The review authors concluded that the prevention of pathological scars remains an area of active research, and that to date there is only weak clinical data to substantiate the efficacy of products that claim to prevent and treat scars. Due to the significant medical implications of pathological scars, they advocate for more and better clinical studies with a one-year follow-up.

In the meantime, based on the available evidence, they recommend using silicone gel products, which have minimal adverse effects. They suggest that, for this use, silicone gel sheets should be applied for twelve hours a day for two to three months after the injury. For large scars or those in an area where a sheet won't work, silicone gel can be used instead.

Side Effects/Risks

Potential adverse reactions to scar therapy products include itchy rash (contact dermatitis), hives (urticarial eruptions) and skin irritation.

Bottom Line on Scar Therapy

If you have a raised red scar, especially one that runs laterally across your body above an area of lymphedema, the scar could be impeding your lymph flow and preventing you from getting the best outcomes from your lymphedema therapies. Talk with your lymphedema therapist about silicone gel sheets or another treatment for your scar, or ask for a referral to a trusted colleague who is trained in scar therapy. In addition to the products mentioned here, manual scar treatments can help improve scar texture and appearance. If you are scheduled for surgery in a lymphedema-sensitive area, ask your surgeon or rehab therapist about using silicone gel sheets or their preferred treatment to help prevent pathological scar formation.

References for Scar Therapy

Chan J. 2017. "Noonan Syndrome." DermNet. Accessed June 22, 2025. https://dermnetnz.org/topics/noonan-syndrome.

Tran B, Wu JJ, Ratner D, Han G. 2020. Topical Scar Treatment Products for Wounds: A Systematic Review. *Dermatol Surg* 46 (12): 1564–71.

Yoong NKM, Numan H. 2022. "Keloid and Hypertrophic Scar." DermNet. Accessed June 22, 2025. https://dermnetnz.org/topics/keloid-and-hypertrophic-scar.

Stress Reduction

What Is It?

Stress reduction involves intentional practices to reduce the impact of emotional stress on your body. Common strategies include mindfulness-based practices, such as meditation (see page 44), yoga (page 61) and deep breathing (page 83). Potential outcomes are a calmer mind, relaxed muscles, improved sleep, lower blood pressure and heart rate, reduced cortisol levels and improved quality of life.

> **Technical Breakdown**
> Cortisol, the primary stress hormone, can be measured in the blood and tracked over time. Heart rate variability is another way to measure stress; wearable devices such as smart watches can measure heart rate variability and provide feedback about your stress levels. High blood pressure is another indicator of stress. Practicing stress reduction regularly is good for your health.

Lymphedema-Specific Research

In an Austrian study, seventy-one patients with a BMI above 25 (meaning they were classified as overweight or obese) were admitted to an in-patient rehabilitation center to improve their lymphedema or lipedema (Loibnegger-Traußnigh 2023). All were given complete decongestive therapy, including manual lymphatic drainage and physical therapy, plus nutrition counseling and psychological interventions as part of the standard rehabilitation care. Thirty-six patients received additional stress management training consisting of five 45-minute meetings in groups of seven to nine participants over three weeks.

By the end of their stay, all of the participants had lost weight. That outcome was expected, since the goal had been to reduce lymphedema swelling, but the group that received the additional stress management training lost significantly more than the control group, even when considering the weight of the edema loss. This result may be credited to a session on mindful eating practices that was given as part of the stress management training. The patients in the stress reduction group were also fitter—being able to walk a greater distance in a six-minute walk test—which the authors attributed to the motivational boost provided by the meetings.

Oddly, when twenty-eight of the participants were given follow-up questionnaires about their perceived stress, those in the control group reported greater improvements than those in the stress reduction group (perhaps they were now more aware of their stress). However, chronic stress had decreased more in the stress reduction group.

Side Effects/Risks

None were noted, but with any psychological therapy, there is a risk of painful or traumatic memories resurfacing.

Bottom Line on Stress Reduction

The Austrian in-patient program sounds like an excellent holistic approach to lymphedema and lipedema, and all of the patients in the Loibnegger-Traußnig study appear to have benefitted. It seems sensible to include stress management and mindful eating training in any health program, though it is unclear whether these interventions have any direct (or indirect) impact on lymphedema. You could argue that weight loss and improved fitness can be expected to yield beneficial lymphedema outcomes, but no data was collected to demonstrate the validity of that hypothesis.

References for Stress Reduction

Loibnegger-Traußnig K, Schwerdtfeger AR, Flaggl F. 2023. Effects of a Stress Management Training in Patients with Lymphedema and Obesity During Rehabilitation. *Eur J Health Psychol* 30 (3): 126–37.

Taping

What Is It?

Taping, also known as athletic taping or Kinesio taping, involves the application of stretchy athletic tape to a treatment area. It stimulates the skin to assist in pain relief, help increase the contraction of a weak muscle, or inhibit muscles that are too tight (Kinesio, n.d.). One popular brand, Kinesio tape, was developed in 1973 by chiropractor Dr. Kenzo Kase to treat sports injuries. The original tape was polymer elastic strands wrapped in 100% cotton, which allowed moisture to evaporate. Today, the tape can be cotton or synthetic.

Taping is common in lymphedema; in fact, there are training courses for lymphedema therapists to become certified in its use.

> **Anecdotal Report**
>
> "I use Kinesio tape on almost every lymphedema patient. It's fabulous, and 95% of my patients love it. I also tape my ortho patients with total knee replacements. It's so versatile. I've taught patients to tape themselves. It's a great carry-over."
>
> —Ryan Schumacher, PT, CLT, Froedtert Health, Milwaukee, Wisconsin

Lymphedema-Specific Research

Taping is the most studied of all the complementary therapies. It has been cited in lymphedema research since around 2006, and there are multiple studies and meta-analyses. One of the more recent meta-analyses included seven randomized controlled trials (Marotta 2023). The reviewers concluded that taping, as a complement to conventional rehabilitative approaches, might improve upper limb volume in patients in the early phases of breast cancer–related lymphedema. The positive effects of taping may be due in part to improved microcirculation in the space between cells, which increases blood and lymphatic flow.

A review and meta-analysis evaluating three complementary therapies—low-level laser (page 241), Endermologie (page 212) and taping—concluded that "Kinesio taping [and low-level laser] are beneficial for lymphedema because they stimulate lymphatic movement and lymphangiogenesis" and that Kinesio taping is efficacious for managing early-stage lymphedema (Wahid 2024).

> **User Experience**
>
> "Taping has helped me when travelling, especially when flying."
>
> —Willa, British Columbia (full-body lymphedema tarda)

Anecdotal Report

"I have incorporated Kinesio taping with many of my lymphedema patients, with mixed reviews and results. For a primary lymphedema patient with leg swelling, a two-week trial showed no change. However, I have observed good results when using Kinesio taping with secondary lymphedema patients for face, hand and breast swelling. Some patients continue to request intermittent taping even after over a year of trials. They report that this approach helps to reduce the severity of their lymphedema and provides a less restrictive alternative to compression therapy. It is especially favored when outdoor temperatures are warm, and compression garments become too hot to tolerate. All of these patients had stage 2 lymphedema."

—**Dawn F. Brinkman, CLT-LANA, Florida**

Side Effects/Risks

Taping was well tolerated in the Marotta meta-analysis. However, any skin treatment has the potential to provoke a sensitivity reaction. Not everyone is a candidate for taping: It should not be used for injuries unless they are properly diagnosed; it should not be used by people with a fever; it is not recommended over broken or damaged skin; and caution is advised for people who are pregnant or have thrombosis or a heart condition (Thysol, n.d.).

Bottom Line on Taping

Taping is very well researched, safe and well tolerated, and it may help reduce arm volume for patients in the early stages of breast cancer–related lymphedema. Keep in mind that athletic tape varies widely. It can be pre-stretched with different directions of stretch, and the thread count affects the amount of lift. How you apply it and the number of pieces you use is also important and must be part of an individualized treatment plan. Consult your lymphedema therapist for a plan that includes the type of tape, the number of strips, the location of application, the length of time to wear the tape and instructions on how to safely remove it.

References for Taping

Kinesio. n.d. "Our History." Accessed January 3, 2025. https://kinesiotaping.com/about/our-history/.

Marotta N, Lippi L, Ammendolia V, et al. 2023. Efficacy of Kinesio Taping on Upper Limb Volume Reduction in Patients with Breast Cancer-Related Lymphedema: A Systematic Review of Randomized Controlled Trials. *Eur J Phys Rehabil Med* 59 (2): 237–47.

Thysol. n.d. "Kinesiotape Precautions and Contraindications." Accessed January 3, 2025. https://www.thysol.us/kinesiology-tape-instructions/contraindications/

Wahid DI, Wahyono RA, Setiaji K, et al. 2024. The Effication of Low-Level Laser Therapy, Kinesio Taping, and Endermology on Post-Mastectomy Lymphedema: A Systematic Review and Meta-Analysis. *Asian Pac J Cancer Prev* 25 (11): 3771–79.

Tuning Fork

What Is It?

A tuning fork is a two-pronged metal device that resonates at a specific frequency when struck and can produce a pure and consistent tone. It began as a musical instrument and was adopted into medicine in 1546. It has come to have a variety of medical uses, including observing sound conduction through bone to detect bone fractures and distinguishing different types of hearing loss (Eraniyan 2024). Tuning fork therapy is sometimes called sound healing, and a tuning fork is also used in a form of energy medicine called biofield tuning, which uses the energy field around the body to stimulate healing (Jain 2023).

Lymphedema-Specific Research

There is no lymphedema-specific research on tuning forks. Practitioners extol the benefits of their tuning fork therapy for lymphedema on several websites, but none of them supports their claims with links to research.

> **Technical Breakdown**
> The tuning fork is not the only vibration therapy. Others include music medicine (page 253), deep oscillation (see Hivamat, page 230), singing bowls (page 50), vibration plates (page 270), and ultrasound (page 265). Even far-infrared sauna (page 218) can be considered a form of vibration therapy, as it can cause water molecules to vibrate. Proponents of vibration therapies claim that vibrations can disrupt fibrotic adhesions and release the trapped fluid pockets.

Side Effects/Risks

None noted.

Bottom Line on Tuning Forks

Tuning forks resonate at different frequencies depending on their size and could conceivably benefit lymphedema via vibration and bioresonance. Although there are lymphatic practitioners who currently use tuning forks, I was not able to locate any published evidence to validate this work. Research on tuning fork therapy for lymphedema would be welcome, especially if it can define the most effective treatment parameters, such as pitch, duration and location.

References for Tuning Forks

Eraniyan K, Ganti L. 2024. History and Evolution of the Tuning Fork. *Cureus* 16 (1): e51465.

Jain S, McKusick E, Ciccone L, et al. 2023. Sound Healing Reduces Generalized Anxiety During the Pandemic: A Feasibility Study. *Complement Ther Med* 74 (June): 102947.

Body Work Summary

The body work category varies greatly, from newer experimental strategies such as the Circle of Healing to established and well-researched therapies such as taping. The tables that follow summarize the evidence for their use to treat lymphedema.

Therapy	What It Is	Claims	Lymphedema Research	Results	Side-Effects/Risks
Ai chi	Tai chi performed in water	Balances and stretches the meridians	One study of ai chi versus conventional aqua therapy with 18 participants	Greater volume reduction immediately after class	Feeling cold
Aqua therapy	Exercises done in a pool	Applies hydrostatic pressure to the whole body	Four studies and one review with 134 participants	Significant arm volume reduction, more than seen in land-based exercise	Potential risk of flare if water is too hot
Art therapy	Creative expression of feelings and emotions	Provides a medium for therapy and healing	Two collage studies, one with 7 participants and one with 19	Group support, empowerment, courage, feeling less confused and alone, reframing of negative experiences	None noted
Circle of Healing	A structured small-group program with relaxation, deep breathing and more	Harnesses the immune system's role in healing	One study with 32 participants	Greater weight loss and improved RoM, mood, QoL, bioimpedance and general health	None noted
Deep breathing	Deep breaths that expand the diaphragm	Reduces stress, anxiety, heart rate and blood pressure	One study of 38 women with post–breast cancer lymphedema	Reduced volume, heaviness, tightness, and pins and needles	Note noted
Dry brushing	The use of a bristle brush on dry skin	Lymphatic detoxification	None	n/a	Infection if used over a wound
Dry needling	Acupuncture needles used to stimulate trigger points	Eliminates tension via stimulation of trigger points	One case study of a cancer patient with lymphedema	Improved pain	Potential for implant punctures
Foam roller	Compressed foam in a tube shape	Myofascial release, sports injury rehabilitation, treats pain and proprioception	None	n/a	Contraindicated with wounds and fractures; caution with inflammation
Lidong needling therapy	Acupuncture + body movement	Stimulates trigger points to eliminate tension	One study of 73 patients with breast cancer lymphedema	Reduced swelling and perceived swelling	Potential for skin infection

n/a = not applicable; QoL = quality of life; RoM = range of motion

Therapy	What It Is	Claims	Lymphedema Research	Results	Side-Effects/Risks
Music therapy	Using music as an aid in psychological therapy	Offers mental, emotional, social, cognitive and physical benefits	None	n/a	May trigger uncomfortable or painful memories
Pilates	Resistance training and stretching, synchronized with breathing	Rehabilitation	One study with 60 participants of Pilates versus a home exercise program	Significant improvements in lymphedema, pain, RoM, QoL, grip strength, and social anxiety	None noted
Progressive muscle relaxation	Contraction and relaxation of muscles in a specific sequence	Relieves tension in the body and stimulates the sympathetic nervous system	One study of 31 women with post–breast cancer lymphedema	Significant reductions in anxiety and depression, nonsignificant reduction of lymph volume	None noted
Pyro-drive jet injector	A needle-free injection device	Enables lymph drainage via clefts formed between collagen fibers	One animal study	Reduction of lymphedema	Minimal tissue damage
Rebounding	A mini trampoline	Exercise with less joint impact	None	n/a	Falls
Reflexology	Acupressure applied to the hands or feet	The Reflexology Lymph Drainage protocol mimics MLD	Three studies, with a total of 54 participants	Improvements in lymphedema, pain, mobility, stress, self-confidence, body image and well-being	Minor and transient discomforts
Scar Therapy	Various modalities to reduce pathological scars	Improvement in scars can lead to improvement in lymphedema	None	Mixed results in non-lymphedema patients	Itchy rash, hives and skin irritation
Stress reduction	Psychosocial strategies to reduce physiological stress	Calms the mind, relaxes muscles, improves sleep and lowers blood pressure	One study of lymphedema and lipedema in 71 patients	Greater weight loss, greater distance walked in 6 minutes, reduced chronic stress	Potential for traumatic memories to resurface
Taping	Stretchy adhesive tape for the skin	Lifts the skin to allow for lymph flow	Multiple studies and meta-analyses	Improved lymphedema volume in early phases, improved interstitial microcirculation	Potential for skin reactions
Tuning fork	A two-pronged metal device that resonates at a specific frequency	Vibrations can disrupt fibrotic adhesions and release the trapped fluid pockets	None	n/a	None noted

n/a = not applicable; MLD = manual lymphatic drainage; QoL = quality of life; RoM = range of motion

Part Three
Natural Health Products

Introduction to Natural Health Products

Natural health products are "naturally occurring substances that are used to restore or maintain good health," such as vitamins and minerals, herbal remedies, probiotics and traditional Chinese and Ayurvedic medicines (Health Canada 2016). They are generally considered safe, though, like any ingested or topical substance, there are some potential risks, including allergic reactions and interactions with other medicines.

If you google "supplements for lymphedema," you will see many results. The vast majority have never been included in any research, though claims like "clinically proven" might give you the impression that they have been. The studies that do exist are often small and of poor quality, sometimes lacking blinding or controls. This section discusses natural health products that have specifically been tested for their use in treating lymphedema, in either human or animal trials, plus a few others—omega-3 fatty acids, ginger and Pycnogenol—that I decided to include because of their popularity among lymphedema patients and therapists, despite there being no lymphedema-specific research that I could find. I also analyze the benzopyrone class as a whole to help you understand the terms "alpha-benzopyrone," "gamma-benzopyrone," "flavonoids" and so on, since there are several natural health products from this group.

Each country has its own guidelines for the oversight of natural health products. In the United States, the Food and Drug Administration (FDA) considers them foods, and therefore does not regulate them as it does prescription medications, stating that they are "not authorized to review dietary supplement products for safety and effectiveness before they are marketed" (FDA 2022). This has been the case since 1994, when the Dietary Supplement Health and Education Act was modified. Since then, the number of supplements on the market has exploded. The FDA does publish information to educate consumers about supplement safety, identify unsafe or illegal products and remove them from the market, and provide alerts for consumers. But they do not ensure that a product contains what the label says, or that it provides the intended outcome.

Health Canada, through the Natural and Non-prescription Health Products Directorate (NNHPD), has a mandate to oversee non-prescription drugs and natural health products. All such products must have a license before they can be sold in Canada. To get a license, the manufacturer must supply the ingredient list, source, dose, potency and recommended uses. After issuing a license, Health Canada will assign the product a Natural Product Number (NPN) (Health Canada 2016).

To help you find a safe product for your needs, several reputable sources provide information on supplements and their interactions, risks and considerations:

- Memorial Sloan Kettering Cancer Center: mskcc.org
- National Institutes of Health, Office of Dietary Supplements: ods.od.nih.gov
- Mayo Clinic: mayoclinic.org
- United States Pharmacopoeia: quality-supplements.org
- Operation Supplement Safety: opss.org
- Government of Canada, Licensed Natural Health Products Database: health-products.canada.ca/lnhpd-bdpsnh/

These are also two excellent subscription websites that offer valuable information:

- Natural Medicines Comprehensive Database: naturalmedicines.therapeuticresearch.com
- Consumer Lab: consumerlab.com

There are times that I cited the Natural Medicines Database in this section. As such, they are included in the reference lists, but the exact links will only be accessible to members.

Technical Breakdown

Pharmaceuticals and natural health products are treated very differently by government regulators. The research and development required to bring a new pharmaceutical to market is extensive. There is a structured process that includes gaining an understanding of how the drug works at a molecular level, then animal testing and finally human clinical trials. If a drug is found to be safe and effective, it must then be approved by government regulatory agencies. As a reward for its investment in research and development, the pharmaceutical company is granted a 20-year patent, allowing it to recoup the investment and fund new drug trials. When the patent expires, generic drugs can be developed to mimic the original.

An herb in its natural form cannot be patented unless it is significantly modified or part of a specific formulation. Because there is no way to recoup the cost of research on herbal remedies, they unfortunately remain under-investigated.

If you're considering a supplement, your pharmacist is a good resource and can answer questions and tell you whether there are any potential interactions between the supplement and your medications. Here are some questions to ask them, or another health professional, about natural health products for lymphedema:

- Are there any safety concerns associated with this product?
- What are the side effects?
- Are there contraindications with any drugs, supplements or foods?
- Are there contraindications for diseases or medical conditions?
- What is the recommended dose and administration?

It's important to note that although a particular herb may be used to prepare, say, two different gels, tinctures or extracts, the manufacturers may have standardized different active ingredients. (To standardize means to ensure an ingredient is included at a specific level.) For example, horse chestnut seed contains many natural compounds, and products that include extract of horse chestnut are standardized for different ingredients:

Oxerutins are the active ingredient in Venoruton and Paroven; escin is the active ingredient in Venostasin and Essaven Gel. In addition, a product may be available in different forms, such as a cream for topical use, a tablet and a liquid extract.

In a review of research on botanicals for lymphedema published between 2004 and 2012, commissioned by the American Lymphedema Framework and the International Lymphedema Framework (Poage 2015), the authors concluded that:

- Botanicals may be more effective in cases of lymphedema that arise from venous insufficiency.
- It is best to choose botanical products from Germany, where more testing is done.
- Any product that has not been evaluated by the FDA should be avoided.
- More research is needed before any botanicals can be confidently recommended as a treatment for lymphedema.

All of these factors must be considered when you are deciding what supplement, if any, to try for your lymphedema. While the sales pitch for many of these products can be compelling, most are overhyped and unsupported by research. Ask your medical team and other people with lymphedema what their experience with a supplement has been, but keep in mind that everyone's lymphedema is unique, and results may vary.

Before seeking treatment from a health practitioner who works with supplements, it's best to research them too. Some practitioners may be involved in multilevel marketing or commission-based incentives to sell certain supplement brands. It's okay to ask about your practitioner's financial stake in the products they are selling. If they do profit from the sale of supplements, it doesn't necessarily mean you shouldn't follow their recommendations, but take their financial interest into account and use your best judgment.

If you participate in a trial of a natural health product, do some baseline observations and measurements at the outset so you can objectively evaluate whether the product has benefited you.

Survey Says

In my survey of complementary therapy use, natural health products were the least-used category. Of the eighteen people who had used one, the most popular natural health product was omega-3 fatty acids, which were used by ten respondents (56%). Four respondents (22%) had tried Pycnogenol, and three (17%) had tried serrapeptase or homeopathy. Fifteen of the products reviewed here had not been tried by any respondents.

References for Natural Health Products

Food and Drug Administration (FDA). 2022. "Information for Consumers on Using Dietary Supplements." Accessed September 27, 2024. https://www.fda.gov/food/dietary-supplements/information-consumers-using-dietary-supplements.

Health Canada. 2016. "About Natural Health Products." Accessed August 27, 2024. https://www.canada.ca/en/health-canada/services/drugs-health-products/natural-non-prescription/regulation/about-products.html.

Poage EG, Rodrick JR, Wanchai A, et al. 2015. Exploring the Usefulness of Botanicals as an Adjunctive Treatment for Lymphedema: A Systematic Search and Review. *PM&R* 7 (3): 296–310.

Astragalus & Peony

What Are They?

Astragalus and peony are two commonly used edible medicinal herbs with a long history of use in traditional Chinese medicine. More recently, Chinese researchers learned that each of these herbs contains an important chemical (Chiu 2020)—gallic acid in peony (*Paeoniae rubra*) and calycosin in astragalus (likely *Astragalus radix*, though it's not clear from the write-up). Preparing these two plant extracts together was meant to mimic the prescription drug Ubenimex (also known as bestatin, a protease inhibitor), which was used in a clinical trial of lymphedema as it is anti-inflammatory and antifibrotic (Eiger 2023).

Lymphedema-Specific Research

In a small pilot study of nine women who had had post-mastectomy lymphedema for two to nineteen years, the herbs were prepared in powdered form and taken orally six days a week for six months (Chiu 2020). Water displacement measurements and quality of life questionnaires were completed monthly.

At the end of the study, the women's body weight had stayed the same or gone down slightly. Lymphedema volume, as measured by water displacement, was mixed: It decreased in four participants, was stable in two and increased in two (the ninth patient did not return for the final six-month measurement). The average was a reduction of 94 milliliters (3.2 ounces). There was no significant change in hand grip strength, and no change in tonometer readings (a measure of tissue tension/fibrosis).

The women's quality of life had improved significantly. Most encouraging were reports of "less heaviness," "less congestion," "increased comfort" and "reduced tingling." Although there was no objective change in function, some participants reported that their limb appeared lighter and was less clumsy. Overall, patient satisfaction was very high.

Due to the mixed results with volume but positive patient reports, the authors speculated that the herbal combination's main effects were flow facilitation and reduced inflammation and fibrosis. They recommended ongoing study in larger trials with more sophisticated measurements.

Side Effects/Risks

None noted.

Bottom Line on Astragalus & Peony

When a combination of astragalus and peony was tested to see if it could mimic the effects of the prescription drug Ubenimex, patients provided positive reports despite a lack of clearly measurable improvements. More research is warranted. The formulation seems to have been prepared specifically for this study and is not a commercially available product, so even if results were stronger, it would be difficult to recommend at the current time.

References for Astragalus & Peony

Chiu TW, Kong SL, Cheng KF, Leung PC. 2020. Treatment of Post-mastectomy Lymphedema with Herbal Medicine: An Innovative Pilot Study. *Plast Reconstr Surg Glob Open* 8 (6): e2915.

Eiger BioPharmaceuticals. 2023. "Ubenimex in Adult Patients with Lymphedema of the Lower Limb (ULTRA)." Accessed August 8, 2025. https://ClinicalTrials.gov/show/NCT02700529

Benzopyrones

What Are They?

Benzopyrones are naturally occurring substances from a variety of plants. They have important effects on microcirculation (Michelini 2019) and were originally used to treat vascular conditions such as peripheral vascular disease, as they had been shown to decrease the permeability of blood vessels and reduce pooling (Badger 2004). Despite that history of use, it's important not to simply extrapolate findings from vascular studies to lymphedema: "It must be kept in mind that the histological structure of lymphatic vessels is completely different from that of blood vessels" (Bruns 2004). For example, much higher doses of benzopyrones are needed for lymphedema than for venous disease (Badger 2004).

There are two types of benzopyrones: alpha and gamma. The alpha-benzopyrones have two main pharmacological effects: activating contraction of the lymphangions and activating the macrophages to break down proteins (Michelini 2019). Coumarin (see page 118) is an example of an alpha-benzopyrone. The gamma-benzopyrones, also called flavonoids, play an important role in anti-exuding and membrane stabilization (Michelini 2019). Rutin, hesperidin and diosmin are gamma-benzopyrones. Flavonoids have pigments, including yellow, red and blue, that can be seen in the plants that contain them, such as blueberries, strawberries, bananas and citrus fruits. Parsley, onions, and tea also contain flavonoids (Haytowitz 2006).

Natural health products that have been developed with benzopyrones include Daflon 500 (page 132), which contains diosmin and hesperidin; Cyclo 3 Fort (page 130), which contains hesperidin; Lysedem, which contains coumarin (page 124) and trox-erutin; and Meliven 3 (page 152), which contains coumarin and rutin. They are believed to reduce fluid infiltration into the tissues, and thereby reduce pain, as well as to increase macrophage activity and break down extracellular proteins, reducing the formation of fibrotic tissue (Badger 2004).

Lymphedema-Specific Research

A thorough review of fifteen studies, including non-English and unpublished papers, determined that, unfortunately, the trials did not strengthen the argument for using benzopyrones to treat lymphedema, and that it was impossible to draw conclusions about their effectiveness (Badger 2004).

All but two of the studies in the Badger review included John Casley-Smith and/or Judith Casley-Smith as an author. The husband-and-wife duo, who are the founders of a well-regarded Australian training school for lymphedema therapists, had previously published a review of data from studies of 628 patients using oral and topical benzopyrones, in which they concluded that benzopyrones increased the fluid reductions achieved by complex physical therapy by 150% to 300% (Casley-Smith 1996).

Side Effects/Risks

Little is known about the long-term use of benzopyrones, but they are known to be damaging to the liver, so caution is recommended (Badger 2004).

Bottom Line on Benzopyrones

All benzopyrones belong to the same family of compounds, so keep in mind that they are all connected as you read my chapters on products containing them. A 2004 review on benzopyrones for lymphedema concluded that further research is needed and caution is required, but as this review is over twenty years old, an updated meta-analysis would be very welcome.

References for Benzopyrones

Badger C, Preston N, Seers K, Mortimer P. 2004. Benzo-pyrones for Reducing and Controlling Lymphoedema of the Limbs. *Cochrane Database Syst Rev* 2004 (2): CD003140.

Bruns F, Büntzel J, Mücke R, et al. 2004. Selenium in the Treatment of Head and Neck Lymphedema. *Med Princ Pract* 13 (4): 185–90.

Casley-Smith JR, Casley-Smith JR. 1996. Treatment of Lymphedema by Complex Physical Therapy, with and Without Oral and Topical Benzopyrones: What Should Therapists and Patients Expect. *Lymphology* 29 (2): 76–82.

Haytowitz DB, Bhagwat S, Harnly J, et al. 2006. "Sources of Flavonoids in the U.S. Diet Using USDA's Updated Database on the Flavonoid Content of Selected Foods." USDA Agricultural Research Service. Accessed October 2, 2024. https://www.ars.usda.gov/ARSUserFiles/80400525/articles/aicr06_flav.pdf.

Michelini S, Fiorentino A, Cardone M. 2019. Melilotus, Rutin and Bromelain in Primary and Secondary Lymphedema. *Lymphology* 52 (4): 177–86.

Coumarin

What Is It?

Coumarin is a sweet-smelling compound in the benzopyrone family (see page 122). It is found in many plants, including tonka beans (*Coumarouna odorata*), sweet clover (*Melilotus officinalis*) and cassia (Chinese cinnamon, Saigon cinnamon). Cassia, the type of cinnamon found at the grocery store, contains up to 1% coumarin. Ceylon cinnamon, which has a strong, hot flavor and is used to make cinnamon candies and gum, has only trace amounts.

Coumarin was used as a flavoring agent and perfume for many years, until reports of associated liver toxicity accumulated (Health Canada 2024). The European Food Safety Authority (EFSA) established a tolerable intake of 0.1 milligram per kilogram of body weight per day for coumarin in food (EFSA 2008).

Many natural health products—including supplements for lymphedema—contain coumarin, either alone or in combination. The manufacturers of these products claim that they stimulate lymphatic function and activate contractions of the lymphangions, thereby reducing edema and inflammation (Michelini 2019).

> **Technical Breakdown**
> To calculate a safe intake of coumarin, you need to know your weight in kilograms. If you know your weight in pounds, divide it by 2.2. For example, 200 pounds ÷ 2.2 = 91 kilograms. A safe intake is 0.1 milligram per kilogram per day. For a 91-kilogram person, this would be 0.1 × 91 = 9.1 milligrams per day. The amount of coumarin in cassia cinnamon is up to 1% (Wang 2013), so 1 teaspoon of ground cinnamon, which weighs 5 grams, could contain as much as 0.05 grams (50 milligrams) of coumarin. If you weigh 200 pounds and consume a teaspoon of cinnamon, you are five times over your daily level. However, it's not likely that you will consume even 1/5 teaspoon of cinnamon a day, so most people are within the safe intake level. If you are shaking a bit of cinnamon onto your cereal, you are well within the safe limit.

Lymphedema-Specific Research

Coumarin is one of the more promising supplements. According to a review of herbal products for lymphedema, it has been studied the most, with eight trials of coumarin being used either alone or as part of a blend (Sheikhi-Mobarakeh 2020). The results from these eight studies—summarized below and in the table on page 128—were mostly positive, with reports of volume reduction and/or symptom improvement.

Study #1: Pecking 1990

This randomized double-blind study was published in French, with only an abstract available in English. The study found improvement in mild lymphedema when coumarin was used in addition to physiotherapy, but details are lacking in the abstract.

Study #2: Casley-Smith, Jamal and Casley-Smith 1993

This randomized double-blind trial, which took place in India, studied 163 patients with filarial lymphedema with elephantiasis (see "Technical Breakdown," page 133).

There were four treatment groups, each of which took a different combination of supplements:

- Coumarin + diethylcarbamazine (to kill the microfilariae)
- Placebo + diethylcarbamazine
- Coumarin + placebo
- Placebo + placebo

The coumarin dosage was 200 milligrams, twice a day. The patients were followed for two years, but there were several dropouts. Side effects included itching, headache, nausea, diarrhea or constipation, and giddiness, all of which resolved after the first month.

The coumarin + placebo combination led to significant reductions in lymphedema volume, more so than in the placebo-only group or either of the diethylcarbamazine groups. In addition to volume reductions, patients in the coumarin + placebo group reported feeling less swelling and pain, and their inflammation, infections and ulcerations were reduced. Improvement of these symptoms was even higher in the coumarin + diethylcarbamazine group. The authors concluded that coumarin turned a slowly worsening condition into a slowly improving one.

Study #3: Casley-Smith, Morgan and Piller 1993

Thirty-one patients with post-mastectomy arm lymphedema and twenty-one patients with leg lymphedema of various causes were given, in random order, 400 milligrams of coumarin per day for six months and placebo for six months. While they were taking the placebo, their lymphedema often got worse, especially in the arm. When they were taking coumarin, lymphedema arm volume as compared with healthy arm improved from an average of 46% larger to 26% larger. For those with leg lymphedema, volume improved from 25% larger to 17% larger. In addition, their skin softness improved, their skin temperature was lowered, and acute inflammatory issues were reduced. Pain and limb mobility improved, as did feelings of hardness, tightness, tension, swelling and heaviness. Ninety-three percent of the patients preferred the coumarin to the placebo.

The side effects of mild nausea or diarrhea experienced by some patients in this trial improved within the first month.

STUDY #4: CASLEY-SMITH, WANG, ET AL. 1993

This study included 104 Chinese men and women with filarial lymphedema with elephantiasis in one leg. Sixty-four of the participants took two 200-milligram coumarin tablets per day; the remainder took a placebo. The study went on for just over a year, with measurements taken every three months. There was no other treatment used, not even compression garments. A unique grading system for filarial lymphedema was created for the study (the details are provided in the article). At the end, the total reduction of lymphedema was 100% for grade 1, 95% for grade 2, and 45% for grades 3 to 5. In addition, patients reported symptom improvement and fewer complications—most notably fewer cellulitis outbreaks.

For the patients in this trial, side effects included dizziness, sleepiness, nausea, diarrhea and skin rash, none of which were severe enough for the patient to drop out, and all of which resolved after one month.

STUDY #5: CHANG 1996

Sixty patients with leg lymphedema from a variety of causes were randomly assigned to receive either a placebo or 400 milligrams of coumarin per day for a year. After six months, compression garments and heat therapy, provided via microwave (see page 251), were added to the treatment. Eight patients dropped out of the study, including six from the treatment group. Two reported that they were cured—one after one month, and one after five months.

In the first six months, the coumarin on its own reduced volume by 20% and improved circumference, mobility and feelings of swelling, pain and heaviness. In the second six months, some but not all of the patients in the coumarin group made further improvements. Several reported new hair growth on the affected leg, which was interpreted as improved skin condition. Nodules reduced or disappeared, warts became smaller, skin elasticity and softness improved, patients regained the ability to sweat, and knee mobility improved. By comparison, the placebo group did not improve.

The authors concluded that coumarin was effective at stimulating macrophage activity, which may have reopened lymphatics that were blocked by filaria and fibrosis.

STUDY #6: VETTORELLO 1996

In this open-label trial, for which only the abstract is available in English, seventy-six patients with lower leg lymphedema were given manual lymphatic damage and a supplement composed of coumarin, ginkgo biloba and melilotus (sweet clover). After six to eight months, there was significant improvement in lymphedema circumference, pain, heaviness and episodes of infection.

STUDY #7: BURGOS 1999

For this Spanish study, seventy-seven women with post–breast cancer lymphedema received either 90 or 135 milligrams per day of Lysedem, a blend of coumarin and troxerutin, for twelve months. Lysedem is a sustained-release formulation, which is reported to improve bioavailability. According to the study authors, these were the two most common dosages of Lysedem used in Europe at the time.

In both dosage groups, lymphedema volume decreased steadily, with no statistically significant difference between the groups. The patients also saw improvement in hardness, heaviness, sensation of edema and neurological signs. After twelve months, lymphedema volume had reduced by 15% in the 90-milligram group, and 72% of the patients deemed the efficacy of the treatment either good or excellent. In the 135-milligram group, lymphedema volume had reduced by 13%, and 69% of the patients felt that the treatment's efficacy was good or excellent. The authors concluded that Lysedem was an effective complement to physical therapy and compression bandaging in improving quality of life.

Notably, eleven of the original seventy-seven participants dropped out due to adverse events (stomach pain, headache, nausea, or vomiting). Those who remained noted only mild side effects, which included stomach pain or heaviness, headache, increased menstrual flow and spotting between periods.

Study #8: Loprinzi 1999

One hundred and forty women with arm lymphedema following breast cancer received either a placebo or 200 milligrams of coumarin twice a day for six months, then switched to taking the other for six months. After six months of the placebo, arm volume increased by an average of 21 milliliters (0.7 ounces); after six months of coumarin, it increased by an average of 58 milliliters (2.0 ounces). The authors concluded that coumarin was not effective, and although it was generally well tolerated, 6% of the patients developed liver toxicity.

Side Effects/Risks

Despite the generally positive lymphedema results, there are multiple side effects associated with coumarin, though most seem to resolve within the first month. The most serious risk is liver toxicity. Research is underway on synthetic analogs of coumarin's active ingredients, to produce safer, higher-potency options. Some products are in clinical trials for treatment of breast cancer (Musa 2008). Until they are approved, it would be safer to avoid using coumarin and products containing it if your liver is compromised. Some researchers recommend a genetic screen to determine susceptibility to liver toxicity before using coumarin (Farinola 2005). See the table that follows for a summary of coumarin lymphedema research.

Study	Subjects	Supplement	Outcome	Side Effects/Risks
Pecking 1990	Details not available	Details not available	Improvement in mild lymphedema when coumarin was used in addition to physiotherapy	Details not available
Casley-Smith, Jamal and Casley-Smith 1993	163 patients with filarial lymphedema with elephantiasis	400 mg of coumarin per day, with or without diethylcarbamazine, for 2 years	Volume reduction was best with coumarin alone; symptom improvement was best with coumarin + diethylcarba-mazine	Itching, headache, nausea, diarrhea or constipation, and giddiness, resolved within 1 month
Casley-Smith, Morgan and Piller 1993	31 patients with post-mastectomy lymphedema and 21 with leg lymphedema	400 mg of coumarin per day for 6 months	Improved limb volume and mobility, skin softness and temperature, inflammation, pain, hardness, tightness, tension, swelling and heaviness	Mild nausea or diarrhea, improved within 1 month
Casley-Smith, Wang, et al. 1993	104 patients with filarial lymphedema with elephantiasis	400 mg of coumarin per day	Volume reduction, symptom improvement, less cellulitis, two reports of cure	Dizziness, sleepiness, nausea, diarrhea and skin rash, resolved within 1 month
Chang 1996	60 patients with leg lymphedema	400 mg coumarin per day for 1 year, with added heat therapy for the last 6 months	Improved volume, circumference, mobility swelling, pain, heaviness	Details not available
Vettorello 1996	76 patients with lower leg lymphedema	MLD and a supplement of coumarin + ginkgo biloba + melilotus for 6 to 8 months	Significantly improved circumference, pain, heaviness, and episodes of infection	Details not available
Burgos 1999	77 women with post–breast cancer lymphedema	90 or 135 mg of Lysedem per day for 12 months	Lymphedema volume decreased in both groups, with no statistically significant difference between the dosages; improved hardness, heaviness, sensation of edema and neurological signs	Stomach pain, headache, nausea, or vomiting led 11 women to drop out; the rest had mild side effects
Loprinzi 1999	140 women with arm lymphedema after breast cancer	400 mg of coumarin per day for 6 months	Arm volume increase of 58 ml (2.0 oz)	Liver toxicity in 6% of the women

Bottom Line on Coumarin

Coumarin is the most studied of the potential lymphedema supplements and had its champions in the 1990s, most notably the Casley-Smiths. Of the eight trials reviewed here, seven had positive outcomes, but one study with 140 subjects found coumarin to be ineffective (Loprinzi 1999). There were methodological weaknesses in the published studies, as noted in a 2004 review (Badger 2004).

Despite all the momentum in the 1990s, clinical trials on coumarin appear to have stalled: The last was in 1999. We can remain optimistic that researchers will find a way to unlock coumarin's potential—perhaps in the form of a synthetic alternative—but until they do, it may be wise to avoid coumarin in favor of one of the many complementary therapies without a risk of liver toxicity. If you do decide to try coumarin, or supplement containing coumarin caution is advised. It seems prudent to have genetic testing for susceptibility to liver toxicity, or at the very least have your liver enzymes monitored while you are on this supplement. Don't supplement without discussing with your care team first

References for Coumarin

Badger C, Preston N, Seers K, Mortimer P. 2004. Benzo-pyrones for Reducing and Controlling Lymphoedema of the Limbs. *Cochrane Database Syst Rev* 2004 (2): CD003140.

Burgos A, Alcaide A, Alcoba C, et al. 1999. Comparative Study of the Clinical Efficacy of Two Different Coumarin Dosages in the Management of Arm Lymphedema After Treatment for Breast Cancer. *Lymphology* 32 (1): 3–10.

Casley-Smith JR, Jamal S, Casley-Smith JR. 1993. Reduction of Filaritic Lymphoedema and Elephantiasis by 5,6 Benzo-Alpha-Pyrone (Coumarin), and the Effects of Diethylcarbamazine (DEC). *Ann Trop Med Parasitol* 87 (3): 247–58.

Casley-Smith JR, Morgan RG, Piller NB. 1993. Treatment of Lymphedema of the Arms and Legs with 5,6-Benzo-[alpha]-pyrone. *N Engl J Med* 329 (16): 1158–63.

Casley-Smith JR, Wang CT, Casley-Smith JR, Zi-hai C. 1993. Treatment of Filarial Lymphoedema and Elephantiasis with 5,6-Benzo-alpha-pyrone (Coumarin). *BMJ* 307 (6911): 1037–41.

Chang TS, Gan JL, Fu KD, Huang WY. 1996. The Use of 5,6 Benzo-[alpha]-pyrone (Coumarin) and Heating by Microwaves in the Treatment of Chronic Lymphedema of the Legs. *Lymphology* 29 (3): 106–11.

European Food Safety Authority (EFSA). 2008. Coumarin in Flavourings and Other Food Ingredients with Flavouring Properties—Scientific Opinion of the Panel on Food Additives, Flavourings, Processing Aids and Materials in Contact with Food (AFC). *EFSA Journal* 793 (October): 1–15.

Farinola N, Piller N. 2005. Pharmacogenomics: Its Role in Re-establishing Coumarin as Treatment for Lymphedema. *Lymphat Res Biol* 3 (2): 81–86.

Health Canada. 2024. "Coumarin in Cinnamon-Containing Foods and Vanilla Extracts—April 1, 2014 to March 31, 2015." Accessed October 1, 2024. https://inspection.canada.ca/en/food-safety-industry/food-chemistry-and-microbiology/food-safety-testing-reports-and-journal-articles/coumarin-cinnamon-containing-foods-and-vanilla.

Loprinzi CL, Kugler JW, Sloan JA, et al. 1999. Lack of Effect of Coumarin in Women with Lymphedema After Treatment for Breast Cancer. *N Engl J Med* 340 (5): 346–50.

Michelini S, Fiorentino A, Cardone M. 2019. Melilotus, Rutin and Bromelain in Primary and Secondary Lymphedema. *Lymphology* 52 (4): 177–86.

Musa MA, Cooperwood JS, Khan MO. 2008. A Review of Coumarin Derivatives in Pharmacotherapy of Breast Cancer. *Curr Med Chem* 15 (26): 2664–79.

Pecking A. 1990. Medical Treatment of Lymphedema with Benzopyrones: Experimental Basis and Applications. [In French.] *J Mal Vasc* 15 (2): 157–58.

Sheikhi-Mobarakeh Z, Yarmohammadi H, Mokhatri-Hesari P, et al. 2020. Herbs as Old Potential Treatments for Lymphedema Management: A Systematic Review. *Complement Ther Med* 55 (December): 102615.

Vettorello G, Cerrata G, Derwish A, et al. 1996. Contribution of a Combination of Alpha and Beta Benzopyrones, Flavonoids and Natural Terpenes in the Treatment of Lymphedema of the Lower Limbs at the 2nd Stage of Surgical Classification. [In Italian.] *Minerva Cardioangiol* 44 (9): 447–55.

Wang YH, Avula B, Nanayakkara NP, et al. 2013. Cassia Cinnamon as a Source of Coumarin in Cinnamon-Flavored Food and Food Supplements in the United States. *J Agric Food Chem* 61 (18): 4470–76.

Cyclo 3 Fort

What Is It?

Cyclo 3 Fort is a supplement containing 150 milligrams of butcher's broom (*Ruscus aculeatus*), 150 milligrams of hesperidin methyl chalcone (a synthetic antioxidant) and 100 milligrams of vitamin C (ascorbic acid). It is described as a "venotonic" and "vasculoprotector," meaning it increases venous motility and microcirculation and reduces edema. It is made by the French pharmaceutical company Pierre Fabre.

Technical Breakdown
Hesperidin methyl chalcone is derived from the flavonoid hesperidin (a gamma-benzopyrene), a plant compound found in citrus fruits and thought to decrease microvessel permeability. It is recommended for the treatment of venous circulation issues, such as heavy legs.

Lymphedema-Specific Research

In a double-blinded study at Cognacq-Jay hospital in Paris, fifty-seven patients with lymphedema secondary to breast cancer were treated with either Cyclo 3 Fort or a placebo for three months (Cluzan 1996). They were also given weekly manual lymphatic drainage and had to have been receiving MLD for at least one month prior to enrolling in the study. Each patient took three capsules three times per day for three months.

The patients in the Cyclo 3 Fort group had a significantly greater reduction in arm volume than those in the placebo group, who saw a slight increase in most cases. Reductions in the treatment group were greater in the forearm than in the upper arm. Patients with mild lymphedema appeared to obtain the greatest volume reduction, which may demonstrate that the action is more on the fluid than the fibrotic fat deposits. Body weight did not change.

Side Effects/Risks

Two patients taking Cyclo 3 Fort in the Cluzan trial experienced nausea and abdominal pain and withdrew from the study.

Bottom Line on Cyclo 3 Fort

Cyclo 3 Fort performed well in a relatively large placebo-controlled trial, but it had a greater effect on stage 1 lymphedema and on the forearm, leading the researchers to suggest that its mechanism of action may be more favorable to fluid-dominant lymphedema rather than the more fibrotic tissue that develops in later stages. It's unclear what result a lower dose might yield, as this trial used nine pills per day.

Given that Cyclo 3 Fort has been around since 1959, it's disappointing that there isn't more research on its potential use for lymphedema. In a review examining integrative therapies for breast cancer patients, the American Society of Clinical Oncology (ASCO) concluded that there was insufficient evidence to form a clinical recommendation about using Cyclo 3 Fort to treat lymphedema (Lyman 2018).

References for Cyclo 3 Fort

Cluzan RV, Alliot F, Ghabboun S, Pascot M. 1996. Treatment of Secondary Lymphedema of the Upper Limb with CYCLO 3 FORT. *Lymphology* 29 (1): 29–35.

Lyman GH, Greenlee H, Bohlke K, et al. 2018. Integrative Therapies During and After Breast Cancer Treatment: ASCO Endorsement of the SIO Clinical Practice Guideline. *J Clin Oncol* 36 (25): 2647–55.

Daflon 500

What Is It?

Daflon 500, also known as micronized purified flavonoid fraction (MPFF), contains 450 milligrams of diosmin and 50 milligrams of hesperidin, both bioflavonoids found in citrus fruits. Diosmin is one of the gamma-benzopyrones. Daflon 500 is made by Servier Laboratories in France and appears to have several different brand names, including Arvenum500, Venitol, Capiven, Variton and Detralex (Pecking 1997).

Lymphedema-Specific Research

I found three trials using Daflon 500 to treat lymphedema, described here in chronological order.

STUDY #1: PECKING 1995

I was only able to access the abstract for this open-label pilot study, which took place in France with ten female breast cancer survivors. The women were treated with Daflon 500 pills: two a day for six months. At the end of the study, all patients had a clinical improvement in symptoms, an average limb volume reduction of 6.8% and improved clearance speed of injected colloid as visualized with lymphoscintigraphy. This preliminary study led to a larger blinded study, the results of which were published two years later.

> **User Experience**
> "I have tried both diosmin and serrapeptase with no noticeable benefits."
>
> —Barbara, Illinois (lipo-lymphedema and venous insufficiency)

STUDY #2: PECKING 1997

In this randomized double-blind French trial, ninety-four women with arm lymphedema following treatment for breast cancer took two tablets per day of either Daflon 500 or a placebo for six months. Arm volume was measured every two months, and the patients had a lymphoscintigraphy before starting and at the end of the study. A subset of twenty-four patients with more severe lymphedema were injected with radio tracer colloid and given a lymphoscintigraphy to assess changes in the migration speed of the colloid.

Both the placebo and Daflon 500 groups reported improvements in discomfort, but only the patients taking Daflon 500 reported improvements in arm heaviness. Those with more severe lymphedema who took Daflon 500 had a significantly improved lymphatic migration speed, from 0.26 centimeters per minute to 0.84 centimeters per minute.

The authors attributed the improvement in migration speed of the injected colloid to Daflon 500's lymphagogue and lymphokinetic activity; in other words, there was an increase in lymphatic pumping. They concluded that Daflon 500, at the usual dose of two tablets per day, is highly effective for individuals with severe lymphedema.

STUDY #3: DAS 2003

For this Indian study, twenty-six patients with Bancroftian filarial lymphedema in one leg were randomly allocated to receive 25 milligrams of the antiparasitic drug diethylcarbamazine citrate (DEC) either by itself or with 500 milligrams of Daflon 500. (DEC treats the filarial parasite that causes the lymphedema.) The patients receiving Daflon 500 took two pills a day for fifteen days, then returned to the hospital to be measured. This pattern continued until the patients had completed ninety days of treatment. They continued to return for measurements after 180, 270 and 360 days.

The results showed no improvement in lymphedema when DEC was taken on its own. The group taking DEC + Daflon 500, however, had a 63.8% reduction in volume 360 days after the start of the study (270 days after the 90-day treatment period ended). The authors concluded that Daflon 500 had provided the beneficial effects.

> **Technical Breakdown**
>
> Filarial lymphedema is caused by nematodes (roundworms) from the Filariodidea family. There are three types of filarial worms: Wuchereria bancrofti (90% of cases), Brugia malayi and Brugia timori. After a bite from an infected mosquito, the microscopic larvae make their way to the lymphatic system, where they grow into worms that disrupt the flow of lymphatic fluid. Due to lack of treatment in many tropical countries, the affected limb can grow quite large, which is called elephantiasis. The worms can live for six to eight years, and during their lifetime can produce millions of immature larvae that circulate in the blood (WHO 2025). The treatment for filarial lymphedema includes antiparasitic drugs in addition to complete decongestive therapy.

Side Effects/Risks

In the Das trial, there were no side effects reported. In the 1997 Pecking trial, three patients taking Daflon 500 experienced gastrointestinal side effects (as did four in the placebo group), and five patients in the Daflon 500 group reported "miscellaneous disorders."

Bottom Line on Daflon 500

Daflon 500 was tested in one open-label pilot study and two clinical trials, one for post–breast cancer arm lymphedema and one for filarial leg lymphedema. The results were positive in both trials, but no further studies have been published in English in over two decades, so it's unclear whether Daflon 500 is still relevant for lymphedema. The Natural Medicines database rates Daflon 500 as "possibly ineffective" for lymphedema, which is not exactly a ringing endorsement, although it does add that the supplement is generally well tolerated (NatMed, n.d.).

References for Daflon 500

Das LK, Subramanyam Reddy G, Pani SP. 2003. Some Observations on the Effect of Daflon (Micronized Purified Flavonoid Fraction of *Rutaceae aurantiae*) in Bancroftian Filarial Lymphoedema. *Filaria J* 2 (1): 5.

NatMed. n.d. "Daflon 500 by Servier." Accessed January 10, 2025.https://naturalmedicines.therapeuticresearch.com/Data/Commercial-Products/D/Daflon-500-103440 .

Pecking AP. 1995. Evaluation by Lymphoscintigraphy of the Effect of a Micronized Flavonoid Fraction (Daflon 500 mg) in the Treatment of Upper Limb Lymphedema. *Int Angiol* 14 (3 Suppl 1): 39–43.

Pecking AP, Février B, Wargon C, Pillion G. 1997. Efficacy of Daflon 500 mg in the Treatment of Lymphedema (Secondary to Conventional Therapy of Breast Cancer). *Angiology* 48 (1): 93–98.

World Health Organization (WHO). 2025. "Lymphatic Filariasis." Accessed February 6, 2025. https://www.who.int/news-room/fact-sheets/detail/lymphatic-filariasis.

Escin

What Is It?

Escin (also spelled aescin) is a chemical derived from horse chestnuts (*Aesculus hippocastanum*), the fruit of a deciduous tree native to southeastern Europe. The fruits resemble edible chestnuts but are bitter. Escin has anti-inflammatory and anti-edema properties (Jeong 2023). It is a proven venotonic, meaning it reduces vascular permeability (vein leakiness), thereby reducing the formation of edema (Gallelli 2019). Escin is available in oral and transdermal forms (the latter is delivered through the skin). It is the active ingredient in Reparil, sold as either tablets or a gel by the German pharmaceutical company Madaus.

Lymphedema-Specific Research

In a double-blind trial, sixty-eight women with post–breast cancer lymphedema received either 25 milligrams of escin orally twice a day (50 milligrams total) or a placebo for three months (Hutson 2004). After three months, there was no significant difference in lymphedema, by any measure, between the escin group and the placebo group. The authors concluded that, at this dose, there was no demonstrable significant objective or subjective benefit for arm lymphedema.

The same lead author also published a study proposal on ClinicalTrials.gov, but the full results were not available (ClinicalTrials.gov 2015). Through personal correspondence with the author, I learned that the research team did not see significant change in lymphedema from either horse chestnut seed extract or Pycnogenol (Hutson 2018).

Lymphedema Research in Animals

Rats with lymphedema induced in their tails were divided into five groups to receive either no treatment (the control group) or an escin gel in one of four concentrations: 0.5%, 2%, 10% or 20% (Jeong 2023). The gel was applied evenly along the tail twice a day, using a brush. Treatment started four weeks after the lymphedema induction surgery and continued for four weeks.

After four weeks of treatment, all of the rats that were treated with escin had a significant reduction in swelling: 19% to 27% compared with the control group. There were no significant differences in results for the different concentrations. When the researchers examined skin thickness, the 0.5% escin group did not differ significantly from the control group, but the higher concentrations did. When they compared the number of lymphatic vessels under forty-times magnification, the escin-treated groups all had a greater number of lymph vessels than the control group, with the 2% escin group having the highest number.

The authors speculated that possible mechanisms of action included lymphangiogenesis (formation of new lymph vessels), improved transportation of lymph out of the swollen area, stimulation of blood vessel contractions, which would help blood to return via the venous system, and improvement in lymphatic contractions. They concluded that escin may improve acute secondary lymphedema through a complex set of mechanisms, with the 2% concentration being the most effective, but noted that it's unclear whether the results would apply to chronic or primary lymphedema.

Related Research

Venous insufficiency is a condition in which blood, which should move through the veins in only one direction—toward the heart—can backflow. A meta-analysis of studies that examined horse chestnut seed extract for chronic venous insufficiency in the legs included seventeen randomized controlled trials in which the supplement was standardized for the amount of escin (Pittler 2012). Overall, the trials indicated an improvement in leg pain, swelling and itchiness when the supplement was taken for two to sixteen weeks. When the escin supplement was compared to rutosides (four trials), Pycnogenol (one trial) or compression stockings (two trials), there was no significant difference for leg pain, but escin was superior to Pycnogenol for edema reduction.

Side Effects/Risks

In the 2004 Hutson trial, one patient's breast cancer metastasized, and another participant experienced minor dizziness that resolved with a 50% dose reduction.

Bottom Line on Escin

I am hesitant to recommend any supplement that has been proven for vascular disease, such as escin, for the treatment of lymphedema, especially when the current research is limited. While vascular disease and lymphedema have similarities, they are not the same. Escin might be best indicated for someone with primary lymphedema or lymphedema secondary to peripheral vascular disease (phlebolymphedema). If you have phlebolymphedema, talk to your doctor or pharmacist to see if escin is right for you, but given the limited evidence to date, don't be surprised if their enthusiasm is muted.

References for Escin

ClinicalTrials.gov. 2015. "Horse Chestnut Seed Extract for Lymphedema." Accessed February 8, 2025. https://clinicaltrials.gov/study/NCT00213928.

Gallelli L. 2019. Escin: A Review of Its Anti-Edematous, Anti-Inflammatory, and Venotonic Properties. *Drug Des Devel Ther* 13 (September): 3425–37.

Jeong HH, Kim D, Kim T, et al. 2023. The Role of Escin as a Topical Agent for Lymphedema Treatment in a Rat Model. *Int J Low Extrem Wounds* (August): 15347346231195944.

Hutson PR. 2018. Personal correspondence, June 29, 2018.

Hutson PR, Love RR, Cleary JF, et al. 2004. Horse Chestnut Seed Extract for the Treatment of Arm Lymphedema. *J Clin Oncol* 22 (14 Suppl): 80–95.

Pittler M, Ernst E. 2012. Horse Chestnut Seed Extract for Chronic Venous Insufficiency (Review). *Cochrane Database Syst Rev* 11 (11): CD003230.

Garlive

What Is It?

Garlive is a supplement containing hydroxytyrosol, hesperidin, spermidine and vitamin A, manufactured by the Magi Group in Italy. Hydroxytyrosol is extracted from olive leaves or olive pomace (the parts left over after olive oil is extracted), and it has strong anti-inflammatory and antioxidant effects. Hesperidin is extracted from citrus fruits and is also a component of the supplement Daflon 500 (page 132). Spermidine comes from rice (*Oryza sativa*) and is an anti-inflammatory (Bonetti 2022). Vitamin A is a fat-soluble vitamin found naturally in fish, organ meats, dairy products, eggs, fruits and vegetables. A deficiency of vitamin A is thought to contribute to inflammation (Bhusan 2021). The quantities of each component in Garlive are approximately 250 milligrams of hydroxytyrosol, 200 milligrams of hesperidin, 10 milligrams of spermidine and 0.8 milligram of vitamin A (Bhusan 2021).

Lymphedema-Specific Research

I was unable to locate any human studies using Garlive to treat lymphedema.

Lymphedema Research in Animals

Lymphedema was surgically induced in mice following tail injury (Bhusan 2021). At some time (presumably the same day as the surgery, but it's not specified in the write-up), half of the mice received a dose of Garlive, while the other group served as the control, with no supplements. The supplements were crushed and mixed with distilled water, with each mouse receiving one tablet per day (2.67 milliliters of filtrate, weighing about 30 grams).

Tail circumference was measured daily for twenty days and significantly increased for all of the mice. The mice in the control group had a greater increase in tail volume, which peaked at days ten and eleven and was maintained until day fifteen, when it gradually increased again until day twenty, ending the experiment. In contrast, the mice in the treatment group had a peak tail volume on days six to seven, with a gradual decline thereafter until day twenty. A nonsignificant more rapid increase up to day five was attributed to Garlive boosting the innate immune system, which causes greater swelling in aid of wound healing. There was a significant difference in tail swelling between the two groups, and the tails of the untreated mice had more inflammatory markers, with leukocyte infiltration and collagen deposition.

The authors attributed the inhibition of leukotriene B4, which they stated "is regarded as one of the most important molecules in the pathophysiology of lymphedema," to the hydroxytyrosol component of Garlive. They noted hesperidin's and spermidine's anti-inflammatory and immunomodulatory effects, and credited vitamin A with enhanced lymphatic vessel regeneration. They pointed out that the treatment group's rapid rise in swelling followed by a gradual decline indicates natural wound healing, while the control group's gradual, irreversible increase in swelling is an example of chronic wound healing. They concluded that, based on this successful animal study, their next step is to confirm their findings in human clinical trials.

> **Technical Breakdown**
> Inflammation can be acute (short-term) or chronic (long-term). The acute inflammatory response occurs as a result of injury or infection. White blood cells travel to the area of injury and help to heal it. After several days, the inflammatory cells should disperse. Inflammatory cells that remain in the area after the injury has healed contribute to chronic inflammation, which has been linked to progressive lymphedema, in which fibrotic fatty tissue and thickened skin develop.

Side Effects/Risks

With a single dose of Garlive per day, the mice developed stomach distention, so the dose was divided into two doses per day, at 10:00 a.m. and 5:00 p.m., which resolved the side effect.

Bottom Line on Garlive

I don't recommend food or supplements to humans based only on animal research. This supplement seems promising, but human studies are needed to confirm its safety and efficacy. Based on the Bhusan study, it appears that Garlive may work best as a preventative, if given early enough. I look forward to clinical trials on this promising supplement.

References for Garlive

Bonetti G, Dhuli K, Michelini S, et al. 2022. Dietary Supplements in Lymphedema. *J Prev Med Hyg* 63 (2 Suppl 3): E200–205.

Bhusan Tripathi Y, Pandey N, Mishra P, et al. 2021. Effect of a Dietary Supplement on the Reduction of Lymphedema-Progression in Mouse Tail-Cut Model. *Eur Rev Med Pharmacol Sci* 25 (1 Suppl): 56–66.

Ginger

What Is It?

Ginger is the rhizome (underground stem) of the plant *Zingiber officinale Roscoe*. It is used in fresh, dried and ground forms in cooking, baking and to make tea, and is also available as a supplement. It contains about 400 bioactive compounds, including phenolic compounds, terpenes, lipids and carbohydrates, with four main components being credited for most of ginger's biological effects (Ballester 2022). It has been demonstrated in laboratory and animal research to be a strong antioxidant and anti-inflammatory (Ballester 2022). It is known as an anti-emetic (preventing nausea) and has been studied for this use in humans.

> **User Experience**
> "I just began drinking Traditional Medicinals ginger tea once daily. The tea seems to be helping."
>
> —Anonymous, Massachusetts (uterine cancer–related lymphedema)

Lymphedema-Specific Research

I was unable to locate any studies that used either the food or supplement form of ginger specifically for lymphedema.

Related Research

There are many studies, mostly laboratory and animal research, on ginger's biological effects. A recent systematic review found that certain components in ginger demonstrate efficacy against several inflammatory diseases, including lupus, psoriasis, cancer, Crohn's disease and ulcerative colitis (Ballester 2022).

Another recent systematic review included 109 clinical trials that used powdered ginger, ginger capsules, ginger extracts (some standardized to contain 5% gingerol) or raw ginger in the amount of 2 grams, or ½ teaspoon, per day (Anh 2020). Here are the results:

- Eight of out sixteen trials showed that ginger was beneficial for chemotherapy-induced nausea and vomiting.
- Five out of six studies found that ginger improved menstrual pain.
- There were mixed results on using ginger to treat osteoarthritis.
- Ginger improves blood parameters of cholesterol, fasting blood sugar, hemoglobin A1c, insulin resistance and C-reactive protein.

In their concluding remarks, the authors called for more research with larger sample sizes, consistent evaluation parameters and detailed descriptions of the study's methodology.

Side Effects/Risks

Heartburn (gastroesophageal reflux) was the main side effect reported, occurring at doses from 500 to 2,000 milligrams per day (Ahn 2020).

> **User Experience**
> "I use ginger lozenges if my stomach is upset (happens quite often in the mornings, as my head is draining from my facial lymphedema). I add ginger if I am making a roast or a stir-fry. I grate ahead of time and freeze it, or I grate as I go. It adds flavour but also helps with inflammation. I also drink ginger tea, sometimes with lemon, sometimes with turmeric. Lately I am drinking ginger and turmeric mixed with water to help with inflammation. With the heat in summer, I need all the help I can get."
>
> **—Willa, British Columbia (full-body primary lymphedema tarda)**

Bottom Line on Ginger

Ginger is a spice that has been used in cooking and medicine for generations. It does appear to have anti-inflammatory properties, but it is unclear how that might translate to treating lymphedema. It's also unclear whether culinary intake is sufficient or supplemental doses are needed—and, if so, what the appropriate dosage and standardized ingredients would be. If you are cooking with ginger or drinking ginger tea, there is no reason to stop. If you want to supplement with ginger to evaluate the effect on your lymphedema, be sure to consult with your physician beforehand and monitor changes.

References for Ginger

Anh NH, Kim SJ, Long NP, et al. 2020. Ginger on Human Health: A Comprehensive Systematic Review of 109 Randomized Controlled Trials. *Nutrients* 12 (1): 157.

Ballester P, Cerdá B, Arcusa R, et al. 2022. Effect of Ginger on Inflammatory Diseases. *Molecules* 27 (21): 7223.

Ginkor Fort

What Is It?

Ginkor Fort, also called BN165, is a combination of 14 milligrams of gingko, 300 milligrams of troxerutin and 300 milligrams of heptaminol (Cluzan 2004). Ginkgo (*Gingko biloba*), or maidenhair tree, is a large tree with fan-shaped leaves and radiating veins; it has a long history of use in traditional Chinese medicine (NatMed 2025). Troxerutin is a natural compound in buckwheat, capers, black olives and green tea, among other foods. Heptaminol is a cardiac stimulant and vasodilator. Ginkor Fort is manufactured by Recordati in France and is used to treat venous insufficiency and hemorrhoids. Some studies use the spelling Gingkor Forte (Lyman 2018).

Lymphedema-Specific Research

A preliminary study on Ginkor Fort for lymphedema included forty-eight patients with arm lymphedema secondary to breast cancer treatment (Cluzan 2004). They all agreed to continue with their usual compression garments and manual lymphatic drainage, and were randomly and blindly assigned to one of three groups:

- Two capsules per day of Ginkor Fort (fifteen people)
- Three capsules per day of Ginkor Fort (sixteen people)
- One capsule per day of a placebo (seventeen people)

The results demonstrated why proper dosage is so important. The only group to report a reduction in limb heaviness was the one taking two pills a day, and their reduction was statistically significant. Improvement in tightness was noted in both the two-pills-per-day group and the placebo group. The two-pill group also had a higher and statistically significant increase in lymphatic migration speed (3%), measured by lymphoscintigraphy, as well as less lymphatic stasis and a significant improvement in the lymphatic drainage of the healthy limb. Their lymphedema volume reduced by 1%, while the other groups gained about 1%, though this is considered a nonsignificant finding. Overall, the patients taking two pills per day fared consistently better than those taking three pills a day or a placebo, but no changes in quality of life were quantified.

Related Research

Because Ginkor Fort is known to strengthen veins, increase vessel resistance and reduce permeability, there is more research on its use for venous insufficiency. For example, a review article found that it improved pain, cramps, edema, leg heaviness and bleeding and delayed progression of venous insufficiency with excellent tolerability (Nonikashvili 2022).

Although venous insufficiency and lymphedema are similar conditions, treatment for one should not be assumed to work for the other. However, individuals with phlebolymphedema may wish to discuss the use of Ginkor Fort with their vascular doctor, as improving the underlying venous insufficiency may help.

Technical Breakdown
Phlebolymphedema, a combination of chronic venous insufficiency and lymphedema, is the most common cause of lymphedema in the legs in the Western world. "Phlebo" refers to blood vessels. For example, a phlebotomist is a person who draws blood. "Phlebo-edema" is another word for venous insufficiency. Blood should flow from your feet up your legs toward your heart, but sometimes the valves that prevent the backflow of blood fail, and blood pools in the legs. The lymphatic system tries to help by moving some of the excess fluid out of the legs, but if it also fails, the result is phlebolymphedema.

Side Effects/Risks

In the Cluzan study, Ginkor Fort was well tolerated, with no side effects.

Bottom Line on Ginkor Fort

A review of integrative therapies for cancer survivors by the American Society of Clinical Oncology (ASCO) stated that there was insufficient evidence to form a clinical recommendation regarding the use of Ginkor Fort for lymphedema (Lyman 2018). That seems a reasonable conclusion, since there has been only one study, from 2004. Hopefully, research in this area will resume. If you have phlebolymphedema, you may wish to speak to your vascular specialist about this supplement.

References for Ginkor Fort

Cluzan RV, Pecking AP, Mathiex-Fortunet H, Léger Picherit E. 2004. Efficacy of BN165 (Ginkor Fort) in Breast Cancer Related Upper Limb Lymphedema: A Preliminary Study. *Lymphology* 37 (2): 47–52.

Lyman GH, Greenlee H, Bohlke K, et al. 2018. Integrative Therapies During and After Breast Cancer Treatment: ASCO Endorsement of the SIO Clinical Practice Guideline. *J Clin Oncol* 36 (25): 2647–55.

NatMed. 2025. "Professional Monograph Ginkgo." Accessed February 8, 2025. https://naturalmedicines.therapeuticresearch.com/Data/ProMonographs/Ginkgo.

Nonikashvili Z, Jūratė Gerbutavičienė R. 2022. Ginkgo Biloba, Troxerutin and Heptaminol Chlorhydrate Combined Treatment for the Management of Venous Insufficiency and Hemorrhoidal Crises. *Eur Rev Med Pharmacol Sci* 26 (14): 5200–209.

Goreisan

What Is It?

Goreisan is a traditional Japanese herbal blend of *bukuryo* (hoelen), *takusha* (*Alismatis rhizoma*), *sojutsu* (*Atractylodes lancea rhizome*), *chorie* (polyporus) and *keihi* (cinnamon bark). It is used in Japan, China (where it is called *wullingsan*) and Korea (where it is called *orycogsan*) to treat edema (Yoshikawa 2020). It acts as a mild diuretic. One manufacturer of goreisan is Tsumura & Co. of Japan.

> **Technical Breakdown**
> Kampo, traditional Japanese medicine, evolved from traditional Chinese medicine and was adapted to the Japanese culture and perspective. It includes herbal supplements and natural remedies, including goreisan, to treat illness based on a holistic approach to health.

Lymphedema-Specific Research

In a small pilot study of patients with lower limb lymphedema resulting from gynecological cancer, eight women were treated with compression garments and manual lymphatic drainage, and eleven received the same treatment plus 7.5 grams of goreisan three times a day (Yoshikawa 2020). The participants were in the study between four and fifteen weeks. Selected results were as follows:

Measure	CDT Only	CDT + Goreisan
Body weight	+0.46 kg (+1.0 lbs.)	−1.42 kg (−3.1 lbs.)
Extracellular water/total body water in lymphedema leg	+0.0007	−0.0069*
Lymphedema leg volume	+142 ml	−76 ml
Healthy leg volume	−130 ml	−15 ml

* Statistically significant

The authors concluded that goreisan can alleviate lymphedema symptoms by improving fluid retention, and that CDT + goreisan is more effective than CDT alone.

Side Effects/Risks

No adverse events were noted in the Yoshikawa study, but previously established risks include rash and itching.

Bottom Line on Goreisan

A single small, non-blinded, non-randomized study demonstrated benefits for leg lymphedema when goreisan was used along with CDT to treat eight post–gynecological cancer patients for four to fifteen weeks. It is difficult to make recommendations based on such a limited sample. More research, including randomized, double-blinded controlled trials published in English, would help bolster confidence in the use of goreisan to treat lymphedema.

References for Goreisan

Yoshikawa N, Kajiyama H, Otsuka N, et al. 2020. The Therapeutic Effects of Goreisan, a Traditional Japanese Herbal Medicine, on Lower-Limb Lymphedema After Lymphadenectomy in Gynecologic Malignancies: A Case Series Study. *Evid Based Complement Alternat Med* 2020 (April): 6298293.

Homeopathy

What Is It?

Homeopathy was developed by the German physician Samuel Hahnemann (1755–1843) based on the "law of similars," or "like cures like." The theory proposes that the response produced when a healthy individual ingests a plant, animal or mineral substance offers an indication of the symptoms that substance may treat. For example, a homeopathic preparation derived from onion might be used to treat runny eyes and nose.

Homeopathic remedies are diluted to infinitesimal extracts through a process of diluting and shaking. Low dilutions may contain traces of the original substances; high dilutions contain no trace material but are purported to retain a potent energetic effect. From a biomedical perspective, this theory is considered implausible, and homeopathy is often considered a placebo (Ijaz 2020).

Homeopathy does appear to have a cultural bias. According to Dana Ullman, a researcher from the University of California, Berkeley, around 100 million Europeans are estimated to use homeopathic medicine and a further 100 million people in India depend solely on homeopathy for their health care needs. In France, 44% of health care providers were found to have prescribed at least one homeopathic remedy (Ullman 2021).

Lymphedema-Specific Research

I could find only one study using homeopathy for lymphedema, and it was a case study—which, if you recall the hierarchy of evidence (page 4), is the lowest threshold of evidence (Nwabudike 2022). A seventy-two-year-old Romanian woman had, for four years, been living with renal (kidney) insufficiency and a swollen leg, which had progressed to include large lobules. She was already being treated with 80 milligrams of furosemide diuretic (Lasix) per day. For the study, this was increased to 120 milligrams per day, and the homeopathic product *Apocynum cannabinum* 30CH was added three times a day. (*Apocynum cannabinum*, commonly known as dogbane or Indian hemp, is a poisonous herb used in traditional medicine to treat edema.) She did not use compression, as none was available that fit her.

After three months, the patient's circumference measurements were reduced and her skin looked better. These improvements continued over twenty-three months of monitoring. By the end, her left mid-leg had reduced by 15 centimeters (5.9 inches), her right mid-leg by 21 centimeters (8.3 inches), her left ankle by 2 centimeters (0.8 inch), and her right ankle by 7 centimeters (2.8 inches).

The authors concluded that "the patient responded well to a combination of high dose furosemide and homeopathic medicine." While this is accurate, we cannot know the individual impact of each treatment. Strangely, the authors also stated: "it is unlikely that any placebo effect would play a significant role in the treatment of this case," which seems like bias on their part. I do, though, like their concluding statement, which is a call for further research into the role of integrative therapeutic approaches in the treatment of lymphedema.

> **User Experience**
> "I take one pellet of Apis mellifica 30CH per day—with nothing by mouth for an hour on each side of the pellet. It does seem to bring down the swelling just a bit—maybe a millimeter or two—and I notice my leg is a bit puffier-looking if I miss the pellet."
>
> —Margaret, Colorado (secondary lymphedema of the leg, abdomen and genitals)

Side Effects/Risks

The main risk of homeopathy is the "harm of omission": not receiving proper care when it is used in place of an effective treatment. Homeopathy pills or tinctures themselves have limited side effects, as they do not contain any measurable active ingredients; however, allergic or toxicological side effects are a theoretical possibility, especially when the substance being diluted is toxic. The carrier, which is greater in quantity than the homeopathic substance, may also present a risk for some people; for example, homeopathic pills may contain lactose, and some distillations contain alcohol. Finally, there is a potential risk of contamination.

Technical Breakdown

The placebo effect is real, and it's fascinating. A placebo is a treatment that has no known benefit. In drug trials, it is common for researchers to use a look-alike sugar pill to compare results against the real medication. No matter what symptom is being treated, it seems some people will improve just by taking the placebo—an excellent demonstration of the healing power of the mind. That's why the use of a placebo is important in research: A drug (or other treatment) must outperform the placebo to be considered effective.

Homeopathics are often seen as placebos because they have no detectible active ingredients.

Bottom Line on Homeopathy

There are strong opinions in the medical community on the use of homeopathy. Some go so far as to call it "harm-by-deception," "neglect," "professional misconduct" or "nonsense" (Ijaz 2020), while others come to its defense (Ullman 2021). For an evidence-based practitioner, it is difficult to recommend homeopathy for lymphedema, even as a complementary treatment, and using it in place of conventional therapy could result in the harm of omission.

That said, given the low risks and relatively low cost of homeopathy, the potential harm is minimal. If homeopathy can help a patient harness the healing powers of the mind, then I am in favor of using it, especially if it is part of someone's cultural tradition and belief system. In the end, if the patient improves, does it really matter whether that is due to the placebo effect or the energetic effect of a highly diluted substance?

If you are drawn to homeopathics, seek out someone who can advise you on the right substance and dosage. As with any complementary therapy, monitor your lymphedema and your symptoms to assess if there are measurable benefits. If you don't see an improvement after a reasonable trial period, you can move on and try a different complementary therapy.

References for Homeopathy

Ijaz N. 2020. Paradigm-Specific Risk Conceptions, Patient Safety, and the Regulation of Traditional and Complementary Medicine Practitioners: The Case of Homeopathy in Ontario, Canada. *Front Sociol* 21 (4): 89.

Nwabudike LC, Buzia O, Elisei AM, Tatu AL. 2022. An Integrative Therapeutic Approach to Elephantiasis Nostras Verrucosa: A Case Report. *Exp Ther Med* 23 (4): 289.

Ullman D. 2021. An Analysis of Four Government-Funded Reviews of Research on Homeopathic Medicine. *Cureus* 13 (6): e15899.

Hwanggigyejiomul-tang

What Is It?

Hwanggigyejiomul-tang is a Chinese herbal blend also known as Huangqi Guizhi Wuwu decoction, Huangqi Guizhi Wuwu tang and Huwnggigyejiomul tang (Lee 2024). It is described as "a classic prescription in ancient China, which can be used for diabetic peripheral neuropathy, cervical spondylosis of nerve root type and rheumatoid arthritis" (Wang 2020). In traditional Chinese medicine, it is used to invigorate qi and warm the meridians. From a Western medicine perspective, it is anti-inflammatory, analgesic (pain-relieving) and immune-supportive (Wang 2020). It contains dried astragalus root (*Radix Astragali*), cinnamon twigs (*Ramulus Cinnamomi*) and fresh ginger (*Rhizoma Zingiberis Recens*).

Lymphedema-Specific Research

The good news is that there is a 2024 systematic review and meta-analysis on the use of hwanggigyejiomul-tang for post–breast cancer lymphedema; the bad news is that it was published in Korean (Lee 2024). However, some details are available in English. The meta-analysis included eleven randomized controlled trials. In these studies, the treatment group experienced statistically significant improvements compared with the control group, which was either physical therapy or Western medicine. Outcomes measured included upper arm circumference, upper arm edema grade, shoulder range of motion and the Fugl-Meyer Assessment (which measures joint function, pain, sensation and other clinical evaluations), as well as visual analog scales, presumably of people's subjective experience of their symptoms.

Side Effects/Risks

To the extent that I could read them, there was no mention of side effects or risks in either the Lee review or a systematic review that looked at the use of hwanggigyejiomul-tang for rheumatoid arthritis (Wang 2020).

Bottom Line on Hwanggigyejiomul-tang

The quest to find reliable, safe, effective treatments for lymphedema is worldwide and relies on both ancient practices and modern science to find answers. This should be reassuring if you have lymphedema or work with lymphedema, but of course, we are impatient for answers. Unfortunately, other than the name of this herbal blend, its ingredients and the fact that positive outcomes have been found, I don't know any specifics about hwanggigyejiomul-tang, such as dosage, timing or risks. But astragalus (page 121), cinnamon (which contains coumarin, page 124) and ginger (page 139) are covered in this book. Hopefully, placebo-controlled randomized clinical trials published in English will be forthcoming.

References for Hwanggigyejiomul-tang

Lee Y, Kim Y, Kim Y, Kim K. 2024. Effect of Hwanggigyejiomul-tang on Postoperative Breast Cancer-Related Lymphedema (BCRL): A Systematic Review and Meta-analysis. *J Int Korean Med* 45 (1): 31–54.

Wang L, Fan Y, Xin P, et al. 2020. The Efficacy and Safety of Huangqi Guizhi Wuwu Decoction for Rheumatoid Arthritis: A Protocol for Systematic Review and Meta-Analysis. *Medicine* (Baltimore) 99 (36): e22011.

Hydroxytyrosol

What Is It?

Hydroxytyrosol is extracted from olives, olive leaves, olive pomace or olive mill wastewater. It is also present in extra virgin olive oil. It is a small molecule that quickly penetrates tissues and has been shown to have anti-inflammatory, antioxidant and antimicrobial activities (Bertelli 2020).

> **Technical Breakdown**
> Olive pomace is what remains after the first cold pressing of the olives to extract extra virgin olive oil. The pomace consists of olive pit, skin and pulp, and is sometimes called olive mush.

Lymphedema-Specific Research

I was unable to locate any human lymphedema research using hydroxytyrosol on its own, but I did find case studies of using olive-based skin care products that contain hydroxytyrosol to treat pruritus (itchiness) associated with lymphedema (McCord 2007). Nine patients with lymphedema and morbid obesity who were suffering from pruritus were taught how to use Olivamine-based skin care products: a cleaning lotion, an antimicrobial spray and a protectant paste or skin repair cream. In addition to hydroxytyrosol, the products contained aloe vera leaf juice, niacinamide, pyridoxine and retinyl palmitate. The patients used the products to treat their skin for the next six months, and 95% of the pruritic symptoms resolved quickly, some within a couple of days.

The authors concluded that the Olivamine-based skin care products effectively treated lymphedema-related pruritic symptoms. (*Note:* Although the study reads like an industry-sponsored study, there were no disclosures listed in the paper.)

Lymphedema Research in Animals

A qualitative review of animal and laboratory research on hydroxytyrosol for lymphedema sets forth a hypothesis on how it might work, with some compelling theories on its mechanisms of action (Bertelli 2020). The main theory is that it inhibits the synthesis of leukotriene B4, which is responsible for activating inflammatory cells in lymphedema (de la Puerta 1999). However, this action has only been documented in animal models and in vitro laboratory experiments.

Another potential mechanism of action is its effect on fat cells. Hydroxytyrosol prevents precursor fat cells from forming and encourages mature fat cell breakdown.

Finally, people with lymphedema tend to have a higher level of oxidative stress, which means the body's free radicals and antioxidants are imbalanced, a condition that can lead to further cell and tissue damage. The enzyme cyclooxygenase (COX) plays a key role in activating oxidative stress; therefore, antioxidants that target COX, such as hydroxytyrosol, can reduce lymphedema and relieve associated symptoms.

Hopefully double-blinded research trials in humans can confirm whether these proposed mechanisms of action ring true for humans with lymphedema.

Side Effects/Risks

No side effects or risks were noted in the McCord case studies or the Bertelli review.

Bottom Line on Hydroxytyrosol

Hydroxytyrosol is an intriguing candidate for human lymphedema trials if it can be developed into an oral nutritional supplement. A case series using hydroxytyrosol-containing skin care products demonstrated fast and effective results for lymphedema-related pruritus. Until there is double-blinded research on oral hydroxytyrosol, though, the data is too limited for it to be confidently recommended by evidence-based practitioners.

References for Hydroxytyrosol

Bertelli M, Kiani AK, Paolacci S, et al. 2020. Molecular Pathways Involved in Lymphedema: Hydroxytyrosol as a Candidate Natural Compound for Treating the Effects of Lymph Accumulation. *J Biotechnol* 308 (January): 82–86.

de la Puerta R, Ruiz Gutierrez V, Hoult JR. 1999. Inhibition of Leukocyte 5-Lipoxygenase by Phenolics from Virgin Olive Oil. *Biochem Pharmacol* 57 (4): 445–49.

McCord D, Fore J. 2007. Using Olivamine-Containing Products to Reduce Pruritic Symptoms Associated with Localized Lymphedema. *Adv Skin Wound Care* 20 (8): 441–42, 444–45.

Linba Fang

What Is It?

Linba Fang, also called Aescuven Forte, is a mixture of two traditional Chinese herbal medicines: *ku-shen* (*Sophora flavescens Ait.*) and red sage (*Salvia miltiorrhiza*). It does not have a single manufacturer and is not a branded or patented product but an herbal formulation.

Lymphedema-Specific Research

I was unable to locate any human studies in English on using Linba Fang to treat lymphedema.

Lymphedema Research in Animals

The only research on Linba Fang for lymphedema is a study in which mice with surgically induced tail lymphedema were tube-fed Linba Fang twice a day for either two or four weeks (Luo 2020). The control group did not receive Linba Fang. The treatment groups had a significantly greater reduction in their lymphedema, as well as lower inflammatory blood markers, and those treated for four weeks had better outcomes than those treated for two weeks. The mice treated with Linba Fang also had superior results in reduction of subcutaneous fat thickness, regulatory proteins that indicate fat deposition, subcutaneous fibrotic tissue and collagen, which is needed for fibrosis formation. The authors concluded that Linba Fang was effective against edema, inflammation, fibrosis and fat deposition.

Side Effects/Risks

No side effects were noted in the Luo study.

Bottom Line on Linba Fang

It is promising that, in an animal study, Linba Fang exhibited a multifactorial response by reducing lymphedema swelling, inflammation, fibrosis and fat deposition. However, since it is irresponsible to make recommendations to humans based only on animal research, we will have to wait for human trials to see if the benefits are transferable to people with lymphedema.

References for Linba Fang

Luo Y, Zhao L, Liu NF. 2020. Effects of the Traditional Chinese Medical Prescription Linba Fang as a Treatment for Lymphedema. *Evid Based Complement Alternat Med* 2020 (November): 8889460.

Linfadren

What Is It?

According to Omega Pharma, the Italian manufacturer, Linfadren is a "food supplement based on micronized Diosmin with dried extracts of Meliloto and Uva Ursina . . . that favors the microcirculation and the body fluid drainage" (Omega Pharma, n.d.). Diosmin is a flavonoid found in citrus fruits. Melilotus (sweet clover) contains coumarin, and uva ursi (bearberry) contains arbutin; coumarin and arbutin are the active ingredients. Linfadren is also available as a skin cream made of escin, arnica, coumarin and diosmin.

> **Technical Breakdown**
>
> When it comes to natural health products, oral supplements and topical products, such as skin creams, often have the same active ingredients. But because the route of delivery is different — the ingredients in topical products are absorbed through the skin—it is best practice to have distinct research on each product.

Lymphedema-Specific Research

In a trial conducted at the University of L'Aquila, in Italy, fifty women with breast cancer–related lymphedema received complete decongestive therapy consisting of skin care, manual lymphatic drainage, exercises and compression garments (Cacchio 2019). In addition, half of the women took Linfadren without food twice a day for two weeks, then once a day for four weeks. The patients were evaluated at the beginning and end of treatment, and again three months later. While the women taking Linfadren knew it was a supplement (an "open label" trial), the assessor and the statistician were blinded—they did not know which patients received the supplement and which did not.

At the end of the treatment period, the reduction in excess limb volume was -66.4% in the Linfadren group and -34% in the control group. Three months later, the Linfadren group had continued to improve, with a total -74% reduction, while the control group had regained some excess limb volume and were now at -32%. The Linfadren patients also reported greater functional improvement in their arm, which continued to get better even after they stopped taking the supplement (remember, though, that they knew they were taking it).

Why does Linfadren help? Given that CDT is the gold standard of lymphedema care, what additional assistance is provided by the supplement? As a reminder, lymph is a protein-rich fluid that attracts macrophages, which create an environment that signals the inflammatory cells to build a fibrotic fatty scaffold and to thicken the skin. According to the authors of this paper, Linfadren's mechanisms of action are threefold: The coumarin acts on the interstitial proteins, subjecting them to breakdown (a process called protolysis) by the macrophages; the diosmin acts on the lymphatic system, increasing the oncotic pressure and the frequency and intensity of lymph vessel contractions; and the arbutin has a diuretic effect, reducing fluid retention.

In addition to providing longer-lasting reduction of lymphedema, the breakup of proteins in the lymph fluid may reduce inflammation, fibrotic buildup and bacterial infections.

Side Effects/Risks

In the Cacchio trial, there were no side effects reported after six weeks of supplements. Although coumarin has a documented risk of liver toxicity at a dose of 400 milligrams per day, the amount of coumarin used in this study was well below that level (61.2 milligrams per day for two weeks, then 30.6 milligrams per day for four weeks).

Bottom Line on Linfadren

This multi-action supplement appears to be the true definition of a complementary therapy: When given alongside CDT, it provided enhanced results. While the blend of three active ingredients allows for a lower dose of coumarin that produced no side effects over a six-week trial, further large-scale, double-blinded, randomized controlled trials are needed to confirm that the results are reproducible without harm to the liver.

References for Linfadren

Cacchio A, Prencipe R, Bertone M, et al. 2019. Effectiveness and Safety of a Product Containing Diosmin, Coumarin, and Arbutin (Linfadren) in Addition to Complex Decongestive Therapy on Management of Breast Cancer-Related Lymphedema. *Support Care Cancer* 27 (4): 1471–80.

Omega Pharma. n.d. "Linfadren." Accessed June 21, 2025. https://www.omegapharmasrl.com/en/product/angiology/linfadren/.

Meliven 3

What Is It?

Meliven 3 is a supplement containing 100 milligrams of melilotus (with 20% coumarin), 300 milligrams of rutin and 100 milligrams of bromelain. According to the Italian manufacturer, Natural Bradel, melilotus "is useful for the functionality of the microcirculation and for venous circulation" (Natural Bradel 2025). Bromelain is an enzyme that breaks down protein and is found in pineapple, and rutin is a gamma-benzopyrone (see page 152) found in a variety of fruits and vegetables.

Lymphedema-Specific Research

In an Italian study, fifty women and two men with primary or secondary lymphedema, in stage 1 or 2, were given a supplement containing 100 milligrams of melilotus (with 20% coumarin), 300 milligrams of rutin and 100 milligrams of bromelain (Michelini 2019). Although the authors do not specifically name Meliven 3 as the supplement, what they describe is the exact makeup of this product.

The patients were given one tablet per day for six months. Assessments took place at baseline, at three months and at six months. By three months, 72% experienced less pitting, but the Stemmer sign remained the same as at baseline. Limb circumference reduced by an average of 4% after three months and 6% after six months (with a range of 2% to 12%). But 29% of patients had no reduction in circumference measurements after three months, and about 5% had no change after six months. Skin thickness, measured by ultrasound, decreased in all patients except one, who had an episode of lymphangitis (inflammation of the lymphatic vessels). The average reduction was 8%, with a maximum of 26%. Feedback from the patients included less limitation on activity, improved perceived health status and improved pain. The results did not differ between subjects with primary versus secondary lymphedema.

How does this supplement work? According to analysis put forth by the study authors, melilotus is believed to have a lymphokinetic effect, increasing the contractions of the smooth musculature of the small lymphatic vessels and thus increasing the return of lymphatic fluid to the thoracic duct. Coumarin, which makes up 20% of the melilotus, is proteolytic, meaning it helps to break down the proteins in lymphatic fluid, reducing the concentration of protein and allowing better lymph flow. Rutin is thought to reduce cell permeability (leakiness) and is a powerful antioxidant, protecting cells from DNA damage. Bromelain halves the time it takes to remove proteins from the lymphatic edema and speeds up tissue healing; it is also thought to be helpful in controlling pain in edema conditions.

The authors stated that they intentionally chose patients with stage 1 or 2 lymphedema, as they believed those with more fibrotic disease would not benefit from the lymphokinetic effect of the melilotus. They concluded that the supplement offered valuable help in the clinical control of primary and secondary lymphedema at stages 1 and 2, and in the control of lymph stasis.

This study did have some limitations: The subjects knew that they were receiving the treatment, and there was no control group for comparison. In addition, 29% of the participants had no reduction in volume after three months, which means that remaining on this supplement requires a commitment of time and expense, as patients might be tempted to discontinue a supplement when they don't see results after three months.

See also page 157 for a study using both Procurcuma and Meliven 3.

Side Effects/Risks

There were no side effects noted in the Michelini study, and liver function tests remained unchanged.

Bottom Line on Meliven 3

A single study on an unnamed supplement with ingredients matching Meliven 3 showed a limb volume reduction in 71% of participants by three months and 95% by six months. The patients reported improvements in pain, perceived health status and physical limitations. Skin thickness improved by an average of 8%. Given this multifaceted response, Meliven 3 is a promising supplement, though not every patient was responsive. Future research should include blinding and randomization, and should attempt to determine the ideal candidates for this supplement. For now, the authors of the Michelini study suggest limiting its use to stage 1 or 2 lymphedema.

References for Meliven 3

Michelini S, Fiorentino A, Cardone M. 2019. Melilotus, Rutin and Bromelain in Primary and Secondary Lymphedema. *Lymphology* 52 (4): 177–86.

Natural Bradel. 2025. "Meliven 3." Accessed June 22, 2025. http://www.naturalbradel.com/en/prodotto/meliven-3-food-supplement/.

Omega-3 Fatty Acids

What Are They?

Fatty acids are the building blocks of the fats and oils in our diet. They have carbon chains of various lengths, with or without double bonds. A carbon chain has an alpha and an omega end. An omega-3 fatty acid has a double bond on the third carbon from the omega end, while an omega-9 fatty acid has a double bond on the ninth carbon from the omega end. These different chemical structures behave differently in our body.

Omega-3 fatty acids occur naturally in our food supply. There are three main ones: docosahexaenoic acid (DHA), eicosapentaenoic acid (EPA) and alpha-linolenic acid (ALA). DHA and EPA occur in high amounts in fatty fish such as salmon, sardines, herring, mackerel, rainbow trout and anchovies. ALA is found in walnuts, flax and hemp. All omega-3s are part of an anti-inflammatory eating pattern.

Lymphedema-Specific Research

I was not able to locate any research specifically on lymphedema and omega-3 fatty acids, but there is plenty of human research on issues relevant to lymphedema.

Related Research

A pivotal study published in 2009 identified thirty-six anti-inflammatory and nine pro-inflammatory dietary substances, mainly herbs, spices and nutrients (Cavicchia 2009). One of the top anti-inflammatories was omega-3 fatty acid. A 2014 follow-up study placed omega-3s in the top fifteen anti-inflammatory food components (Shivappa 2014). The literature on diet and inflammation doubles every four years (Hébert 2019), so to say this is a hot topic is an understatement.

What we eat really does make a difference to our inflammation levels, so eating more omega-3-rich foods is a strategy I recommend to my clients and students with lymphedema (for more information, check out my book *The Complete Lymphedema Management and Nutrition Guide* and my program Lymphedema Nutrition School). But what about taking an omega-3 supplement? Does that help?

While many supplements suffer from a lack of studies, omega-3 has had a lot, including multiple meta-analyses on a variety of medical conditions. And yet, to date, there have been no studies of omega-3 supplements (or anti-inflammatory diets) for lymphedema. Here's a summary of some recent related research we do have on omega-3 supplementation:

- A meta-analysis on inflammatory factors in cancer patients found that omega-3 supplementation reduced blood levels of inflammation (Amiri Khosroshahi 2024).
- A meta-analysis on preventing cardiovascular disease found moderate evidence that omega-3 supplements were associated with lower risk of heart attack, death from heart disease and major heart events compared to control groups (Yan 2024).

Side Effects/Risks

The Yan meta-analysis found that omega-3 supplements increased the risk of atrial fibrillation. Overall, they have a good safety profile, but caution is warranted for individuals with bleeding disorders if taking an ethyl ester EPA supplement (Yan 2024). A meta-analysis examining the safety of omega-3 supplementation found increased odds of diarrhea, taste changes and tendency to bleed compared to placebo, but no serious adverse effects (Chang 2023).

Bottom Line on Omega-3 Fatty Acids

The benefits of anti-inflammatory diets are well studied and validated for many different populations. Likewise, there is a mountain of research on omega-3 supplements, with much of it showing benefits, along with some risks. There has yet to be research specifically on either the anti-inflammatory diet or omega-3 supplements for lymphedema, but given omega-3's stable safety profile, there are no major precautions, though users should be aware of a risk of increased bleeding. It's best to confer with your pharmacist, doctor and/or registered dietitian before taking any supplement, to be advised of potential contraindications. If you prefer to get omega-3s from your diet, eat fatty fish at least twice a week (AHA 2024).

References for Omega-3 Fatty Acids

American Heart Association (AHA). 2024. "Fish and Omega-3 Fatty Acids." Accessed December 1, 2024. https://www.heart.org/en/healthy-living/healthy-eating/eat-smart/fats/fish-and-omega-3-fatty-acids.

Amiri Khosroshahi R, Heidari Seyedmahalle M, Zeraattalab-Motlagh S, et al. 2024. The Effects of Omega-3 Fatty Acids Supplementation on Inflammatory Factors in Cancer Patients: A Systematic Review and Dose-Response Meta-Analysis of Randomized Clinical Trials. *Nutr Cancer* 76 (1): 1–16.

Cavicchia PP, Steck SE, Hurley TG, et al. 2009. A New Dietary Inflammatory Index Predicts Interval Changes in Serum High-Sensitivity C-reactive Protein. *J Nutr* 139 (12): 2365–72.

Chang JP, Tseng PT, Zeng BS, et al. 2023. Safety of Supplementation of Omega-3 Polyunsaturated Fatty Acids: A Systematic Review and Meta-Analysis of Randomized Controlled Trials. *Adv Nutr* 14 (6): 1326–36.

Hébert JR, Shivappa N, Wirth MD, et al. 2019. Perspective: The Dietary Inflammatory Index (DII)—Lessons Learned, Improvements Made, and Future Directions. *Adv Nutr* 10 (2): 185–95.

Shivappa N, Steck SE, Hurley TG, et al. 2014. Designing and Developing a Literature-Derived, Population-Based Dietary Inflammatory Index. *Public Health Nutr* 17 (8): 1689–96.

Yan J, Liu M, Yang D, et al. 2024. Efficacy and Safety of Omega-3 Fatty Acids in the Prevention of Cardiovascular Disease: A Systematic Review and Meta-analysis. *Cardiovasc Drugs Ther* 38 (4): 799–817.

Procurcuma

What Is It?

Procurcuma is a supplement composed of 600 milligrams of dry turmeric extract, 100 milligrams of turmeric rhizome powder and 1.9 milligrams of piperine from black pepper (*Piper nigrum*). Made by the Italian company Proeon, it is used to increase intestinal absorption. Curcumin, one of the main active ingredients in turmeric, is a known antioxidant and anti-inflammatory.

Technical Breakdown

Thanks to turmeric's anti-inflammatory action, there are multiple studies on it and its main active ingredient, curcumin. The research suffered a setback in 2013, however, when a prominent cancer researcher and turmeric proponent had their research scrutinized and thirty published papers retracted (Ramesh 2024). This researcher has not published since 2015. When reading research on turmeric and curcumin, pay attention to publication dates and retraction notices.

Lymphedema-Specific Research

In a six-day experiment, forty-one patients with stage 2 and 3 leg lymphedema used the supplements Procurcuma and Meliven 3 (see page 152) along with twenty minutes of MLD, forty minutes of electro-sound lymphatic drainage (see Manutech BH, page 249), multilayer short-stretch bandaging, a low- carbohydrate diet and exercise (Cavezzi 2020). The patients saw a progressive and statistically significant improvement in limb volume and reduced extracellular fluids. While these improvements would need to be maintained over the long term (which presents a different set of challenges), the authors concluded that their intensive short-term CDT and holistic protocol was beneficial.

Side Effects/Risks

According to the manufacturer's website, Procurcuma is contraindicated for those with impaired liver function and biliary tract stones, and there may be additional contraindications with certain medications (Proeon 2025).

Bottom Line on Procurcuma

It is impossible to say what effect Procurcuma had on the patients in the Cavezzi study, as it was only one part of a multimodal six-day approach to treating lymphedema. Clinical trials that test Procurcuma by itself are needed to determine whether it would be a good complementary therapy for lymphedema.

References for Procurcuma

Cavezzi A, Urso SU, Paccasassi S, et al. 2020. Bioimpedance Spectroscopy and Volumetry in the Immediate/Short-Term Monitoring of Intensive Complex Decongestive Treatment of Lymphedema. *Phlebology* 35 (9): 715–23.

Proeon. 2025. "Procurcuma®." Accessed June 22, 2025. https://www.proeon.it/en/integratori-alimentari/procurcuma.

Ramesh S. 2024. "Inside Indian-American Biochemist's 'Haldi Swindle' That Proposed Spice as 'Cancer Hack.'" The Print. Accessed July 2, 2025. https://theprint.in/science/inside-indian-american-biochemists-haldi-swindle-that-proposed-spice-as-cancer-hack/1950784/.

Pycnogenol

What Is It?

Pycnogenol is an herbal supplement made from the dried extract of the bark of the French maritime pine tree (*Pinus pinaster Ait. Ssp. Atlantica*). It has been widely studied for multiple health conditions, with positive results that are mainly attributed to its antioxidant and anti-inflammatory effects on blood circulation (Weichmann 2024).

> **User Experience**
> "When our son was nine years old, a therapist recommended we provide him oral pine bark extract and add a few droppers of a natural detox to his morning and evening beverage. Results were not sufficient for us to justify the continued expense, and our son disliked the taste of the detox formula, so we discontinued after exhausting the second ninety-day supply we had purchased."
>
> —**Anonymous (parent of a child with primary lymphedema in both legs)**

Lymphedema-Specific Research

Despite its popularity, there is no Pycnogenol research specifically for lymphedema, though there are studies on its use to treat swelling, and their results may be transferable to lymphedema.

Related Research

In one study of Pycnogenol for swelling related to air travel, more than 200 participants measured their edema before and after a long-haul flight (Cesarone 2005). Two to three hours before the flight, half of the subjects took two 100-milligram capsules of Pycnogenol with 250 milliliters (1 cup) of water; they took another two capsules six hours later, and one capsule the next day. The remaining subjects followed the same protocol but took a placebo.

Within twelve hours both before and after the flight, Sonosite scanning was performed to study the venous system. Participants were instructed on how to take ankle circumference measurements, which they did before and after the flight. They also answered questions about tolerance to the supplement or placebo.

Edema in the Pycnogenol group increased by 17.9% after the flight, whereas the control group's edema increased by 58.3%. The rate of ankle swelling increased 26% in the Pycnogenol group and 91% in the control group. The authors concluded that Pycnogenol provided subjective and objective improvements in edema following air travel, with no side effects reported.

A review of thirty-nine randomized, double-blind, placebo-controlled clinical trials on Pycnogenol, including over 2,000 subjects, found evidence that it has a beneficial effect on cardiovascular health, chronic venous insufficiency, cognition, joint health, oral health and sports performance (Weichmann 2024). No lymphedema studies were examined in the review.

Side Effects/Risks

None noted.

Technical Breakdown

Why do your ankles swell when you fly? This is a common problem for everyone, not just folks with lymphedema. The swelling is due to lower air pressure, which is measured in atmospheres (ATM). Air pressure at sea level is 1 ATM. At the peak altitude of most airplanes—30,000 to 40,000 feet above sea level—the pressure is about 0.23 ATM; however, the cabin pressure is adjusted so that it is about 0.75 to 0.82 ATM (the equivalent of about 6,000 to 8,000 feet). For many people, the lower air pressure combined with the long sitting time, dry air and salty snacks leads to swelling. Be sure to read about ai chi (page 74) aqua therapy (page 76) and hyperbaric oxygen (page 233), three strategies that use increased pressure to aid lymphedema.

Bottom Line on Pycnogenol

There is no specific evidence to recommend Pycnogenol for lymphedema. That said, if it is being taken for another condition for which it does demonstrate efficacy, such as high blood pressure, high blood cholesterol, diabetes or venous insufficiency, one could reasonably expect that it would not be contraindicated for a comorbidity of lymphedema and may in fact prove beneficial.

References for Pycnogenol

Cesarone MR, Belcaro G, Rohdewald P, et al. 2005. Prevention of Edema in Long Flights with Pycnogenol. *Clin Appl Thromb Hemost* 11 (3): 289–94.

Weichmann F, Rohdewald P. 2024. Pycnogenol® French Maritime Pine Bark Extract in Randomized, Double-Blind, Placebo-Controlled Human Clinical Studies. *Front Nutr* 11 (May): 1389374.

Robuvit

What Is It?

Robuvit is made from the wood of the French oak tree (*Quercus robur*), also called pedunculate oak and English oak. The Swiss company Horphag Research has a propriety extraction and purification method that produces a fine powder. Robuvit is a branded ingredient, which means it is sold to other manufacturers to be incorporated into medicinal products. As a consumer, you can't purchase pure Robuvit from Horphag, but you may be able find it in other products.

Robuvit is high in antioxidants that are also found in wine and spirits aged in oak barrels. As such, humans have been exposed to Robuvit for centuries. At a cellular level, Robuvit is credited with increasing mitochondrial renewal (Weichmann 2021).

Lymphedema-Specific Research

There are three published studies on using Robuvit to treat lymphedema, which I will describe in chronological order.

> **User Experience**
> "Robuvit has been helpful for me."
>
> **—Carleen, Texas (leg lymphedema)**

STUDY #1: BELCARO 2015

In this Italian study, sixty-five patients with single-leg lymphedema were given standard management plus 300 milligrams of Robuvit per day (twenty-three patients), 600 milligrams of Robuvit per day (twenty patients) or no supplement (twenty-two patients) for eight weeks. Standard management included 30 to 40 mmHg compression, exercise, a low-dose diuretic if needed, a low-salt diet, antibiotics for two weeks, daily leg elevation and massage, and skin moisturizing. Here are some of the results reported after eight weeks:

Measure	Standard Treatment Only	300 mg Robuvit	600 mg Robuvit
Leg volume	−6.2%	−15.0%	−18.9%
Edema score	+6.7	+4.3	+3.2
Proteins in interstitial fluid	−14.8%	−29.9%	−36.9%
Skin thickness (pretibial)	−6%	−10.3%	−11.8%
Skin fungal infections	18.1%	4.3%	0

As you can see, those taking 600 milligrams of Robuvit had the greatest reduction in leg volume, proteins in interstitial fluid and skin thickness. They also had no fungal skin infections.

STUDY #2: BELCARO 2018

The aim of this second study was to evaluate whether adding Robuvit to complete decongestive therapy over a two-month period would be more effective than CTD alone. Thirty-three patients with lymphedema were the control group, and another thirty-two took 600 milligrams per day of Robuvit. At the one- and two-month follow-ups, the decrease in volume was significantly greater in the supplement group, with a final reduction in volume after two months of −19.8% (654 milliliters/22 ounces), versus −12.8% (433 milliliters/15 ounces) in the control group. A greater decrease in skin thickness and symptoms was also observed in the Robuvit group.

The authors concluded that CDT combined with self-management can effectively control excess limb volume in post-mastectomy lymphedema, and that supplementation with Robuvit further reduces limb volume.

STUDY #3: HU 2020

This study evaluated the effects of Robuvit in people with diffuse minimal lymphatic retention. Thirty-four women received either standard management (the control group) or standard management plus 300 milligrams per day of Robuvit (the treatment group). After four weeks, the treatment group had significantly reduced edema, as observed via ultrasound, with greater reductions at the more distal locations. The control subjects had no significant changes.

The authors concluded that Robuvit appears to be safe and effective in controlling diffuse minimal lymphatic retention, which they believe indicates a preventative effect.

Side Effects/Risks

No side effects were reported in any of the three studies.

Bottom Line on Robuvit

Despite positive results in three small studies, research has not continued (in English) since the last publication in 2020, which makes it difficult to recommend Robuvit with enthusiasm. And because there is no data on taking Robuvit for longer than eight weeks, we cannot judge its long-term safety or effectiveness. Overall, however, this supplement appears very promising.

References for Robuvit

Belcaro G, Dugall M, Cotellese R, et al. 2018. Supplementation with Robuvit® in Post-mastectomy Post-radiation Arm Lymphedema. *Minerva Chir* 73 (3): 288–94.

Belcaro G, Dugall M, Hu S, et al. 2015. French Oak Wood (Quercus robur) Extract (Robuvit) in Primary Lymphedema: A Supplement, Pilot, Registry Evaluation. *Int J Angiol* 24 (1): 47–54.

Hu S, Belcaro G, Hosoi M, et al. 2020. Prevention of Diffuse, Minimal Lymphatic "Retention" with Robuvit®: A Concept, Supplement Registry Study. *Minerva Cardioangiol* 68 (3): 197–202.

Weichmann F, Avaltroni F, Burki C. 2021. Review of Clinical Effects and Presumed Mechanism of Action of the French Oak Wood Extract Robuvit. *J Med Food* 24 (9): 897–907.

Selenium

What Is It?

Selenium is an essential mineral found naturally in many foods, including Brazil nuts, seafoods and organ meats. It exists in two forms, inorganic and organic, referring to its chemistry, not to organic farming (NIH 2024). Most of the lymphedema research on selenium supplements to date has used the brand Selenase, a supplement containing sodium selenite pentahydrate, used to correct a selenium deficiency when intake from food is insufficient. It is a sterile solution in drinking ampoules of 200 micrograms of selenium in 2 milliliters of saline solution. Selenase is manufactured by the German pharmaceutical and biotech company Biosyn.

> **Technical Breakdown**
> Your daily requirement of selenium is 55 micrograms per day (higher during pregnancy and breastfeeding). One ounce of Brazil nuts (about six to eight nuts) provides 544 micrograms, so just one Brazil nut per day provides your total daily requirement. The upper level of selenium is 400 micrograms per day, so don't overdo your Brazil nut intake.

Lymphedema-Specific Research

Of all the vitamin and mineral supplements for lymphedema, selenium has the greatest number of studies. As an antioxidant with strong anti-inflammatory properties, selenium can improve microcirculation in the area of lymphedema (Kasseroller 2000). Researchers believe that it can help unclog lymphatic capillaries, providing a spontaneous reduction in lymph volume and improving the efficacy of decongestive bandaging.

In addition to the studies discussed below, a trial on sodium selenite was done at Princess Margaret Hospital in Toronto, but the results were not published (University Health Network 2010). However, in a PDF on the Princess Margaret website called "Guide to Lymphedema," there is a mention of selenium in a list headed: "Together we can discuss the less common ways of looking after lymphedema found in the community," which, along with selenium, includes kinesiology taping (see page 108) and hyperbaric oxygen (page 233), among other strategies (Breast Cancer Survivorship Program, n.d.). Below is a description of the research, followed by a summary table.

STUDY #1: KASSEROLLER 2000

This study included 179 women who had had a mastectomy for breast cancer and developed lymphedema as a result. It had been twelve months since their last decongestive therapy session for their stage 1 or 2 lymphedema. After enrolling in the study, the participants were advised to do self-care including hygiene and skin care, were given identical lotions and wrappings, and were advised to follow a low-fat and low-salt diet (for more nutrition advice, read *The Complete Lymphedema Management and Nutrition Guide*). They received decongestive therapy, including compression bandaging and exercise, twice a day for three weeks. They were blinded and randomized to receive either a saline placebo or Selenase in the following amounts:

- **Week 1:** 1,000 micrograms per day (333 micrograms three times a day) before meals.
- **Weeks 2 and 3:** 300 micrograms per day.
- **Remaining 3 months:** 100 micrograms if they weighed less than 70 kilograms (154 pounds) or 200 micrograms if they weighed more.
- The participants in the placebo group received saline in the same solution volumes.

Lymphedema volume reduced by 524 milliliters (17.7 ounces) in the Selenase group, versus 420 milliliters (14.2 ounces) in the placebo group. The Selenase group lost 1.5 kilograms (3.3 pounds), while the placebo group lost 1 kilogram (2.2 pounds). In addition, the Selenase group had greater improvements in nighttime urination, vision, dry skin, mood, skin fold index, skin fold thickness, heat sensitivity in the lymphedema arm, and skin softness in the lymphedema arm, as well as reduced incidence of erysipelas (bacterial skin infection of the dermis layer).

When the Selenase takers compared their current reduction in limb volume to their previous reduction using compression bandaging only, there were mixed results. Two had 14% *less* reduction with compression bandaging + Selenase, but six had a 33% improvement in lymphedema reduction.

In the discussion section of the paper, the authors noted that Selenase is less effective for advanced lymphedema, which can become fibrotic and calcified; it works best for those who have had lymphedema for two years or less. But even in advanced lymphedema, Selenase did still protect against erysipelas and help to soften the limb.

STUDY #2: MICKE 2003

This German study focused on forty-eight patients who had undergone radiation for cancer treatment between two and sixteen months earlier. Twelve had arm lymphedema, and thirty-six had head and neck lymphedema. The participants took Selenase orally once a day for four to six weeks. The dosage was dependent on the patient's size (350 micrograms per square meter of body surface area); on average, it was 500 micrograms per day.

One of the measures used was a visual analog scale. Simply put, the physician and the patient rated their condition on a scale of 0 to 10, with a higher number meaning a lower quality of life. Before the study, the average rating was 7.3±1.9. After selenium treatment, it was 3.0±2.6—demonstrating that they believed their condition had improved.

The authors concluded that "selenium supplementation resulted in a reduction in lymphedema." However, given that there was no control group, the only basis for this assertion is that most people with lymphedema get worse over time, and this group did not.

I did enjoy their analysis of selenium's mechanism of action: Lymphostasis creates more reactive oxygen species (free radicals), and selenium is a strong antioxidant. Many people diagnosed with cancer of the head and neck have low blood levels of selenium (and zinc) and decreased antioxidant enzymes. Selenium "unclogs" lymph capillaries invaded by leukocytes by preventing sticky adhesion molecules from attaching to the lymphatic capillaries. It may also stimulate macrophages ("big eater" immune cells) to break down the excess tissue protein in the lymph fluid.

STUDY #3: BRUNS 2004

Another German study analyzed the outcomes of thirty-six patients with cancer in the head or neck (who appear to be the same participants as in study #2). As with the previous study, all of the participants took Selenase orally once a day for four to six weeks, with the dosage dependent on their size (an average of 500 micrograms per day).

Twenty of the patients had interstitial endolaryngeal edema (swelling of the larynx that makes it difficult to breathe), which is usually treated with a tracheostomy (a surgical procedure that creates an opening in the windpipe to insert a tube for breathing). After selenium supplementation, this group showed a substantial reduction of their endolaryngeal edema, evaluated using an microlaryngoscope (a tube with a camera, inserted down the throat). Thirteen did not require a tracheostomy, five needed a temporary one, and only two needed a permanent tracheostomy.

The remaining sixteen patients were evaluated using two different symptom scoring systems. Ten showed improvements in their lymphedema using the Földi scoring system, and twelve saw improvements using the Miller scoring system. Before and after treatment, patients completed questionnaires on their quality of life, which also improved significantly.

Study #4: Zimmerman 2005

This placebo-controlled, double-blinded, randomized study also took place in Germany. Eighteen men and two women who were about to have neck dissection surgery for squamous cell oral cancer took either a placebo or 1,000 micrograms of sodium selenite (brand unspecified), by IV or by mouth, starting on the day of their surgery and continuing for three weeks. Their lymphedema was measured in the tragus (a part of the ear), nostrils, corner of the mouth and tip of the chin. All measurements were made by the same person, to avoid variation in technique.

The authors looked at several outcomes, including lymphedema measurements and blood levels of selenium and the antioxidant glutathione peroxidase. The patients taking selenium had a more rapid reduction in lymphedema at both one week and two weeks post-surgery. The higher their blood levels of selenium and glutathione peroxidase, the lower the severity of lymphedema.

This paper included a description of fibrosis in lymphedema to explain how selenium helps. When there is an increase in lymphatic fluid in the interstitium (the extracellular spaces outside the blood), protein concentration also increases. The lymph vessels dilate due to the increased workload, and the lymph capillaries become leakier. The increased protein activates fibroblasts—cells that create fibrosis. The fibrosis attracts immune cells that create free radicals, and the free radicals impede the flow of lymphatic fluid by reducing the frequency of contractions and the amount of fluid moved with each contraction. As an antioxidant, selenium can decrease the levels of free radicals.

The authors concluded that sodium selenite is a suitable treatment for secondary lymphedema after oral cancer surgery and is of particular benefit to those who have undergone extensive lymph node removal. They recommend that selenium be started immediately after surgery, and judge that 1,000 micrograms per day should not produce any side effects.

Study #5: Han 2019

This Korean study included twenty-six women with stage 2 or 3 breast cancer–related lymphedema. It was a randomized, double-blinded, placebo-controlled trial—the gold standard in clinical research. The fourteen women in the treatment group received 500 micrograms of Selenase dissolved in 50 milliliters of 0.9% saline by IV five times over two weeks. The twelve women in the control group received an identical volume of saline by IV. All twenty-six women were taught how to do self-MLD.

Of the fourteen women who received selenium, twelve were at stage 3 and two were at stage 2 at the beginning of the study. Nine of the twelve reduced from stage 3 to stage 2 by the end of the two weeks. By one month post-selenium, ten members of that group had achieved and maintained a lower stage. None of the women in the placebo group improved their stage.

The authors concluded that selenium reduced the lymphedema, even though they didn't know exactly how, and that sodium selenite supplementation could be a safe and cost-effective treatment for lymphedema.

Study #6: Lee 2021

The researchers for this study, which also took place in Korea, set out to discover selenium's mechanism of action by performing a secondary analysis of the results from study #5 (Han 2019). They analyzed 107 different metabolites and found a handful that were elevated after selenium supplementation, meaning they could be responsible for the positive effects. For example, the ratio of extracellular water to segmental water (ECW/SW) significantly improved in the Selenase group, correlating with selenium blood levels. This analysis was merely the first phase in mapping out the pathway by which selenium is beneficial; ongoing study is required.

The following table is a summary of the six selenium studies:

Study	Subjects	Dosage	Outcome
Kasseroller 2000	179 women with breast cancer–related lymphedema	• 1000 µg/d for week 1 • 300 µg/d for weeks 2 and 3 • 100–200 µg/d for 3 months	• *Volume:* –524 ml (Selenase) vs. –420 ml (placebo) • *Weight loss:* 1.5 kg (Selenase) vs. 1 kg (placebo) • Improved nighttime urination, vision, dry skin, mood, skin thickness, skin softness, heat sensitivity, erysipelas incidence
Micke 2003	12 patients with arm lymphedema, 36 with head/neck lymphedema	~500 µg/d orally for 4–6 weeks	• Improved lymphedema and QoL
Bruns 2004	36 patients with head/neck lymphedema	~500 µg/d orally for 4–6 weeks	• Improved lymphedema and QoL • Improved airway opening • Fewer tracheostomies
Zimmerman 2005	20 patients with squamous cell oral cancer	1,000 µg by IV or orally for 3 weeks	• More rapid reduction of lymphedema vs. placebo
Han 2019	26 women with breast cancer–related lymphedema	500 µg by IV 5 times over 2 weeks	• 10 out of 14 women taking selenium improved their lymphedema stage vs. 0 in the placebo group
Lee 2021	26 women with breast cancer–related lymphedema	500 µg by IV 5 times over 2 weeks	• Ratio of extracellular water to segmental water (ECW/SW) significantly improved in the Selenase group • ECW/SW correlated with selenium blood levels

µg = microgram; IV = intravenous, QoL = quality of life, "~" = approximately

Side Effects/Risks

Selenase was well tolerated, with no reported side effects. However, vitamin C supplements should not be taken with Selenase, as it can reduce their effectiveness (Kasseroller 2000). Symptoms of excessive selenium supplementation include hair loss and nail brittleness (NIH 2024).

AN IMPORTANT PRECAUTION

Most oncologists don't want their patients to take antioxidants during chemotherapy or radiation because the supplements could inadvertently repair the cancer cells the treatments are designed to damage. There is support for that concern, as a study of breast cancer patients showed that taking an antioxidant supplement before and during cancer treatment increased the risk of recurrence and death by 40% (Ambrosone 2020). Although this study didn't specifically mention selenium, it included vitamins C, A and E, carotenoids and coenzyme Q10, all antioxidants.

In the Zimmerman trial, selenium was taken on the day of cancer surgery and for three weeks thereafter. In most cases, this would not interfere with radiation or chemotherapy, as most oncologists leave at least three weeks for recovery from surgery before providing more treatment (and in many cases, chemo and/or radiation comes before surgery). But it's one more reason to discuss the potential use of selenium with your oncologist or other physician and consider all of the factors in your unique situation. You would not want your antioxidant supplement taken for lymphedema to limit the effectiveness of your cancer treatment.

Bottom Line on Selenium

The six trials on selenium and lymphedema to date all had positive results, but the research seems to be moving incredibly slowly, with only five small studies in twenty-five years, and it's unclear what effect dietary sources of selenium (or supplements other than Selenase) might have on lymphedema. A review published in 2016 concluded that further trials are needed to confirm the results and identify the best dosage and duration of treatment (Pfister 2016).

That said, selenium supplementation seems like a reasonable complementary addition to a lymphedema treatment plan. The brand used in most of the clinical trials was Selenase (sodium selenite pentahydrate), which was chosen intentionally as the selenium compound with the most efficient radical scavengers and a very low toxicity profile (Bruns 2004). If you are considering selenium supplementation, discuss with your physician whether you should have your serum and whole blood selenium levels checked before you begin supplementation, whether oral or IV is the right route for you, and what the best dosing regimen is. Do not exceed the recommended duration of supplementation by your doctor, as selenium toxicity is possible (NIH 2024).

References for Selenium

Ambrosone CB, Zirpoli GR, Hutson AD, et al. 2020. Dietary Supplement Use During Chemotherapy and Survival Outcomes of Patients with Breast Cancer Enrolled in a Cooperative Group Clinical Trial (SWOG S0221). *J Clin Oncol* 38 (8): 804–14.

Breast Cancer Survivorship Program. n.d. "Guide to Lymphedema," page 36. The M. Lau Breast Center, Princess Margaret Hospital, University Health Network. Accessed June 24, 2025. https://www.uhn.ca/PrincessMargaret/PatientsFamilies/Patient_Family_Library/Documents/guide_to_lymphedema.pdf.

Bruns F, Büntzel J, Mücke R, et al. 2004. Selenium in the Treatment of Head and Neck Lymphedema. *Med Princ Pract* 13 (4): 185–90.

Han HW, Yang EJ, Lee SM. 2019. Sodium Selenite Alleviates Breast Cancer-Related Lymphedema Independent of Antioxidant Defense System. *Nutrients* 11 (5): 1021.

Kasseroller RG, Schrauzer GN. 2000. Treatment of Secondary Lymphedema of the Arm with Physical Decongestive Therapy and Sodium Selenite: A Review. *Am J Ther* 7 (4): 273–79.

Lee H, Lee B, Kim Y, et al. 2021. Effects of Sodium Selenite Injection on Serum Metabolic Profiles in Women Diagnosed with Breast Cancer-Related Lymphedema—Secondary Analysis of a Randomized Placebo-Controlled Trial Using Global Metabolomics. *Nutrients* 13 (9): 3253.

Micke O, Bruns F, Mücke R, et al. 2003. Selenium in the Treatment of Radiation-Associated Secondary Lymphedema. *Int J Radiat Oncol Biol Phys* 56 (1): 40–49.

National Institutes of Health (NIH), Office of Dietary Supplements. 2024. "Selenium: Fact Sheet for Health Professionals." Accessed April 21, 2025. https://ods.od.nih.gov/factsheets/Selenium-HealthProfessional/.

Pfister C, Dawczynski H, Schingale FJ. 2016. Sodium Selenite and Cancer Related Lymphedema: Biological and Pharmacological Effects. *J Trace Elem Med Biol* 37 (September): 111–16.

University Health Network, Toronto. 2010. "The Use of Selenium to Treat Secondary Lymphedema—Breast Cancer." Accessed August 8, 2025. https://clinicaltrials.gov/study/NCT00188604?cond=lymphedema&intr=selenium&rank=1.

Zimmermann T, Leonhardt H, Kersting S, et al. 2005. Reduction of Postoperative Lymphedema After Oral Tumor Surgery with Sodium Selenite. *Biol Trace Elem Res* 106 (3): 193–203.

Serrapeptase

What Is It?

Serrapeptase (also called serratiopeptidase) is a proteolytic enzyme, meaning it breaks protein down into its smaller components, facilitating their removal from the body. This property is thought to contribute to its therapeutic effects of reducing inflammation and pain. It is produced by the bacterium *Serratia marcescens*, found in the intestines of *Bombyx mori* silk moths. The enzyme allows the moth to digest and absorb its cocoon.

Serratia was identified as an opportunistic human pathogen in 1959, but production strategies were developed to create a large-scale, safe supply of serrapeptase by creating a mutant strain via ultraviolet radiation and chemical changes (Nair 2022). It is now made by multiple manufacturers.

> **User Experience**
> "I have used serrapeptase for over a year, and it definitely helps with osteoarthritis swelling in my hand that swells due to lymphedema, as well as elbow pain caused by edema. I tried omitting this for two weeks and symptoms returned."
>
> **—Patti, Idaho (breast cancer–related lymphedema)**

Lymphedema-Specific Research

I was not able to locate human lymphedema research using serrapeptase, but found an animal study and related human research.

Lymphedema Research in Animals

In a 2008 study, either subacute or acute inflammation was induced in albino rats (Viswanatha Swamy 2008). To induce subacute inflammation, a sterile cotton pellet soaked in distilled water containing penicillin and streptomycin was implanted in the armpit of rats under anesthesia. After the trial period, the pellet was extracted and weighed to see how many granuloma cells attached to it. Acute inflammation was induced by injecting carrageenan into the hind paw.

The rats were given one of three enzymes—serrapeptase, chymotrypsin or trypsin—half an hour before inflammation induction and then every day for ten days. Saline was used for the control group. Each enzyme was tested at three different dosages, with and without aspirin, to see which would be the most effective anti-inflammatory. The best response to the acute inflammation came from serrapeptase. For the subacute inflammation, the best results came from serrapeptase and chymotrypsin, with or without aspirin. But the dosage was important. None of the enzymes worked at the lowest dosages.

Related Research

There have been a few human, animal and cell studies of serrapeptase. Outcomes relevant for lymphedema include serrapeptase's anti-inflammatory, antifibrotic and antibiotic actions.

ANTI-INFLAMMATORY ACTION

Serrapeptase was first used as an anti-inflammatory in Japan in 1957 (Jadhav 2020). In the normal pathway of inflammation after injury, cyclooxygenase is released to break down arachidonic acid, producing interleukins and prostaglandins, which are responsible for pain and inflammation. Serrapeptase has a high affinity for cyclooxygenase, binding to it and preventing the chain of events that allows pain and inflammation to develop (Nair 2022).

ANTIFIBROTIC ACTION

Lymphedema is both chronic and progressive. Over time, there is a buildup of fibrotic tissue and thickening of the skin, so an important treatment strategy is to delay—or ideally reverse—the progression of fibrosis and skin thickening. Serrapeptase is a known antifibrotic. Might it help?

An open-label pilot study looked at the use of enzymes for idiopathic pulmonary fibrosis (IPF), a progressive disease in which fibrin builds up in the lungs, causing lung tissue to thicken and become stiff, making breathing difficult (Shah 2021). Thirteen people with IPF took oral serrapeptase and nattokinase supplements three times a day as follows:

- **Days 1 to 4:** One Serracor-NK capsule, three times per day.
- **Days 5 to 8:** Two Serracor-NK capsules, three times per day.
- **Days 9 to 92:** Two Serracor-NK capsules, three times per day, plus one Serra Rx260 capsule three times per day (the "therapeutic dose").

The supplements were taken on an empty stomach (one hour before or two hours after a meal), with a cup of water. Because it was an open-label study, the participants knew what supplements they were taking, and there was no placebo or blinding.

After the treatment period, 62% of participants reported a significant improvement in well-being, 15% had no change, and 15% had a reduction in well-being. When it came to shortness of breath, 38% reported a significant improvement, 46% had a small improvement, and 15% reported worsening. In a questionnaire that measured respiratory symptoms, activity and impacts, 46% reported very effective improvement, 8% had moderate improvement, 15% saw slight improvement, and 31% reported a decline.

In describing the reason for the study, the author stated: "Since the factors involved in idiopathic pulmonary fibrosis include chronic inflammation, and uncontrolled healing response, and progressive fibrosis or scarring, treatment with the systemic enzymes serrapeptase and nattokinase is a rational approach." This synopsis makes me wonder if pulmonary fibrosis might be a reasonable stand-in for lymphedema fibrosis, and if serrapeptase would be a "rational approach" for lymphedema too.

Although not every patient improved, the author suggested that, for those who didn't, a longer period of supplementation might be needed, concluding: "The present study suggests that the oral enzyme supplements improve symptoms and the ability to perform activities, and well-being. Further randomized placebo-controlled trials with larger populations and for longer durations are warranted." A funding disclosure noted that the supplements used in the study were provided by AST Enzymes, from Chino, California.

ANTIBACTERIAL ACTION

If you've had cellulitis, you know how scary and uncomfortable it can be. Many people with lymphedema have repeated bouts of cellulitis and live in fear of the next attack. Can serrapeptase reduce infections or help antibiotics work more effectively?

Cellulitis is often caused by the bacteria *Streptococcus pyogenes* or, less frequently, *Staphylococcus aureus* (Burian 2024). As part of the infection process, the bacteria create biofilms to protect themselves. The biofilms can attach to biotic surfaces, like body tissue, or to abiotic surfaces, like a prosthetic device such as an artificial knee or hip. With the biofilms, the bacteria are resistant to your immune system's attacks and can even develop a tolerance to antibiotics given to treat your infection.

Just as serrapeptase helps a silkworm break out of its cocoon, it breaks up the bacteria's protective biofilms, allowing antibiotics to penetrate into the pathogenic bacteria. In a study of both methicillin-susceptible and methicillin-resistant *Staphylococcus aureus*, serrapeptase was effective in inhibiting the formation of biofilms (Jadhav 2020).

OTHER ACTIONS

Serrapeptase is also linked to wound healing, mucus reduction and prevention of clotting. I won't go into detail on these actions, as my focus is on using serrapeptase for lymphedema-related issues, but the sources in the references have more information if you're interested.

Side Effects/Risks

If you are taking blood thinners, such as aspirin, Plavix or Brilinta, speak with your health care provider before taking proteolytic enzymes, as the additional blood-thinning effect of serrapeptase may be too much for you (Shah 2021). For the same reason, you would need to stop serrapeptase two weeks before any surgery, to avoid excessive bleeding.

In the Shah study, the enzymes were introduced gradually to prevent "minor symptoms of intestinal cleansing" . . . so don't be too far from home if you are trying these for the first time. Starting with a lower dose and working up is likely prudent.

Bottom Line on Serrapeptase

Serrapeptase has several modes of action. The three that are relevant to lymphedema are its anti-inflammatory, antifibrotic and antibacterial effects. Currently, there are no human studies on its use in lymphedema, but animal and related research suggests that this supplement is promising, especially for people with chronic infections, fibrosis or inflammation. More research is needed to fully understand serrapeptase's efficacy and safety. If you are considering using it, speak with your health care provider first to determine if it is the right treatment for you.

References for Serrapeptase

Burian EA, Franks PJ, Borman P, et al. 2024. Factors Associated with Cellulitis in Lymphoedema of the Arm—An International Cross-Sectional Study (LIMPRINT). *BMC Infect Dis* 24 (1): 102.

Jadhav SB, Shah N, Rathi A, et al. 2020. Serratiopeptidase: Insights into the Therapeutic Applications. *Biotechnol Rep* (Amsterdam) 28 (October): e00544.

Nair SR, C SD. 2022. Serratiopeptidase: An Integrated View of Multifaceted Therapeutic Enzyme. *Biomolecules* 12 (10): 1468.

Shah N. 2021. Effects of Systemic Enzyme Supplements on Symptoms and Quality of Life in Patients with Pulmonary Fibrosis—A Pilot Study. *Medicines* (Basel) 8 (11): 68.

Viswanatha Swamy AH, Patil PA. 2008. Effect of Some Clinically Used Proteolytic Enzymes on Inflammation in Rats. *Indian J Pharm Sci* 70 (1): 114–17.

Sulfuretin

What Is It?

Sulfuretin is a naturally occurring flavonoid (see Benzopyrenes, page 122) and is one of the main active ingredients found in Chinese lacquer tree (*Toxicodendron verniciflumm*, formerly *Rhus verniciflua*), which grows in and around China, Japan, Korea and India. It is also called Japanese lacquer tree, Japanese sumac and varnish tree. It produces a sap that gives a glossy and durable finish to dishes, musical instruments, jewelry and other consumer goods. Sulfuretin is used in nutritional supplements for its anti-inflammatory, antifibrotic and antioxidant activity (Roh 2017). It is produced by several manufacturers.

Lymphedema-Specific Research

I was unable to locate any human studies using sulfuretin to treat lymphedema.

Lymphedema Research in Animals

To date, there is one animal study of sulfuretin for lymphedema, which tested the supplement to see if it could prevent lymphedema from developing after it was surgically induced in mice (Roh 2017). This was a unique protocol, as most studies of natural health products are tested as treatments for existing lymphedema, not as preventatives. The group treated with sulfuretin did indeed exhibit a reduction in lymphedema formation.

Side Effects/Risks

None noted.

Bottom Line on Sulfuretin

Sulfuretin has been tested only in mice and therefore cannot yet be recommended as a treatment for humans with lymphedema. It offers interesting potential as a preventive, which suggests a basis for studies to see if it can help prevent postsurgical lymphedema.

References for Sulfuretin

Roh K, Kim S, Kang H, et al. 2017. Sulfuretin Has Therapeutic Activity Against Acquired Lymphedema by Reducing Adipogenesis. *Pharmacol Res* 121 (July): 230–39.

Synbiotics

What Are They?

Synbiotics are a combination of probiotics (live beneficial bacteria) and prebiotics (fermentable fibers). Probiotics are live microorganisms that, when eaten in a large enough quantity, provide a health benefit (FAO/WHO 2002). When you search for a list of probiotics, you are often given a list of fermented foods, but while all probiotics are made from fermented foods, not all fermented foods contain probiotics. Some food processes, such as heating or pasteurizing, destroy the live microorganisms; some bacteria do not survive in a high enough quantity by the food's expiry date; some do not survive stomach acid; and some don't reach the intestines in a large enough number to provide a health benefit. Unfortunately, there aren't good labeling laws to tell us which fermented foods contain probiotics, but the most reliable source is yogurt labeled "probiotic."

Prebiotics are fibers that healthy microbiota can ferment, providing nourishment for the beneficial bacteria so they can thrive. Prebiotic fibers are found in a variety of foods, including asparagus, onions and wheat bran. While all prebiotics are fibers, not all fibers are prebiotic. There are five criteria that determine whether a fiber is a prebiotic (Markowiak 2017):

1. It can withstand food processing.
2. It resists full digestion in the upper gastrointestinal tract.
3. It reaches the colon, where it is fermented by beneficial bacteria.
4. The fermentation results in an improvement in the host's immune function.
5. Beneficial intestinal bacteria grow or increase their activity.

While probiotics and prebiotics have both food and supplement sources, "synbiotics" generally refers to supplements and not a combination of pre- and probiotic foods, such as yogurt and bananas. As the name implies, the pre- and probiotics in a synbiotic have a symbiotic relationship: The benefits of the combination are greater than the sum of the benefits of the individual components. Synbiotics are made by multiple manufacturers, with various types and quantities of prebiotics and probiotics.

> **Technical Breakdown**
> On a supplement label, you may see prebiotic fibers listed as fructooligosaccharides, galactooligosaccharides, or xylooligosaccharides. While these long, difficult-to-pronounce chemical names might seem scary, they all occur naturally in food such as bananas, onions, milk, and corncobs. Another popular prebiotic supplement is inulin, which is made from chicory root.

Lymphedema-Specific Research

A group of researchers in Iran published four studies on lymphedema and synbiotic supplements.

Study #1: Vafa, Haghighat, et al. 2020

Eighty-eight women with breast cancer–related lymphedema in one arm were put on a low-calorie diet to promote weight loss. Half took a placebo, and the other half took a synbiotic supplement for ten weeks. The researchers measured and compared their starting and ending body weight, percentage of body fat and waist circumference, as well as blood levels of:

- **TNF-alpha:** A pro-inflammatory protein.
- **Leptin:** A "hunger hormone" made by fat cells and intestinal cells. Elevated leptin can increase TNF-alpha and edema. As you lose fat, leptin levels reduce, which can stimulate an increase in appetite.
- **Interleukin-1beta:** A pro-inflammatory protein.
- **High-sensitivity C-reactive protein (hs-CRP):** An indicator of inflammation.

As shown in the table below, after ten weeks, the synbiotic group had a significant reduction in TNF-alpha and leptin compared to the control group. Lymphedema volume was also significantly reduced compared to baseline in the synbiotic group, but not in the control group. There were no significant differences between the groups in body weight, body fat percentage, waist circumference, interleukin-1beta or hs-CRP.

Measure	Synbiotic Group	Control Group
Body weight	–3.1%*	–2.2%*
Body fat %	–2.6%*	–1.9%*
Waist circumference	–3.7%*	–3.7%*
TNF-alpha	–5.6%**	+5.3%
Leptin	–25.6%**	–20.5%
Interleukin-1beta	–8.4%*	–5.0%*
High-sensitivity C-reactive protein	–3.1%	–2.7%
Lymphedema	–37%*	–21%

* Statistically significant compared to baseline
** Statistically significant between the two groups

The synbiotic supplement used in this study was LactoCare, manufactured by Zist Takhmir in Iran. Its components are 10^9 CFUs (colony-forming units) of *Lactobacillus acidophilus*, *Lactobacillus rhamnosus*, *Lactobacillus bulgaricus*, *Bifidobacterium breve*, *Bifidobacterium longum* and *Streptococcus thermophiles*, and 38.5 milligrams of fructooligosaccharides. The study showed that adding this supplement to a low-calorie diet reduced inflammation and lymphedema more than the diet alone.

STUDY #2: VAFA, ZARRATI, ET AL. 2020

This study included the same eighty-eight women as study #1, plus forty-five age-matched controls. The participants completed Lymphedema Life Impact Scale (LIIS) questionnaires. There was a significant difference in LIIS scores between the diet + synbiotic group and the diet-only group compared to the age-matched controls, indicating that the low-calorie diet improved quality of life. When comparing the two diet groups—the women who received the synbiotic versus the placebo—quality of life scores were better in the synbiotic group, but not significantly. The researchers concluded that a low-calorie diet + synbiotics improved quality of life more than the diet alone, but not in a statistically significant way, and that adding a dietitian consultation to lymphedema management may provide superior results.

STUDY #3: NAVAEI 2020

In this study, the same eighty-eight women had their oxidative markers measured and compared at the beginning and end of the ten weeks to see if antioxidant capacity improved with the synbiotic supplement. Specifically, the researchers measured malondialdehyde, superoxide dismutase, glutathione peroxidase and total antioxidant capacity.

Malondialdehyde, a reactive oxygen species, indicates the presence of oxidative stress. At the end of the study period, malondialdehyde levels were lower for those on the synbiotic supplement than for the placebo group. Superoxide dismutase, an antioxidant that combats oxidative stress, was significantly elevated compared to baseline in the supplement group, and not significantly different compared to baseline in the placebo group—another positive result of the synbiotic. Levels of glutathione peroxidase, another protective enzyme, did not change significantly in either group. Total antioxidant capacity was significantly increased compared to baseline in both groups; this improvement was attributed to the diet that all the women were on.

Overall, it appears that a synbiotic supplement added to a low-calorie diet benefits antioxidant capacity more than the diet alone, but more research of this nature is needed.

STUDY #4: SANEEI TOTMAJ 2022

Like study #1, this one looked at inflammatory markers in the same eighty-eight subjects, but it focused on different blood measures: interleukin-10 (IL-10), an anti-inflammatory messenger; transforming growth factor beta (TGF-β), a measure of inflammation; vascular endothelial growth factor (VEGF), which promotes the growth of new lymph and blood vessels; and adiponectin, a hormone that was shown in mice to reduce lymphedema.

At the end of the study period, IL-10 and VEGF were reduced in the placebo group but not in the synbiotic group. These were seen as positive results for the synbiotic group, as IL-10 is anti-inflammatory and the growth of new lymph vessels (promoted by VEGF) is considered a positive outcome in this context. TGF-β and adiponectin both increased compared to baseline in the synbiotic group, but were not significantly different between the two groups after ten weeks.

The researchers concluded that "synbiotic supplementation can be effective in improving health status in breast cancer lymphedema patients."

Side Effects/Risks

There were no side effects reported in these studies, but probiotics have potential side effects of diarrhea, gas and upset stomach. They are generally not recommended when you are immunocompromised, such as during chemotherapy treatment, or if you have a damaged heart valve (Cleveland Clinic 2022). If you cannot take probiotics for these or other reasons, you can take a prebiotic instead of a synbiotic, or avoid supplements and rely on pre- and probiotic foods in your diet.

Bottom Line on Synbiotics

Four studies published by the same research team in Iran focused on eighty-eight overweight women with breast cancer–related lymphedema. The women who took a synbiotic supplement showed improvements in some inflammatory markers, leptin, antioxidants and lymphedema volume compared to placebo. This is promising, but one thing to consider is that people from different parts of the world have different microbiota, so it would be great if this research were repeated in North America to see if the results can be reproduced, and with what formulation. If you decide to try a synbiotic supplement, choose a formulation similar to the one used in these studies, which included six different probiotic species along with prebiotic fiber.

It is unclear what effect a diet high in pre- and probiotics might have on lymphedema. If you prefer to get them from diet, choose foods with active bacteria, such as yogurt and kefir, along with plenty of fruits, vegetables, whole grains, herbs and spices. Read more about nutrition for lymphedema in *The Complete Lymphedema Management and Nutrition Guide*.

References for Synbiotics

Cleveland Clinic. 2022. "Acidophilus." Accessed September 22, 2025. https://my.clevelandclinic.org/health/drugs/22650-acidophilus.

Food and Agriculture Organization of the United Nations and World Health Organization (FAO/WHO). 2002. "Guidelines for the Evaluation of Probiotics in Food: Report of a Joint FAO/WHO Working Group on Drafting Guidelines for the Evaluation of Probiotics in Food." London, Ontario, Canada, April 30 and May 1. Accessed July 30, 2025. https://isappscience.org/wp-content/uploads/2019/04/probiotic_guidelines.pdf.

Markowiak P, Śliżewska K. 2017. Effects of Probiotics, Prebiotics, and Synbiotics on Human Health. *Nutrients* 9 (9): 1021.

Navaei M, Haghighat S, Janani L, et al. 2020. The Effects of Synbiotic Supplementation on Antioxidant Capacity and Arm Volumes in Survivors of Breast Cancer-Related Lymphedema. *Nutr Cancer* 72 (1): 62–73.

Saneei Totmaj A, Haghighat S, Jaberzadeh S, et al. 2022. The Effects of Synbiotic Supplementation on Serum Anti-Inflammatory Factors in the Survivors of Breast Cancer with Lymphedema following a Low Calorie Diet: A Randomized, Double-Blind, Clinical Trial. *Nutr Cancer* 74 (3): 869–81.

Vafa S, Haghighat S, Janani L, et al. 2020. The Effects of Synbiotic Supplementation on Serum Inflammatory Markers and Edema Volume in Breast Cancer Survivors with Lymphedema. *EXCLI J* 19 (January): 1–15.

Vafa S, Zarrati M, Malakootinejad M, et al. 2020. Calorie Restriction and Synbiotics Effect on Quality of Life and Edema Reduction in Breast Cancer-Related Lymphedema, a Clinical Trial. *Breast* 54 (December): 37–45.

Unguentum Lymphaticum

What Is It?

Unguentum Lymphaticum is an ointment created by a German pharmaceutical company. At the time of publication, their website had gone offline, and it is unclear whether this product is still being made. Nevertheless, I'm including it in case it becomes available again in the future.

The ingredients in Unguentum Lymphaticum are digitalis, calendulin, hyoscyamine, colchicine and podophyllin. According to the company's former website, it is used for vascular disease and acute and chronic painful alterations of the blood and lymph vessels, including lymph nodes and vascular spasms. It works by activating macrophages, accelerating lymph flow and stimulating the immune cells in the skin.

Lymphedema-Specific Research

In a Polish study on thirty-three patients with leg lymphedema, Unguentum Lymphaticum was applied to the entire skin area of the foot and calf, rubbed for five minutes, then wrapped in gauze soaked in more of the ointment (Olszewski 2002). This was done every day for one week, three weeks or twelve weeks, with a different number of sessions depending on group assignment.

Participants reported a sensation of skin warming while receiving the treatment. After three weeks, several patients noted skin softening and a reduction in the time it took for pitting to refill and be indistinguishable. Skin biopsies revealed stimulation of keratinocytes and immune cells, leading the authors to conclude that the product is useful in chronic lymphedema with inflammation.

It's important to note that patients with hyperkeratosis were excluded from the study. Also, many of the outcomes were microscopic findings. For example, there was an increase in the density of macrophages ("big eater" immune cells), which would typically be considered an inflammatory response. So it is difficult to interpret what exactly caused the clinical improvements the researchers observed.

This paper cited two older studies of Unguentum Lymphaticum for lymphedema. I could not access them, but they are included in the references below (Casley-Smith 1983 and Cluzan 1996).

Side Effects/Risks

No side effects were reported other than temporary redness of the skin. There are no known drug interactions. Unguentum Lymphaticum is contraindicated for people with multiple sclerosis or who are allergic to the preservative methyl 4-hydroxybenzoate.

Bottom Line on Unguentum Lymphaticum

The decades-old research on this ointment appears promising, but more current studies would be reassuring, and it is unclear whether this product is still available.

References for Unguentum Lymphaticum

Casley-Smith JR. 1983. Electron Microscopy of the Effects of Unguentum Lymphaticum on Acute Experimental Lymphedema and Various High-Protein Edemas. *Lymphology* 16 (4): 233–42.

Cluzan R, Pecking A, von Keudell CH, et al. 1996. "Randomized Double Blind Placebo-Controlled Prospective Clinical Trial Documenting the Therapeutic Efficacy of Unguentum Lymphaticum on Patients with Secondary Arm Lymphedema After Mastectomy by Lymphoscintigraphy with 99mtc Marked Rhenium Sulphur Colloid." (Abstract.) European Group Lymphology, Rome.

Olszewski WL, Kubicka U. 2002. The Effects of Unguentum Lymphaticum on Skin in Patients with Obstructive Lymphedema of the Lower Extremities. *Lymphology* 35 (4): 171–81.

Vitamin D

What Is It?

Vitamin D, also known as the sunshine vitamin, is a fat-soluble vitamin that can be made in the skin after exposure to UVB radiation, which converts the skin's pre-vitamin D_3 to vitamin D_3.

The season, the time of day, cloud cover, smog, skin melanin content, skin color, sunscreen and age affect the amount of vitamin D you can form from sunshine. It's also worth noting that UVB light does not penetrate glass, so you can't absorb it through a window. The recommended amount of sun exposure for forming vitamin D from UVB rays is five to thirty minutes between 10:00 a.m. and 4:00 p.m., two to seven days per week, to the face, arms, hands and legs, without sunscreen (NIH 2022).

Vitamin D is also available in food sources such as fatty fish (trout, salmon, tuna, mackerel), fish liver oils, beef liver, egg yolks and cheese. Mushrooms exposed to UVB light can also be sources of vitamin D. The recommended daily intake is 15 micrograms (600 IU) for adults up to age seventy, and 20 micrograms (800 IU) for adults over seventy (NIH 2022). Supplements can be in the form of D_2 (ergocalciferol) or D_3 (cholecalciferol), with D_3 being more effective at increasing blood vitamin D levels than D_2 (NIH 2025).

Lymphedema-Specific Research

I located three human observational studies looking for a correlation between vitamin D blood levels and lymphedema, as well as one animal clinical trial exploring that relationship.

STUDY #1: ÖZGAN 2019

This case-control study, conducted in Turkey, included eighty women with breast cancer–related lymphedema and eighty healthy controls. Blood tests for 25-hydroxyvitamin D_3, calcium, phosphorus, alkaline phosphatase and parathormone levels were compared. The test for 25-hydroxyvitamin D_3 is a good one to measure overall vitamin D status and is used to detect deficiencies of vitamin D. Blood tests were done only in summer or autumn, to control for seasonal variations. A comparison between the two groups revealed that the women with lymphedema had lower vitamin D blood levels than age-matched healthy controls.

For this study, "normal vitamin D" was defined as more than 29 nanograms per milliliter (ng/ml), "insufficient vitamin D" was 20–29 ng/ml, and "vitamin D deficiency" was less than 20 ng/ml. Of those with lymphedema, 15% had normal vitamin D, 60% had insufficient vitamin D, and 25% had vitamin D deficiency (in other words, 85% were below normal). In the control group, 21% of the women had normal vitamin D, 41% had insufficient vitamin D, and 38% had vitamin D deficiency (79% were below normal). Vitamin D levels were significantly lower in cases of stage 3 lymphedema compared to stage 1, as well as in older women, those who had cancer for longer and those with more severe cancer.

STUDY #2: DORUK ANALAN 2020

The goal of this study was to evaluate blood levels of vitamin D (25-hydroxyvitamin D_3) in relation to the presence and severity of lymphedema, pain, disability and function after treatment for breast cancer. Seventy-one women were included, of whom thirty-seven had lymphedema and thirty-four served as controls. The study found no correlation between vitamin D blood levels and the presence of lymphedema or the levels of pain, disability or physical functioning. The authors did note that most of the women with lymphedema in this study had only low-grade lymphedema, which may have affected the results. No mention was made of the time of year that the blood draw took place.

STUDY #3: KARAKILIÇ 2025

A third study, also done in Turkey, included 603 women, with 201 from each of three cohorts: those with breast cancer–related lymphedema, those with breast cancer but no lymphedema and age-matched healthy controls. The researchers performed a chart audit to access blood tests of 25-hydroxyvitamin D_3. Only blood tests done in June, July or August were retrieved. As shown in the table that follows, a cohort comparison revealed significantly reduced vitamin D levels in women with lymphedema compared to both breast cancer survivors without lymphedema and healthy controls, with the healthy controls having the highest vitamin D levels. There was also a strong negative correlation between vitamin D level and lymphedema stage, meaning the lower the vitamin D level, the worse the lymphedema.

Vitamin D	Breast Cancer + Lymphedema	Breast Cancer Only	Healthy Controls
Normal	1.5%	7%	26%
Insufficient	3%	21%	29%
Deficient	95.5%	72%	44%

Lymphedema Research in Animals

Forty-five Sprague-Dawley rats had surgery to remove a popliteal lymph node and an inguinal fat pad containing an inguinal lymph node, and to dissect the main lymphatic duct from the neurovascular bundle (Aksöyler 2024). One week later, the researchers applied a single dose of radiation therapy (20 Gy) to the surgical region. The rats were randomly assigned to receive either no supplement (the control group), both pre- and postoperative calcitriol—the active form of vitamin D (1,25-dihydroxy vitamin D_3)—or only postoperative calcitriol.

Following the treatment, the study authors used micro-computed tomography to calculate limb volume and fluorescence lymphatic imaging to detect lymphedema. The control group had a 75% lymphedema incidence rate, while both calcitriol groups had only a 25% incidence. The calcitriol groups also had an increase in M2 macrophages and newly formed lymphatic vessels, while the control group had elevated M1 macrophages and collagen. M1 macrophages promote inflammation and tissue damage, while M2 macrophages have anti-inflammatory effects.

Side Effects/Risks

No side effects were noted, but the human research was correlation studies, not clinical trials. Side effects of excess vitamin D intake include nausea, vomiting, muscle weakness, confusion, pain, loss of appetite, dehydration, excessive urination, thirst and kidney stones (NIH 2022). The upper level for vitamin D intake from both food and supplements together is 100 micrograms (4,000 IU) per day.

Bottom Line on Vitamin D

Two out of three human correlation studies found a relationship between vitamin D insufficiency or deficiency and the presence of lymphedema in breast cancer survivors. The third study included patients with less severe lymphedema and may not have controlled for the month that the blood testing was done. These findings do not prove that low vitamin D causes lymphedema, or that vitamin D can be used as a treatment for lymphedema, only that there is an association, or correlation, between low vitamin D and lymphedema. The mechanism of action that has been suggested to explain the relationship is that vitamin D suppresses pro-inflammatory cytokines and can reduce chronic inflammation (Karakiliç 2025).

The animal study provides proof of concept that vitamin D in the form of calcitriol supplementation may reduce lymphedema development in surgery and radiation recipients, which may be of particular interest as a risk reduction strategy for oncology patients.

Assessing vitamin D blood levels and advising patients on vitamin D supplementation and/or dietary sources is already a common practice for registered dietitians and physicians. If additional research confirms a relationship between vitamin D and lymphedema, vitamin D supplementation may become standard practice for all at-risk individuals. Vitamin D supplementation is easy, low-cost, low-risk and accessible, so get your vitamin D blood levels checked and, if they're low, start trying to boost them with supplements and/or dietary sources. Consult a registered dietitian if you have questions. Health Canada currently recommends that all Canadians over the age of two supplement with 10 micrograms (400 IU) of vitamin D every day, in addition to dietary sources (Health Canada 2022).

Further research would be most welcome to confirm the impact of this simple, cost-effective and accessible intervention on lymphedema risk and management.

References for Vitamin D

Aksöyler D, Kozanoğlu E, Korkut M, et al. Evaluation of the Effectiveness of Active Vitamin D Use in Experimental Rat Lymphedema Model. Medicina (Kaunas). 2024 Nov 1;60(11):1788.

Doruk Analan P, Kaya E. The Effect of Serum 25(OH)D3 Level on Breast Cancer-Related Lymphedema. Lymphat Res Biol. 2020 Feb;18(1):22-26.

Health Canada. Vitamin D. Last updated May 2, 2022. Accessed Sept 5, 2025 https://www.canada.ca/en/health-canada/services/nutrients/vitamin-d.html

Karakilic GD, Selcuk MA. The Effect of Vitamin D Levels on Breast Cancer-Related Lymphedema. Lymphology. 2025;58(2):56-65.

NIH. Vitamin D. Last updated Nov 8, 2022. Accessed Sept 4, 2025. https://ods.od.nih.gov/factsheets/VitaminD-Consumer/#:~:text=of%20COVID%2D19.-,What%20is%20vitamin%20D%20and%20what%20does%20it%20do?,off%20invading%20bacteria%20and%20viruses.

NIH. Vitamin D Fact Sheet for Health Professionals. Last updated June 27, 2025. Accessed Sept 4, 2025. https://ods.od.nih.gov/factsheets/VitaminD-HealthProfessional/

Özcan DS, Dalyan M, Ergül S, et al. Evaluation of Vitamin D Levels in Patients with Breast Cancer-related Lymphedema: An Observational Cross-sectional Study. Turk J Osteoporos. 2019 Dec 12;25(3):105-110

Wobenzym N

What Is It?

Wobenzym N is a supplement containing five different enzymes—pancreatin, papain, bromelain, trypsin and chymotrypsin—and the flavonoid rutin. It is made by Mucos Pharma in Germany and distributed by Douglas Laboratories in the US. The manufacturer's website says it "can accelerate the healing of inflammatory injuries and diseases such as activated osteoarthritis, phlebitis or swelling after injury" (Mucos Pharma, n.d.). The distributor's brochure states that Wobenzym N "promotes lymphatic drainage" and "supports healthy tissue fluid levels" (Douglas Labs 2017). There are two additional Wobenzym formulations, Wobenzym Plus and Wobenzym PS, but according to the brochure, only Wobenzym N is used for lymphatic health. Older research on this supplement simply uses the name Wobenzym.

Lymphedema-Specific Research

There is very little published in English on Wobenzym for lymphedema. One German study with an English abstract included fifty-five women with arm lymphedema, who received "manual machine lymph drainage" (I'm not exactly sure what that is), exercised and took either a diuretic or Wobenzym (Korpan 1996). After seven weeks, arm volume, skinfold thickness and arm circumference were all significantly improved in the Wobenzym group compared to the diuretic group. In addition, more patients taking Wobenzym reported improvements in pain than those taking diuretics.

Technical Breakdown

I asked AI why manufacturers don't conduct more research on their natural health products. Its answer seemed logical: Clinical research is very expensive, and if a product is already selling well, the return on investment may not justify the cost. By contrast, pharmaceutical companies must provide research and get approval from a national health agency before their drug is made available to patients and prescribers.

Related Research

In a double-blind, placebo-controlled trial, 150 adults with knee osteoarthritis were randomly assigned to Wobenzym (52 patients), 150 milligrams of the non-steroidal anti-inflammatory drug diclofenac (46 patients) or a placebo (52 patients) for twelve weeks (Bolten 2015). The dosage of Wobenzym was two tablets, three times per day. In addition, if the pain became unbearable, patients were allowed to take 500 milligrams of paracetamol (acetaminophen) and record how often it was required.

Pain scores improved with both Wobenzym and diclofenac compared to placebo; the median scores for reduction of pain were −33% and −28% respectively. All three groups, including the placebo group, reported improvements in knee joint stiffness. Those on Wobenzym required, on average, only a half tablet of the rescue medication paracetamol over twelve weeks, while the placebo users took an average of ten paracetamol tablets over twelve weeks.

The authors divulged their conflict as employees of the manufacturer, but noted that theirs was the first placebo-controlled trial of Wobenzym. They concluded that Wobenzym may be as effective as diclofenac in relieving pain and increasing function in adults with moderate to severe osteoarthritis of the knee, although they admitted that further study is needed, including trials lasting longer than twelve weeks.

Side Effects/Risks

Wobenzym's safety profile appears to be good, with limited side effects. The Bolten study did report that sixteen people dropped out due to adverse reactions, but did not specify which treatment group they were in or what the reactions were; they later stated that the adverse event profile of Wobenzym was similar to that of placebo.

Bottom Line on Wobenzym N

Wobenzym N may have similar mechanisms of action as serrapeptase, but whereas serrapeptase is a single enzyme, Wobenzym N combines five different ones. A thirty-year-old study on Wobenzym for lymphedema yielded positive results; sadly, research in this area does not seem to have continued. Wobenzym was also tested in a placebo-controlled trial of knee osteoarthritis, with a good outcome on pain reduction over twelve weeks.

With only one study available, it's difficult to get too excited about this product for lymphedema treatment, but the fact that it has been on the market for over fifty years suggests a long track record of safety and efficacy. Its use as an anti-inflammatory and for relief of joint pain are certainly relevant for some lymphedema patients.

References for Wobenzym N

Bolten WW, Glade MJ, Raum S, Ritz BW. 2015. The Safety and Efficacy of an Enzyme Combination in Managing Knee Osteoarthritis Pain in Adults: A Randomized, Double-Blind, Placebo-Controlled Trial. *Arthritis* 2015: 251521.

Douglas Laboratories. 2017. "Clinically Researched Wobenzym®." Accessed June 26, 2025. https://www.douglaslabs.com/media/DL_Wobenzym_Brochure.pdf.

Korpan MI, Fialka V. 1996. Wobezyme and Diuretic Therapy in Lymphedema After Breast Operation. [In German.] *Wien. Med Wochenschr* 146 (4): 67–72; discussion 74.

Mucos Pharma. n.d. "Wobenzym®." Accessed June 26, 2025. https://www.wobenzym.de/arzneimittel/wobenzym.

Natural Health Products Summary

This is a very broad category, including enzymes, herbs, spices, traditional Chinese medicines, minerals, fatty acids, vitamins and synbiotics. There appears to be growing interest in natural health products, so hopefully new human trials will pick up where past research left off, as several of these supplements seem promising.

Some of the existing trials had quite long study periods—six months for Daflon 500; one year plus an additional one-year follow-up for coumarin. While it's great to know the long-term effects of a product, the extended study periods may hint at a need to be patient when taking these supplements and expect a slow, gradual improvement (still, better than a slow worsening).

In the tables that follow, the statement "None noted" in the Side Effects/Risks column does not necessarily mean there are no concerns related to the supplement—just that no adverse reactions were reported in the research I've reviewed. Before trying any natural health product, talk to your pharmacist about contraindications and interactions with the medications you are taking.

Therapy	What It Is	Claims	Lymphedema Research	Results	Side Effects/Risks
Astragalus + peony	Edible medicinal plants	Mimics the drug Ubenimex; anti-inflammatory, antifibrotic	One pilot study of 9 women post–breast cancer	Reduced water displacement in 4, stable in 2 and increased in 2; less heaviness, congestion and tingling; improved comfort and QoL	None noted
Benzopyrones	A class of naturally occurring chemicals	Reduces the permeability of blood vessels	One meta-analysis of 15 studies	Further research is needed; caution is required	Liver damage
Coumarin	A benzo-pyrone from tonka beans and cassia cinnamon	Stimulates lymphatic function, reduces inflammation and edema	Eight studies, and two reviews, with a total of 651+ participants	Improved volume (up to 100%), cellulitis, skin softness, skin temperature, pain, hardness, mobility and heaviness	Liver toxicity
Cyclo 3 Fort	A supplement with butcher's broom, hesperidin methyl chalcone and vitamin C	Increases venous motility, decreases microvessel permeability, reduces edema	One study of 57 women post–breast cancer	Reduced lymphedema volume (up to 23%)	Nausea and abdominal pain
Daflon 500	A supplement with diosmin and hesperidin	Stimulates lymphagogue and lymphokinetic activity	Two studies of 10 and 94 women post–breast cancer and one study of 26 people with filarial lymphedema	Improved limb volume (up to 64%), arm heaviness and lymphatic migration speed	GI symptoms, "miscellaneous disorders"
Escin	A component of horse chestnut	Anti-inflammatory, anti-edema, venotonic	One study of 68 women post–breast cancer and one animal study	No improvement in human study; reduced swelling and increased lymph vessel growth in rats	Dizziness, metastatic disease
Garlive	A supplement with hydroxy-tyrosol, hesperidin, spermidine and vitamin A	Anti-inflammatory, antioxidant, boosts the innate immune system	One animal study	Rapid swelling to day 5, peak volume at day 6 or 7, then a gradual decline and reduced swelling overall	Stomach distention of mice on a single dose per day

QoL = quality of life; GI = gastrointestinal

Therapy	What It Is	Claims	Lymphedema Research	Results	Side Effects/ Risks
Ginger	The rhizome of *Zingiber officinale Roscoe*	Anti-inflammatory	None	n/a	Heartburn
Ginkor Fort	A supplement with gingko biloba, troxerutin and heptaminol	Strengthens veins, increases vessel resistance and reduces permeability	One study of 48 women post–breast cancer	Two pills per day improved limb volume (by 1%) heaviness, tightness lymphatic stasis, migration speed and drainage	None noted
Goreisan	A traditional Japanese herbal blend	Mild diuretic	One study of 19 woman post–gynecological cancer	Improved weight loss, extracellular water and lymphedema volume	Rash and itching
Homeopathy	A dilution of a plant, animal or mineral substance	*Apocynum cannabinum* reduces edema	One human case study using *Apocynum cannabinum* + diuretic	Lymphedema improved, but unclear whether homeopathy or diuretic was responsible	Harm of omission, low risk of allergic reaction
Hwanggigye-jiomul-tang	A blend of astragalus, cinnamon and ginger	Anti-inflammatory, analgesic	One systematic review and meta-analysis of eleven randomized controlled trials	Improved upper arm circumference, edema, shoulder range of motion, Fugl-Meyer assessment and visual analog scales	None noted
Hydroxytyrosol	An olive extract	Anti-inflammatory, antioxidant, antimicrobial	Case studies of 9 people with morbid obesity, pruritus and lymphedema	Olivamine-based skin care products improved pruritus	None noted
Linba Fang	A mixture of two traditional Chinese herbal medicines	Anti-inflammatory, antifibrotic	One animal study	Improved lymphedema	None noted
Linfadren	Micronized diosmin with dried extracts of melilotus (20% coumarin) and bearberry (10% arbutin)	Improves microcirculation and fluid drainage	One study of 50 women post–breast cancer	CDT + Linfadren improved volume (up to 74%) after 6 weeks of treatment and 3 months later	None noted, but risk of liver toxicity at high doses

n/a = not applicable; CDT = complete decongestive therapy

Therapy	What It Is	Claims	Lymphedema Research	Results	Side Effects/Risks
Meliven 3	A supplement with melilotus (20% coumarin), rutin and bromelain	Improves microcirculation and venous circulation	One study of 50 women and 2 men with primary or secondary lymphedema	Slight to no volume reduction; decreased skin thickness and functional improvements	Believed ineffective for stage 3 or higher
Omega-3 fatty acids	EPA, DHA and ALA	Anti-inflammatory	None	n/a	Increased bleeding and atrial fibrillation
Procurcuma	A supplement with dry turmeric extract, turmeric rhizome powder and piperine	Antioxidant, anti-inflammatory	One study on Procurcuma + Meliven for 41 people with leg lymphedema	Improved lymphedema as part of a multimodal 6-day treatment	Contraindicated with impaired liver function, biliary tract stones
Pycnogenol	An extract from the bark of the French maritime pine tree	Antioxidant, anti-inflammatory	None	Reduced edema during air travel in people without lymphedema	None noted
Robuvit	A powder made from French oak wood	Antioxidant, anti-inflammatory, increases mitochondrial renewal	Three studies on various lymphedemas with a total of 164 participants	Reduced limb volume (up to 19.8%), skin thickness and fungal skin infections	None noted
Selenium	An essential mineral	Antioxidant, anti-inflammatory, unclogs lymphatic capillaries	Six studies of cancer survivors with a total of 309 participants (five studies specified Selenase)	Improved lymph volume, weight loss, nighttime urination, vision, dry skin, mood, skin thickness, heat sensitivity, infections and blood antioxidant levels, and fewer tracheostomies	None noted
Serrapeptase	A proteolytic enzyme from the GI tract of silkworms	Anti-inflammatory, antifibrotic, antibiotic	One animal study	Reduced inflammation	Blood thinning, minor GI symptoms
Sulfuretin	An extract from the Chinese lacquer tree	Anti-inflammatory, antifibrotic, antioxidant	One animal study	Prevented lymphedema from developing after surgery	None noted
Synbiotics	A combination of prebiotics and probiotics	Restores gut health, anti-inflammatory	Four studies on the same group of 88 breast cancer survivors	Improved lymphedema (37%), inflammation and antioxidant levels	Diarrhea, gas, upset stomach

n/a = not applicable; GI = gastrointestinal

Therapy	What It Is	Claims	Lymphedema Research	Results	Side Effects/Risks
Unguentum Lymphaticum	An ointment containing digitalis, calendulin, hyoscyamine, colchicine and podophyllin	Accelerates lymph flow, stimulates immune cells in the skin	One study of 33 people with leg lymphedema	Skin softening, improved pitting refill	Temporary redness
Vitamin D	A fat-soluble vitamin	Anti-inflammatory	Three human observational studies and one animal clinical trial	Two observational studies found an association between vitamin D and lymphedema	Excess associated with nausea/vomiting and other symptoms
Wobezym N	A supplement with 5 enzymes and rutin	Promotes lymphatic drainage	One study of 55 women with arm lymphedema	Improved arm circumference, volume, skin fold thickness and pain	None noted

Part Four
High-Tech Devices

Introduction to High-Tech Devices

My definition of "high tech" is pretty simple: If you have to plug it in or it requires batteries, it's included here. There is quite an array of devices, but I'll do my best to explain how each one works and what makes it unique. As a reminder, inclusion in this book does not mean I endorse a product. As usual, I will focus on the published evidence as it relates to lymphedema; where that is not available, I will share evidence from related areas of study.

One thing to keep in mind is that technology changes quickly. Models, features and designs are ever-evolving—the polar opposite of the traditional medicines. For that reason, I've included only the most recent research where there are multiple studies. Since it can be challenging to stay up-to-date on the latest version of a technology, seek out advice from a lymphedema therapist who uses the product and has direct contact with a representative from the company that makes it.

The studies that test heat as a treatment for lymphedema—such as Fizyoflug, microwave therapy, far-infrared sauna and electric blankets—are contesting a widely held belief in the North American lymphedema community that heat is not safe for people with lymphedema. These therapies may require more extensive research before they can overcome that preconception and be accepted. It reminds me of research on exercise for breast cancer survivors. Experts believed that strenuous exercise would lead to lymphedema until, in 1996, a boat full of brave volunteers tested that premise in a dragon boat called *Abreast in a Boat* (McKenzie 1998). Since then, hundreds of studies have been done on exercise for lymphedema, and it is now one of the four cornerstones of complete decongestive therapy. Regardless of how the research on heat therapies turns out, I want to acknowledge the bravery it takes—from both researchers and especially participants—to challenge current standards in order to seek evidence-informed solutions.

Developing new technologies to treat lymphedema is a truly global quest. For example, the Hivamat is from Germany, the Manutech BH and Linforoll are from Italy, the RianCorp LTU-904 low-level laser is from Australia, the far-infrared sauna prototype tested for lymphedema is from China, Endermologie is from France, RAGodoy is from Brazil, Vacumed is from Germany, Fizyoflug is from Turkey, the Novin 710L faradic current device is from Iran, the BEMER is from Liechtenstein, the Dolphin Neurostim is from Canada, and the CVAC and Dayspring are from the United States. It's reassuring to know that there are investigators around the world working to find innovative complementary therapies for lymphedema.

The downside of this worldwide effort is that it may be challenging to get access to the latest devices. High-tech health devices must be approved by government authorities, and manufacturers are required to submit them for approval in each country. For that reason, not every device mentioned here is available everywhere. (In fact, there seem to be strong regional preferences for the types of technologies favored.) To find out if a medical device is approved in the US, search at https://www.accessdata.fda.gov/scripts/cdrh/devicesatfda/index.cfm; in Canada, check the database at https://health-products.canada.ca/mdall-limh/prepareSearch?type=active.

Once a technology is approved in a particular country, it takes time for therapists to become aware of it, get trained on it and adopt it as part of their practice. If you are a patient, ask your lymphedema therapist which high-tech devices they have that might be appropriate for you. If you are a therapist and are interested in getting trained on one of these devices, your best bet is to reach out to the manufacturer to find out how to go about it.

High-tech devices can be expensive, but unlike most traditional medicines or natural health products, there may be insurance coverage for them—either to buy them or to be treated with them by your therapist. Check your plan to see what is covered and what isn't.

SURVEY SAYS

Among the forty survey respondents, thirty (75%) had tried a high-tech device. The most popular high-tech therapy was pneumatic compression pumps, used by twenty-one respondents (70%), followed by vibration plates, with thirteen users (43%), then low-level laser and infrared sauna, each with five users (17%). Eighteen of the devices had not been used by any of my respondents. I've included their comments throughout this section where appropriate.

References for High-Tech Devices

McKenzie DC. 1998. Abreast in a Boat—A Race Against Breast Cancer. *CMAJ* 159 (4): 376–78.

BEMER Therapy

What Is It?

BEMER is a medical device that provides pulsed electromagnetic field therapy (PEMFT). It is thought to work by increasing nitric oxide formation, which dilates microvessels and increases flow (Biermann 2020). The technology is available in different forms, such as a handheld device, a pad (B.Pad) and a Velcro-fastened body wrap. It is made by Innomed International in Liechtenstein. According to the brand's website, it can "improve microcirculatory blood flow by up to 30%" (BEMER Group, n.d.). But I did not find any studies listed on the website that used the product in a clinical setting.

Lymphedema-Specific Research

A unique study set out to test the effect of PEMFT on lymphatic microcirculation compared to conventional manual lymphatic drainage during supermicrosurgery (Biermann 2020). Before the operation, ten patients with leg lymphedema (four primary and six secondary) were injected with indocyanine green, allowing the surgeon to see the lymphatic vessels and the flow of lymph fluid, which is otherwise clear. During the procedure, the patients' lymphedema leg was placed on a B.Pad, which looks like a thick mat but has the PEMFT embedded between the layers of fabric. The pad was placed beneath the sterile operating room table cover and turned on for two minutes at the highest intensity. There was a two-minute pause, then the patient received MLD, starting at the foot.

Video of the lymph fluid movement—as seen through a fluoroscopic microscope that tracks the movement of the green-tinted lymph—was recorded before and after each treatment. The researchers then calculated the change in light intensity seen on the videos. Light intensity increased 79% for the MLD and 2% for the BEMER therapy.

The authors concluded that they saw no change in the lymphatic flow during the PEMFT phase, while there was a significant alteration with conventional MLD. They recommended further studies with longer PEMFT application times to see if that could allow for improvements in lymphatic flow.

Technical Breakdown

Supermicrosurgery, done under thirty times magnification with specialized instruments, connects delicate lymphatic vessels to blood vessels (a lympho-venous anastomosis, or LVA) to improve lymphedema. It can be a treatment for lymphedema or a preventative measure during cancer surgery when lymph nodes are removed. When performed as a preventative, it is called LYMPHA (lymphatic microsurgical preventive healing approach).

Side Effects/Risks

None noted.

Bottom Line on BEMER Therapy

A study that gave patients a two-minute exposure to BEMER during supermicrosurgery was unable to demonstrate a benefit. Future research with longer exposure times may yield better outcomes, but for now there is no compelling published research that would encourage evidence-based practitioners to recommend this treatment. Although the product's website does not list any side effects or contraindications, suggesting it has a low risk profile, a cost-benefit analysis needs to take into account the device's price, which is several thousand dollars.

References for BEMER Therapy

BEMER Group. n.d. "What Is Bemer?" Accessed July 27, 2025. https://bemergroup.com/en_CA/human-line/home.

Biermann N, Ruewe M, Zeman F, et al. 2020. The Influence of Pulsed Electromagnetic Field Therapy on Lymphatic Flow During Supermicrosurgery. *Lymphat Res Biol* 18 (6): 549–54.

Chi Machine

What Is It?

The Sun Ancon Chi Machine looks like a small box with two ankle cradles. You lie on your back, place your ankles in the half circles and turn on the timer, and the device moves back and forth in an "undulating 'goldfish' motion," acting as an aerobic exerciser that delivers both elevation and passive side-to-side movement (Harvest Haven 2025). It moves at 140 swings per minute, with a 10% (12-degree) swing angle (Moseley 2004). It was invented by Japanese scientist Keiichi Ohashi and is distributed by Hsin Ten Enterprise in Taiwan.

> **User Experience**
>
> "I still use my Chi Machine. The effect is similar to a vibration plate, except you are lying down and the speed is preset. It is very relaxing. The cost of the Chi Machine makes getting a vibration plate more affordable."
>
> **—Willa, British Columbia (full-body primary lymphedema tarda)**

Lymphedema-Specific Research

Thirty people diagnosed with secondary leg lymphedema were given a Sun Ancon Chi Machine for home use (Moseley 2004). They used it every morning and evening for three weeks, starting with five-minute sessions and increasing by three minutes every few days until they were at twelve minutes per session. Measurements were taken at baseline, weekly throughout the three-week trial and at a one-month follow-up.

Lymphedema was measured by perometry (limb volume), bioimpedance (extracellular fluid) and tonometry (tissue stiffness/fibrosis), and eight subjects also had lymphoscintigraphy (to view lymph flow). After three weeks, there was a median reduction of 300 milliliters (10.1 ounces) in leg volume, of which a median of 100 milliliters (3.4 ounces) returned by the one-month follow-up. Extracellular fluid was reduced by a median of 120 milliliters (4.1 ounces) in the leg and 300 milliliters (10.1 ounces) in the body as a whole, with most of the loss maintained at the one-month follow-up. No change in tissue fibrosis was noted in the tonometry measurements. Of the eight participants who had lymphoscintigraphy, three showed an improvement in dermal backflow, while the other five had no change.

When asked to describe their symptoms, subjects reported a significant reduction in pain, tightness, heaviness, skin dryness and perceived leg size. Body weight also reduced by an average of 0.5 kilograms (1.1 pounds), which remained stable at the one-month follow-up, with body fat down between 0.71% and 0.79%.

The study authors concluded that the Sun Ancon Chi Machine was effective at reducing total leg volume, leg fluid, whole-body extracellular fluid, body weight and participants' subjective symptoms. However, it should be noted that there was no control group in this trial.

Side Effects/Risks

Participants in the Moseley trial noted knee pain (17%), dizziness (8%) and neck pain (10%). These issues were resolved by putting a pillow under the knees and neck. A further 8% complained that the ankle moldings weren't comfortable, which was solved by using a sheep skin for padding on the lower legs.

Bottom Line on Chi Machine

The Chi Machine seems so simple, yet it was surprisingly effective in short treatment sessions in several measures, including lymph volume, extracellular fluid, body weight, body fat and subjective satisfaction. It seems like a combination of the RAGodoy passive movement machine (see page 261) and a vibration plate (page 270). Because you use it lying down, with your legs elevated, it takes advantage of gravity, in addition to vibration, to help move the lymph up the legs. This treatment is very time-efficient, with only five- to twelve-minute sessions, twice a day, required to see results. Since the user can purchase their own device, it may also be cost-effective, as it does not require repeat clinic visits. The user would need to be able to lie flat on the floor or a hard surface, which may present limitations for some.

The one aspect of this device that gives me pause is that the only study on it is over two decades old—if it's so effective, why hasn't it caught on or been the subject of more research? While it could simply be a marketing issue, new research would be very welcome before folks invest in the product. That said, if you can lie on your back and have no joint issues that might make it painful, this device has potential for leg lymphedema.

References for Chi Machine

Harvest Haven. 2025. "The Chi Machine." Accessed June 28, 2025. https://www.harvesthaven.com/collections/health-aids-and-devices/products/the-chi-machine.

Moseley AL, Piller N, Esterman A, Carati C. 2004. The Sun Ancon Chi Machine Aerobic Exerciser: A New Patient Focused, Home Based Therapy for People with Chronic Secondary Leg Lymphedema. *Lymphology* 37 (2): 53–61.

Chinese Heat Therapy

What Is It?

Chinese heat therapy uses a semicircular wooden device fitted with multiple light bulbs. A person with lymphedema can place their affected limb under the device to receive an at-home heat treatment. The radiant heat comes from sixteen light bulbs of 100 watts each. The temperature can be controlled between 45°C and 50°C (113°F and 122°F) by turning on or off some of the bulbs. It is easy to make yourself, affordable and transportable.

The device is widely used in China and was brought to India by Dr. Tambwekar, a plastic surgeon in Mumbai. I've included it in "High-Tech Therapies" because it needs to be plugged in, but in terms of its mechanical sophistication, it is lower-tech than other devices in this section.

Lymphedema-Specific Research

I found two Indian studies using Chinese heat therapy. One thing that struck me about the write-up of the second study was its opening statement: "Heat therapy is a well-known conservative management for lymphoedema" (Kulkarni 2010). This is a different perspective, as in North America, heat is warned against for lymphedema. However, in researching this book, I've discovered many heat therapies, including a detailed review paper (Hill 2024).

STUDY #1: GOGIA 2009

This study was conducted in India, where they refer to the Chinese heat therapy device as "the apparatus." Patients with filarial lymphedema (see "Technical Break-down," page 133) initially received two weeks of three different treatments: Chinese heat therapy, pneumatic compression pump (see page 256) and faradic currents (page 222). After that, they were allocated to only one therapy, which continued until lymphedema measurements plateaued, with the typical timeline being three to six months (the maximum was eighteen months).

The results demonstrated that compression pump therapy was superior to heat therapy. In fact, it was superior to combined treatments with all three therapies. Patients who used Chinese heat therapy achieved an average of 31% volume reduction, with a corresponding softening of the skin.

STUDY #2: KULKARNI 2010

This study also took place in India. Six patients with filarial lymphedema of the leg were given instructions on how to build the heat therapy device using plywood, hinges, light bulbs and regulators. There is a photo of the device in the study write-up. The patients were measured before therapy, which consisted of up to thirty minutes inside the device. In addition, they took a micronized flavonoid tablet (see Daflon 500, page 132) and elevated their leg on a regular basis.

The results—reported as a summary, rather than for each individual in the case study—were overall reductions of up to 30% of the original volume after three months of treatment.

Side Effects/Risks

None were noted in the Gogia and Kulkarni studies, but burns are a potential risk.

Bottom Line on Chinese Heat Therapy

Controlled clinical trials would need to be conducted before this treatment can be recommended with confidence. Although the Gogia study had comparison groups, the treatment durations varied, and the Kulkarni study lacked blinding, a control group and details about what other types of treatments the subjects were receiving. Also, these studies were done on filarial lymphedema, which is caused by a mosquito-borne parasite common in tropical climates. A major concern with filarial lymphedema is recurrent attacks of streptococcal lymphangitis, for which heat therapy may play a role that isn't applicable to lymphedema from other causes.

References for Chinese Heat Therapy

Gogia SB, Appavoo NC, Mohan A, Kumar MB. 2009. Comparative Results of Non-Operative Multi-modal Therapy for Filarial Lymphoedema. *Indian J Plast Surg* 42 (1): 22–30.

Hill JE, Whitaker JC, Sharafi N, et al. 2024. The Effectiveness and Safety of Heat/Cold Therapy in Adults with Lymphoedema: Systematic Review. *Disabil Rehabil* 46 (11): 2184–95.

Kulkarni AA, Abhyankar SV, Chaudhari GS, et al. 2010. Simple and Effective Method of Heat Therapy in Lymphoedema. *Indian J Surg* 72 (1): 64–65.

CO_2 Laser

What Is It?

The CO_2 (carbon dioxide) laser, also called an ablative CO_2 laser, is a medical device used to remove damaged outer layers of the skin. According to the American Board of Cosmetic Surgery, it treats "scars, warts, wrinkles, and other deeper skin flaws" (ABCS 2021). It produces infrared light in the range of 9,000 to 12,000 nanometers of wavelength. Treatment with a CO_2 laser is different from low-level laser therapy (see page 241). There are two main types of CO_2 lasers: traditional and fractional. A traditional CO_2 laser removes the entire top layer of skin and is the more aggressive therapy. A fractional CO_2 laser treats a smaller, targeted area. CO_2 lasers are made by several different manufacturers.

Lymphedema-Specific Research

There are multiple case studies of using CO_2 laser to treat lymphedema. I'll describe the most recent ones.

Case Study #1: Robinson 2018

This study, from the University of Texas's Department of Dermatology, involved a fifty-seven year-old morbidly obese woman with elephantiasis nostras verrucosa. She'd had "failed prior treatment with compression and lymphatic massage in the three years prior." She received three treatments, six to eight weeks apart, of ablative CO_2 laser therapy on her right thigh, to a depth of 700 to 2,100 microns. The laser used was the UltraPulse CO_2. After each treatment, she took antibiotics and applied vitamin A and D ointment to her skin twice a day until the next laser treatment. She experienced a significant improvement in the appearance of her skin and the amount of lymphorrhea (lymphatic leakage through the skin).

Technical Breakdown

Elephantiasis nostras verrucosa is the most severe form of lymphedema, with disfiguring changes in skin appearance, including discoloration and multiple papules, nodules and warts.

Case Study #2: Sancho 2019

These studies, which took place in Spain, followed a seventy-six-year-old man with a history of heart failure, obesity and prostate cancer and a seventy-three-year-old woman with obesity, diabetes and venous insufficiency. Both received topical numbing, followed by treatment with a 10,600-nanometer CO_2 laser. Afterward, they received oral antibiotics for two weeks and were instructed on proper wound cleaning. The patients were extremely satisfied with the significant improvement in their skin's appearance (before and after photos are available in the paper).

Six months after the procedure, there had been no relapse of the skin lesions. The authors noted that, since the underlying lymphedema was still present, the lesions might return, but said the risk could be lessened with compression garments, proper hygiene, weight loss, walking, leg elevation and use of skin moisturizer containing keratolytic ingredients (such as salicylic acid, urea, lactic acid and glycolic acid) to prevent excess buildup of the outer layer of skin.

Case Study #3: Menzer 2022

This publication describes two patients: a sixty-one-year-old woman with cervical cancer and lymphangiectasia (dilation of lymphatic vessels) and a thirty-two-year-old woman with lower leg lymphedema following inguinal lymph node dissection and radiation for melanoma on her right shin. I'll focus on the lymphedema patient.

The woman was using her compression garments consistently and also receiving manual lymphatic drainage, but her lymphedema had plateaued. After a local anesthetic of lidocaine, she was given a CO_2 laser treatment, then her skin was treated with a 50:50 mixture of white vinegar and warm water. She received a total of ten treatments over three years.

Following the first treatment, the patient reported increased flexibility and softness of the scar. After four treatments, she had a decrease in leg circumference from 30 to 23 centimeters (11.8 to 9.1 inches), which the authors believed may have been due to the CO_2 laser softening the scar and fibrosis in the area of the femoral vein, resulting in less venous compression. They concluded that fractional CO_2 laser therapy may be a promising treatment for lymphedema and lymphorrhea but noted that post-procedure wound care is essential.

Side Effects/Risks

No adverse effects were reported in any of the case studies. While it appears that numbing is needed prior to the procedure, the Menzer study noted that there is minimal post-procedure pain because the treatment seals nerve endings. Protection from the sun may be required for up to a year following the procedure (ABCS 2021).

Bottom Line on CO_2 Laser

I often see posts from lymphedema therapists discussing the challenges of advanced, treatment-resistant cases of lymphedema. These case studies, which demonstrate the efficacy of the CO_2 laser, remind us that dermatologists can play an important role in lymphedema management. If you see yourself or one of your patients reflected in these case studies, you might consider a referral to a dermatologist who uses CO_2 lasers as part of their treatment plans.

References for CO_2 Laser

American Board of Cosmetic Surgery (ABCS). 2021. "Laser Skin Resurfacing: Top 8 Things You Need to Know." Accessed June 20, 2025. https://www.americanboardcosmeticsurgery.org/skin-resurfacing/the-top-8-things-you-need-to-know-about-laser-skin-resurfacing/.

Menzer C, Aleisa A, Wilson BN, et al. 2022. Efficacy of Laser CO2 Treatment for Refractory Lymphedema Secondary to Cancer Treatments. *Lasers Surg Med* 54 (3): 337–41.

Robinson CG, Lee KR, Thomas VD. 2018. The Successful Treatment of Elephantiasis Nostras Verrucosa with Ablative Carbon Dioxide Laser. *J Cutan Med Surg* 22 (6): 611–13.

Sancho AQ, Cura LRD, Alonso SA, et al. 2019. Treatment of Elephantiasis Nostras Verrucosa with CO2 Laser. *Indian Dermatol Online J* 10 (6): 704–6.

CVAC Therapy

What Is It?

CVAC, which stands for "Cyclic Variations in Adaptive Conditioning," is a medical device that looks like a fully enclosed single cockpit and simulates multiple altitude changes in rapid succession. It is made by CVAC Systems, whose website describes it as "whole-body adaptive cellular conditioning" that will "optimize overall performance" (CVAC, n.d.). The technology is targeted toward athletic recovery, diabetic neuropathy, chronic obstructive pulmonary disease, traumatic brain injury and concussion. CVAC Systems claims its device "provides the benefits of traditional aerobic and anaerobic exercise without the joint stress and physical exertion that can be associated with these activities" (CVAC, n.d.).

Lymphedema-Specific Research

I was unable to locate any studies using this technology on individuals with lymphedema as their primary complaint.

Related Research

In a pilot study of four men and six women with adiposis dolorosa, a rare disorder in which the patient has painful nodular fat, fatigue, difficulty losing weight, inflammation, lymphedema, lipedema and nerve pain, the participants completed twenty to forty minutes of CVAC therapy a day for five days, with most doing two twenty-minute sessions a day (Herbst 2010). During each session, the pressure cycled 300 to 500 times, simulating altitudes of up to 3,200 meters (10,498 feet). For comparison, Denver, Colorado, known as the mile-high city, is at 1,609 meters (5,280 feet). Each twenty-minute session provided a cumulative change in altitude of 365,760 meters (1,200,000 feet).

In responding to the McGill Pain Questionnaire—used to assess the quality and intensity of pain—the participants reported a significant reduction in "current pain severity" after five days of treatment, but no change in pain quality or in worst or least pain. However, when they rated their pain on a scale of 0 to 10, their average, highest and lowest pain levels were all significantly reduced on day five. There was also a significant reduction in the patients' tendency to catastrophize their pain.

There was no change in their physical functioning, pain disability index or sleep quality, but a significant increase in their mental functioning. They lost weight, but their fat mass increased while their non-fat mass decreased, which can indicate loss of muscle; in this case, however, because bioimpedance measurements indicated less body water, some of the weight loss was thought to be from reduced edema fluid. The multiple changes in external pressure also acted like compression, reducing the participants' lymphedema, which the authors hypothesized played a role in the reduced pain.

The authors noted that their patients did not start to report reduced pain until day three or four, so it would not be reasonable to expect improvement after a single session. They recommended randomized controlled trials on using CVAC therapy for adiposis dolorosa and painful lipedema. Although they didn't mention trials for lymphedema, this therapy seems like it might also be a good candidate for lymphedema treatment, especially where lymphedema is accompanied by pain or lipedema.

Side Effects/Risks

No side effects were reported in the Herbst study, but two participants reported difficulty with equalizing ear pressure, which limited the number of sessions they could complete.

Bottom Line on CVAC Therapy

The CVAC device's multiple pressure changes may reduce lymphedema and associated pain, but before it can be recommended with confidence as a treatment for lymphedema, it should be studied specifically for that condition. In any case, there are only fifteen clinics listed on the manufacturer's website in the United States and one in Canada that offer CVAC therapy at the time of writing. Time will tell if this device becomes more widely available as a complementary therapy for lymphedema.

References for CVAC Therapy

CVAC. n.d. "Optimal Cellular Conditioning" and "Solutions for Wellness." Accessed January 11, 2025. https://cvacsystems.com/ and https://cvacsystems.com/solutions-for-active-lifestyles/.

Herbst KL, Rutledge T. 2010. Pilot Study: Rapidly Cycling Hypobaric Pressure Improves Pain After 5 Days in Adiposis Dolorosa. *J Pain Res* 3 (August): 147–53.

Dayspring

What Is It?

The Dayspring is a non-pneumatic compression pump made by Koya Medical. The company describes it as "an FDA-cleared, prescription-only, active gradient sequential compression treatment indicated for lymphedema, venous insufficiency, and reducing wound healing time. . . . It is the first and only wearable, dynamic active compression system that is not plugged into the wall" (Koya Medical 2022). As such, it allows you to walk around and perform many of your usual activities while it is working.

The Dayspring includes a small controller that you wear with a cross-body strap. It resembles a wearable heart monitor. The sleeve component looks similar to a Velcro compression garment. Rather than pneumatic compression, it uses its patented Flexframes, which "contract and relax to provide pressure using energy from a current that flows through the resistance of the shape memory alloy material with a temporal modulation" (Rockson 2022).

Lymphedema-Specific Research

Even though the Dayspring pump is new, several studies on its use for lymphedema have already been published.

STUDY #1: ROCKSON 2022

In this randomized crossover trial, fifty women with breast cancer–related lymphedema were enrolled from five different locations in the US. For the first twenty-eight days, twenty-three of the women used the Dayspring pump for one hour a day, and the others used a pneumatic compression pump for one hour a day. For the next twenty-eight days—known as the washout period—all fifty women refrained from using any compression pump. Then the women switched pumps: Those who had used the Dayspring used a pneumatic pump, and vice versa.

At the end of each twenty-eight-day pumping period, the volume difference between the healthy arm and lymphedema arm was calculated and compared to baseline. In both pumping periods, the lymphedema arm volume of the Dayspring users reduced by 65%, while that of the pneumatic pump users reduced by just 28%. The overall response rate was significantly higher for the Dayspring (88%) than for the pneumatic compression pump (42%). All of the patients said they were able to be active while using the portable pump, and 90% were either somewhat or very satisfied with it.

Notably, at the end of the washout period, swelling had returned to levels comparable to baseline for all of the women, which tells us that ongoing pump use—whether pneumatic or non-pneumatic—is needed to maintain results.

Between Professionals
When I worked as a home care dietitian, I visited many patients who received food via a feeding tube. The equipment usually included a pump that controlled the amount of feeding that dripped through. When given the choice between a traditional pump, which needed to be secured to an IV pole, and a portable device they could carry around with them, everyone chose the portable device. I suspect the same benefit of improved mobility may be a big selling feature for the Dayspring portable lymphedema pump.

STUDY #2: ROCKSON 2023

This subanalysis of study #1 included only the fourteen participants who were sixty-five years or older (the average age was seventy-two). The seniors who used the Dayspring portable pump experienced a 100.3% decrease in edema and significant improvement in quality-of-life scores, while the traditional pneumatic pump resulted in an edema decrease of 2.9% and no improvement in quality of life.

The authors hypothesized that the results were more dramatic with the Dayspring pump because participants reported greater adherence, using it, on average, for twenty-eight hours—consistent with the instruction to use it one hour a day for twenty-eight days. The pneumatic compression pump was used, on average, for thirty-five minutes a day.

STUDY #3: BARFIELD 2025

A total of seventy-one patients with primary or secondary lymphedema in one or both legs participated in this crossover study. The protocol began with thirty days without pump use, then ninety days of using either the Dayspring or a pneumatic compression pump. This was followed by a thirty-day washout period (no pump), then another ninety days of pumping with the alternate device. The patients were instructed to pump once a day for at least sixty minutes.

Measurements were taken after each phase. After ninety days of Dayspring pumping, the average reduction in limb volume was 300 milliliters (10.1 ounces), which was significantly greater than the average reduction of 62 milliliters (2.1 ounces) after 90 days of pneumatic compression pumping. There was also a significant improvement in quality of life after Dayspring pumping that was not seen after pneumatic pump treatment. There was no significant difference between the two pumps in foot measurements.

Compliance with pumping was also significantly better when the patients were using the Dayspring pump: an average of 90% of days, versus 60% for the pneumatic compression pump. When asked about their preferences at the end of the trial, 78% of the participants preferred the Dayspring, while 22% preferred the pneumatic compression pump. There were no instances of cellulitis, ulceration or hospitalization during the Dayspring phase; in the pneumatic pump phase, there were three cases of cellulitis, one case of ulceration and eight hospitalizations.

In the discussion section, the authors pointed out two features of the Dayspring that may explain the beneficial findings. First, the higher use of the product: 90% compliance means participants used their pump on eighty-one out of ninety days. Second, since the person can be mobile while pumping, muscle and joint contractions may amplify the work of the gradient sequential compression provided by the pump. Especially important is using the calf muscle, which increases injection fraction and improves the flow of blood through the veins in the leg.

User Experience

"I used a pneumatic pump for seven years, and while it did help, it was cumbersome and uncomfortable to use. I recently purchased a Dayspring non-pneumatic device and am very pleased with the ease of using it and the results. I can put it on and walk around. No discomfort at all—actually, it feels very good, like manual lymphatic massage."

—Kate, Washington (phlebolymphedema in both legs)

Side Effects/Risks

In the Rockson and Barfield trials, there were no serious adverse events recorded for the Dayspring pump, and none of the participants had additional or worsening swelling as a result of using the pump.

Bottom Line on Dayspring

The Dayspring non-pneumatic compression pump seems to have been very well received upon its introduction to the market. Its portability and high adherence rates compared to pneumatic compression pumps will likely make it a desirable complementary therapy—especially if insurance companies find positive cost-effectiveness data, as they did for pneumatic pumps (see page 256). I suspect we'll be hearing a lot more about this exciting innovation.

References for Dayspring

Barfield M, Winokur R, Berland T, et al. 2025. Results from a Comparative Study to Evaluate the Treatment Effectiveness of a Nonpneumatic Compression Device vs an Advanced Pneumatic Compression Device for Lower Extremity Lymphedema Swelling (TEAYS Study). *J Vasc Surg Venous Lymphat Disord* 13 (1): 101965.

Koya Medical. 2022. "Dayspring® by Koya." Accessed June 30, 2025. https://assets-global.website-files.com/60afbb3a71afb687c88000e3/664f9682591e6571def6d1c5_FAQS-M-2022L-Rev%20C.pdf.

Rockson SG, Skoracki R. 2023. Effectiveness of a Nonpneumatic Active Compression Device in Older Adults with Breast Cancer-Related Lymphedema: A Subanalysis of a Randomized Crossover Trial. *Lymphat Res Biol* 21 (6): 581–84.

Rockson SG, Whitworth PW, Cooper A, et al. 2022. Safety and Effectiveness of a Novel Nonpneumatic Active Compression Device for Treating Breast Cancer-Related Lymphedema: A Multicenter Randomized, Crossover Trial (NILE). *J Vasc Surg Venous Lymphat Disord* 10 (6): 1359–66.e1.

Dolphin Neurostim

What Is It?

The Dolphin Neurostim is a handheld device that provides DC microcurrents at the level of a "gentle whisper," according to the manufacturer's website (Dolphin Neurostim 2025). Although it is a high-tech device, it can be applied using traditional knowledge of acupressure points, creating a hybrid therapy known as microcurrent point stimulation or electro-acupuncture. It can also be applied directly to scars. The Canadian manufacturer sells kits with either one or two devices, along with optional vagus nerve stimulation pads and ear clips.

Lymphedema-Specific Research

To date, there has been no research published on the use of the Dolphin Neurostim in individuals with lymphedema.

Related Research

Two areas of interest for lymphedema for which there is research on the Dolphin Neurostim are pain management and scar therapy (see page 102). One study included fifty-one patients who had had chronic nonspecific pain for at least three months and had a visible scar from either surgery or trauma (Gokal 2017). The goal was to investigate whether microcurrent applied to scars could help with chronic pain. Scar locations included abdomen, knee, hernia, ankle, breast, neck, wrist and hand. Pain scores were recorded immediately before and after treatment, and again forty-eight hours later.

For the treatment, two Dolphin Neurostim devices were applied ½ inch (1.3 centimeters) apart and held in place for 30 seconds, then moved down the length of the scar until the entire scar was treated. The average treatment duration was 30 minutes (patients with longer scars would have longer treatment). One Dolphin device was set to a negative pole, and the other was set to a positive-negative pole to push negatively charged current back and forth through the positively charged scar tissue.

Immediately after treatment, the patients' pain scores had reduced by an average of 59% compared to pre-treatment levels. When they were questioned about their pain forty-eight hours later, the scores reduced a further 34% from the post-treatment level, for a total reduction of 73% compared to pre-treatment levels. There was no correlation between the location of the scar and the change in pain scores. The study made no mention of any effect on the scar itself, so we don't know whether the treatment softened it or aided in lymph flow through the scar area.

The authors concluded that microcurrent point stimulation via the Dolphin Neurostim provided a statistically significant reduction in initial pain levels, with a further reduction forty-eight hours later, and that their results help to validate the potential use of this therapy for scars and chronic pain.

Side Effects/Risks

None noted.

Bottom Line on Dolphin Neurostim

The Dolphin Neurostim was shown in one study to improve chronic pain for patients with a visible scar. Yet to be researched is the effect such treatment might have on the scar itself and on the underlying lymphatic vessels and lymphedema. For individuals with lymphedema secondary to surgery or trauma, and who have a visible scar, there may be additional benefits to lymphatic flow as the scar is treated. This would be an interesting area of study for future research.

References for Dolphin Neurostim

Dolphin Neurostim. 2025. "What Is the Dolphin Neurostim?" Accessed July 2, 2025. https://www.dolphinmps.ca/what-is-dolphin-neurostim/.

Gokal R, Armstrong K, Duant J. et al. 2017. The Successful Treatment of Chronic Pain Using Microcurrent Point Stimulation Applied to Scars. *Int J Complement Alt Med* 10 (3): 00333.

Electric Blanket

What Is It?

This is not a medical device, just a regular electric blanket consisting of a fabric sleeve with internal heating coils. You plug the blanket into an outlet and set the desired temperature. Electric blankets are generally used in cold climates to keep you warm while you are sleeping or to warm the bed before you get in. There are multiple manufacturers of electric blankets.

Lymphedema-Specific Research

In a Brazilian study, seven participants received mechanical lymph drainage via the RAGodoy device (see page 261), with or without an electric blanket (Mariana 2011). The use of heat did not affect the results, either positively or negatively.

Side Effects/Risks

No side effects were noted in the Mariana study, but electric blankets can cause burns. There is concurrently no consensus on the use of heat in lymphedema, and many warn of its dangers; however, one review of heat and cold therapies found no negative effects from heat (Hill 2024).

Bottom Line on Electric Blankets

A small study on using an electric blanket along with RAGodoy mechanical lymph drainage found no benefit over using the RAGodoy at room temperature. While no side effects were noted, caution is recommended when using heat with lymphedema.

References for Electric Blankets

Hill JE, Whitaker JC, Sharafi N, et al. 2024. The Effectiveness and Safety of Heat/Cold Therapy in Adults with Lymphoedema: Systematic Review. *Disabil Rehabil* 46 (11): 2184–95.

Mariana VF, de Fátima GG, Maria Pde G. 2011. The Effect of Mechanical Lymph Drainage Accompanied with Heat on Lymphedema. *J Res Med Sci* 16 (11): 1448–51.

Electronic Moxibustion

What Is It?

Moxibustion (see page 46), the heating of acupressure points, is traditionally done by burning ground dried mugwort to generate heat. A more modern practice is to use an electronic device to create heat, either with or without mugwort. Electronic moxibustion, also called smokeless moxa, has the benefits of limiting burns and noxious smoke (mugwort has a very strong smell when burned) and faster heating. According to traditional Chinese medicine, moxibustion improves circulation of qi and blood (Han 2020). There are multiple manufacturers of electronic moxibustion devices.

Lymphedema-Specific Research

A small clinical trial on electronic moxibustion used a device called Cettum, made by K-medical Co. in South Korea, where the study took place (Han 2020). Based on the description in the study, the device does not appear to contain mugwort. It is described as a cube-shaped apparatus with a base embedded in an electrical board controlled by a heat sensor. It is attached to acupressure points and secured with double-sided tape. At the push of a button, the temperature rises as high as 45°C (113°F), similar to the temperature of conventional moxibustion. The device can be raised up to 1 centimeter (0.4 inch) above the skin to prevent burns.

In this pilot trial, ten breast cancer patients with lymphedema received electronic moxibustion sessions, each lasting thirty minutes, twice a week for eight weeks. Treatment was given on six acupressure points on both the affected and unaffected arm. After each treatment, participants could wear a compression sleeve as usual, which most did only on days when the arm felt heavy. When the treatment period ended, there was a further four weeks of follow-up.

At the end of the treatment period, the mean difference in circumference between the healthy arm and lymphedema arm was down by 2.9 centimeters (1.1 inches)—a significant reduction. Circumference was reduced by 15% at week five, by 38% at week nine and by 29% at the end of the follow-up period. Bioimpedance values did not change significantly. Shoulder flexion and internal rotation improved significantly during the treatment period, but the results did not last over the four weeks of follow-up. Self-reported arm stiffness improved, but quality of life scores did not (the authors believed that might be because the questions did not cover milder symptoms such as stiffness and discomfort). Even so, the patients said they would recommend the treatment.

Technical Breakdown
Bioelectrical impedance analysis (BIA), sometimes called bioimpedance, is a measuring tool that requires you to stand on or hold a metal contact while a weak electrical current is sent through your body. The device measures the resistance as the current travels through your body, then calculates the percentage of body water, fat and muscle. BIA devices are used in gyms and fitness centers to allow people to see the changes in their muscle and fat as they exercise (someone who exercises regularly may not see a change in their weight, but may have less body fat and more muscle, which the BIA can measure). A simple scale would miss these changes. When used for lymphedema, BIA can demonstrate changes in the amount of body water.

Why would a study find a reduction in lymphedema circumference but no change in bioimpedance? There are several possibilities: The fluid may have been redistributed within the body but not removed from it; the treatment may have compressed the limb without affecting the fluid volume; or the treatment may have affected the limb's fat or muscle but not its fluid volume. Finally, the circumference measurement relies on the user to use the same tension with the tape measure and to place the tape measure in the same location with each measurement, opening up the possibility of user error or even bias.

Side Effects/Risks

The risks of moxibustion include skin burns. Although the risk is purported to be lower with electronic moxibustion than with traditional moxibustion, one participant in the 2020 Han trial did report a mild burn.

Bottom Line on Electronic Moxibustion

Electronic moxibustion is a small device that can be placed on the skin over acupressure points to provide heat. To date, its efficacy for lymphedema has been tested in only one small non-blinded, non-controlled trial, which demonstrated reduced limb circumference but no change in bioimpedance. Patients did self-report improvement in arm stiffness, but their quality of life scores did not change. Based on this study alone, it would be premature to recommend electronic moxibustion to treat lymphedema, especially given the risk of burns.

References for Electronic Moxibustion

Han K, Kwon O, Park HJ, et al. 2020. Electronic Moxibustion for Breast Cancer-Related Lymphedema: A Pilot Clinical Trial. *Integr Cancer Ther* 19 (October): 1534735420962854.

Endermologie

What Is It?

Endermologie is also known as depressomassage, vacuotherapy, endermotherapy, vacuum suction therapy and lipomassage. The handheld device is manufactured in France by LPG Medical. It has two motorized cylindrical skin rollers, which are applied to the limb by a trained therapist. The device picks up and massages the skin inside the two rollers. There are different-size treatment heads, which can be changed depending on the area being treated. Endermologie is FDA-approved for the treatment of cellulite and is commonly used in the cosmetic industry for body sculpting and cellulite treatment (Moseley, Esplin, et al. 2007).

Lymphedema-Specific Research

There are six studies and one review of Endermologie for lymphedema. I have summarized the results of the studies below and in a table that follows.

STUDY #1: CAMPISI 2002

In this early study, twenty people with arm and leg lymphedema who were one to three months post-microsurgery received twenty-five minutes of treatment, three times a week, for five weeks. Before and after photos showed improvements in limb size, and volume reduced by 5% to 10%. Ultrasound revealed decreased fibrosis and skin thickness. Lymphoscintigraphy showed reduced dermal backflow. Laser Doppler imaging showed increased blood microcirculation. The authors concluded that Endermologie, along with physical therapies, was helpful after microsurgery to reduce and soften fibrosis.

Study #2: Moseley, Esplin, et al. 2007

The goal of this study was to find the best treatment protocol for lymphedema. Funded by LPG Medical through Flinders Consulting, it included thirty-four women with post–breast cancer lymphedema and fibrosis. The first protocol, tested on twenty-four women, included twenty-five minutes of Endermologie treatment, starting with the area of the lungs on the back of the body on the lymphedema side. This treatment led to significant volume reductions, but the researchers developed a second protocol to see if they could achieve even better results. It was tested on ten women, used a larger treatment head and included thirty minutes of treatment, starting with the armpit on the non-affected side and finishing with extra time spent clearing the back.

Immediately after treatment (for both protocols), the patients were given a gauze sleeve, high-density foam rubber and two to three layers of short stretch bandaging and were asked to wear this overnight if they could tolerate it. Both protocols were performed four days a week, with three days free from bandaging. Each lasted four weeks.

Here are the results, measured by bioimpedance:

- **Protocol #1:** Treatment that started on the back resulted in a limb volume reduction of 182 milliliters (6.1 ounces) and a trunk volume reduction of 342 milliliters (11.5 ounces).
- **Protocol #2:** Treatment with a larger treatment head that started at the unaffected armpit and finished with extra time on the back resulted in a limb volume reduction of 216 milliliters (7.2 ounces) and a trunk volume reduction of 290 milliliters (9.8 ounces).

The second protocol provided superior results. Both groups reported improvement in fibrotic tissue and significant improvement in ratings of heaviness, tightness, tissue hardness and limb size. Both groups had small increases in upper arm volume after the first treatment, but they reduced as treatment continued. There were some complaints, including increased thirst and urination (which could indicate that the lymph was draining) and difficulty sleeping with the arm bandaged.

One month after treatment, there was some refilling, but arm volume was still less than pre-treatment levels. An important conclusion was that therapists should emphasize the importance of continuing self-management after Endermologie treatment ended.

There was no control group for this study, so we don't know what benefit Endermologie treatment provides compared to multilayer compression bandaging alone, or what the benefit would be without multilayer bandaging afterward.

Study #3: Moseley, Piller, et al. 2007

Another study funded by LPG Medical through Flinders Consulting included thirty women with breast cancer–related arm lymphedema, who were randomized to receive either MLD (twenty patients) or Endermologie (ten patients) four days per week for four weeks. Compression bandaging was applied after each treatment. After four weeks of treatment, the patients were given a new compression garment to wear.

Both groups saw volume reductions: 140 milliliters (4.7 ounces) for the MLD group, and 186 milliliters (6.3 ounces) for the Endermologie group. One month post-treatment, some of the reduction remained: 106 milliliters (3.6 ounces) for the MLD group and 142 milliliters (4.8 ounces) for the Endermologie group. In addition, both groups had reductions in heaviness, tightness and hardness.

The authors made a couple of interesting observations. First, the volume reductions in the Endermologie group occurred within the first two weeks; for this reason, the authors recommended two weeks as the minimum treatment duration. Second, the MLD group had a greater reduction in truncal lymphedema and less refilling at one-month post-treatment.

STUDY #4: MOHAMED 2011

Forty women with arm lymphedema following breast cancer surgery were divided into two groups. The first group received twenty minutes of Endermologie treatment to the back, upper arm, forearm and hand, twice weekly for four weeks, plus compression bandaging. The second group received compression bandaging only. Circumference measurements decreased in both groups, but more in the Endermologie group. In addition, the women that received Endermologie reported improved range of motion, pain and softening of fibrotic tissue.

STUDY #5: AHMED 2013

For this Egyptian study, forty women with post–breast cancer lymphedema were randomly divided into two groups. Both groups were treated with MLD, pneumatic compression pump, short stretch bandages, and exercise two times a week for four weeks. One group also received Endermologie treatment. Comparing pre-treatment to post-treatment, both groups demonstrated a highly significant decrease in pain, limb volume and shoulder function, but the results were higher for the Endermologie group. The author concluded that the study added support for using Endermologie as an accredited physical therapy for lymphedema.

STUDY #6: ZIETHAR 2021

This interesting protocol compared two complementary therapies head-to-head: low-level laser (see page 241) versus Endermologie. Thirty women with post–breast cancer lymphedema were randomly assigned to either thirty minutes of Endermologie or twenty minutes of low-level laser (904 nanometers). Both groups received treatment three times per week for six weeks, and everyone also received CDT, including MLD, compression bandaging, range of motion exercises, hygiene and skin care.

Both groups saw a significant decrease in limb volume and circumference compared to pre-treatment: 18.5% for the Endermologie group, and 8.4% for the laser group. The authors concluded that Endermologie was more effective than low-level laser in reducing limb circumference and volume in post-mastectomy lymphedema. However, it's unclear why the treatment lengths were different, with the Endermologie group receiving a total of 180 minutes more treatment time over six weeks.

The six studies are summarized in the following table:

Study	Subjects	Results
Campisi 2002	20 people post-microsurgery	Improved fibrosis, skin thickness, dermal backflow and blood microcirculation
Moseley, Esplin, et al. 2007	34 women post–breast cancer	Significant volume reduction, improvement in fibrotic tissue, significant improvement in heaviness, tightness, tissue hardness and limb size
Moseley, Piller, et al. 2007	30 women post–breast cancer	Volume reduction superior to MLD
Mohamed 2011	40 women post–breast cancer	Improved circumference, range of motion, pain and fibrotic tissue
Ahmed 2013	40 women post–breast cancer	Improved pain, volume and shoulder function, superior to MLD alone
Ziethar 2021	30 women post–breast cancer	Improved volume and circumference, superior to low-level laser

MLD = manual lymphatic drainage

REVIEW #1: WAHID 2024

A review that included three of the studies discussed above (Moseley, Esplin, et al. 2007; Mohamed 2011; Ahmed 2013) examined low-level laser (page 241), Kinesio taping (page 108) and Endermologie (which the authors spelled "endermology"). The authors concluded that there was more significant clinical improvement in limb volume in the Endermologie groups than in the control groups.

Side Effects/Risks

No serious side effects were noted, but one study reported increased thirst and urination.

Bottom Line on Endermologie

This cosmetic device is making a breakthrough into the medical management of lymphedema, and it seems promising. Six small studies show that Endermologie treatment is well tolerated by individuals with lymphedema, with no serious side effects. Research has been published as recently as 2021, and at least one study is currently underway (Malloizel-Delaunay 2019).

Where Endermologie is available, practitioners may be more accustomed to cosmetic applications such as body sculpting and cellulite treatment, which is not ideal; working with a practitioner who understands lymphedema would be preferable. If you decide to try Endermologie, the recommendation based on available research to date is a minimum of two weeks of treatment, with four weeks being ideal. As with any complementary therapy, and for optimal results, continue with conventional therapies like compression, skin care and MLD and discuss with your lymphedema therapist.

References for Endermologie

Ahmed ET. 2013. Endermologie Technique Versus Decongestive Lymphatic Therapy on Post-mastectomy Related Lymphedema. *J Nov Physiother* 3 (3): 1000155.

Campisi C, Boccardo F, Zilli A, et al. 2022. LPG® Technique in the Treatment of Peripheral Lymphedema: Clinical Preliminary Results and Perspectives. *Eur J Lymphology* 10 (35–36): 16.

Malloizel-Delaunay J, Chantalat E, Bongard V, et al. 2019. Endermology Treatment for Breast Cancer Related Lymphedema (ELOCS): Protocol for a Phase II Randomized Controlled Trial. *Eur J Obstet Gynecol Reprod Biol* 241 (October): 35–41.

Mohamed F, Abol-Atta H. 2011. Effectiveness of Endermologie Technique in Post-Mastectomy Lymphedema. *Med J Cairo Univ* 79 (2): 1–4.

Moseley A, Esplin M, Piller NB, Douglass J. 2007. Endermologie (with and Without Compression Bandaging)—A New Treatment Option for Secondary Arm Lymphedema. *Lymphology* 40 (3): 129–37.

Moseley A, Piller N, Douglass J, Esplin M. 2007. Comparison of the Effectiveness of MLD and LPG Technique. *Wounds Int J* 2 (2): 30–36.

Wahid DI, Wahyono RA, Setiaji K, et al. 2024. The Effication of Low-Level Laser Therapy, Kinesio Taping, and Endermology on Post-Mastectomy Lymphedema: A Systematic Review and Meta-Analysis. *Asian Pac J Cancer Prev* 25 (11): 3771–79.

Ziethar MMA, Waked IS, Toson RA, Sherif RRA. 2021. Endermologie Versus Low Level Laser Therapy on Post Mastectomy Lymphedema. *Med J Cairo Univ* 89 (4): 1359–66.

Extracorporeal Shock Wave Therapy

What Is It?

Extracorporeal shock wave therapy (ESWT) delivers high-energy sound waves by two mechanisms: 1) a focused shock wave with a single pulse and a wide frequency range, or 2) a radial shock wave with energy dissipated over a large area. Low-energy ESWT helps tissues regenerate by increasing stem cell activity, promoting endothelial angiogenesis (the regrowth of cells that line the inside of blood vessels), regulating inflammation, relieving pain and preventing soft-tissue fibrosis (Tsai 2021). ESWT has been used in physiotherapy for decades for the treatment of bone spurs, plantar fasciitis and other conditions, but the first study for lymphedema was in 2010 (Michelini 2010). There are multiple manufacturers of ESWT devices.

Technical Breakdown

Some ESWT devices deliver a focused beam of acoustic waves to one pinpoint area —described as a "laser beam"—while others deliver a low-intensity, broadly focused wave, described as a "flashlight." As you research this therapy, pay attention to the type of device used, the depth of penetration into the skin and whether it delivers radial or focused wave patterns.

Lymphedema-Specific Research

A recent systematic review collected studies of extracorporeal shock wave therapy on patients with breast cancer–related lymphedema (Tsai 2021). It included eight studies—six randomized controlled trials and two prospective pilot studies—all relatively small studies ranging from twenty to sixty participants. A total of 193 patients had participated in the randomized controlled trials. Five of the trials used ESWT + CDT, and one compared ESWT to CDT. The treatments were given two to three times per week, for a maximum of sixteen sessions.

Following the review, four of the studies were included in a meta-analysis, which found that when ESWT was used as a complementary therapy to CDT, there was superior improvement in arm volume, skin thickness and shoulder range of motion versus CDT alone. But the authors stated that current evidence is still of low methodological quality, and that there is not enough evidence to support the use of ESWT as a replacement for CDT.

Lymphedema Research in Animals

Animal and cell studies on lymphatic tissue have shown that extracorporeal shock wave therapy can promote lymphangiogenesis—the growth of new lymph vessels (Tsai 2021).

Side Effects/Risks

No adverse effects were reported in the studies, but contraindications do exist and ESWT is not recommended if you have metastatic disease, for treatment over ischemic tissue, where vascular disease is present, where there is an infection, or if you take blood thinners (FDA 2005). This is not a complete list of contraindications; discuss this therapy with your lymphedema therapist before using it. If you are a practitioner, you may want to read the research on the specific device you have to determine whether this treatment is appropriate for your patients.

Bottom Line on Extracorporeal Shock Wave Therapy

Physiotherapists have used extracorporeal shock wave therapy for decades to treat bone spurs, plantar fasciitis and other conditions. When used in conjunction with CDT, it has been shown in a few small studies to have superior results over CDT alone, with improvements in arm volume, skin thickness and shoulder range of motion for women with post–breast cancer lymphedema. Although there are some contraindications, ESWT is a promising lymphedema therapy, and hopefully more research on its use for this population will be forthcoming.

References for Extracorporeal Shock Wave Therapy

Food and Drug Administration (FDA). 2005. "Summary of Safety and Effectiveness Data for Orthospec Orthopedic ESWT." Accessed September 25, 2024. https://www.accessdata.fda.gov/cdrh_docs/pdf4/P040026b.pdf.

Michelini S, Cardone M, Failla A, et al. 2010. Treatment of Geriatrics Lymphedema with Shockwave Therapy. *BMC Geriatr* 10 (Suppl 1): A105.

Tsai YL, I TJ, Chuang YC, et al. 2021. Extracorporeal Shock Wave Therapy Combined with Complex Decongestive Therapy in Patients with Breast Cancer-Related Lymphedema: A Systemic Review and Meta-analysis. *J Clin Med* 10 (24): 5970.

Far-Infrared Sauna

What Is It?

A far-infrared (FIR) sauna uses light from the far end of the spectrum to generate heat. Because far-infrared light can penetrate your skin, it heats your body directly, whereas a Swedish sauna uses heat to warm the air, which warms you up as you sit in it. In an far-infrared sauna, you will still sweat, and your heart rate will increase, but these effects happen at a lower air temperature: The temperature inside a far-infrared sauna is typically 43°C to 57°C (110°F to 135°F), versus the 80°C to 100°C (150°F to 195°F) of a traditional sauna.

Lymphedema-Specific Research

All of the research I could find on treating lymphedema with far-infrared rays used a device made in Shanghai that generates infrared radiation with 6.0 and 14.0 micromolar wavelengths, using a ring of eight far-infrared quartz lamps surrounded by a stainless steel casing (Li, Xu, et al. 2017; Li, Zhang, et al. 2017; Li 2018; Xia 2022). It is not a full-body device; only the lymphedema limb (either the arm or the leg) goes inside. During treatments, the device is set to maintain 42°C (107.6°F), to achieve a skin temperature of 39.5±0.5°C (103±1°F).

Technical Breakdown
Infrared rays can be near infrared (short wavelength) or far infrared (long wavelength). The far-infrared region of the light spectrum lies beyond the red end of the visible range. Far-infrared rays penetrate our skin layers and resonate with water and organic molecules in our body, making them potentially beneficial for all living beings.

STUDY #1: LI, XU, ET AL. 2017

This study included sixty-four women who had been treated for gynecological cancer (31% cervical, 8% ovarian and 61% endometrial) and had had stage 2 or 3 lymphedema in one leg for at least one year. In addition, the women had had an outbreak of dermatolymphangioadenitis—inflammation and infection of the skin over the lymphedema tissue—at least once in the previous year. The symptoms of dermatolymphangioadenitis are pain, red rash (erythema), red streaks that align with the superficial lymphatics, lymph node swelling and fever.

The women received five far-infrared treatments per week for four weeks. During each treatment, the affected leg was kept in the device for two hours. Before treatment, the mean frequency of dermatolymphangioadenitis was three times per year. Afterward, the mean frequency reduced to less than once per year. The majority of the women (78%) had no episodes of dermatolymphangioadenitis in the year after treatment. Tightness, heaviness, pain, hardness, soreness, discomfort, heat, fullness, tingling, limb weakness, numbness and quality of life scores also improved significantly after treatment. Changes in blood and lymph inflammatory markers could be interpreted as improvements in immune dysfunction.

User Experience
"For my personal edema issues, I exercise and use an infrared sauna daily. Compression pumps, infrared sauna and vibration plates are something I use in my practice that have proven to assist in the edema management of my clients. The infrared sauna and vibration plate therapy are provided free to my clients following their one-hour hands-on therapy session."

—**Anonymous, Illinois (lymphedema therapist with primary lymphedema of the leg)**

Study #2: Li, Zhang, et al. 2017

Thirty-two people with stage 2 or 3 lymphedema in the arm (eleven participants) or leg (twenty-one participants), along with repeated episodes of cellulitis, were treated with far-infrared radiation for two hours a day, five days a week, for four weeks. The treatment reduced the weight of the fluid in the lymphedema limb, the circumference measurements, the thickness of the skin and subcutaneous tissue, and the amounts of fluid, fat, protein and hyaluronan in the limb. (Hyaluronan, or hyaluronic acid, is one of the main components of interstitial tissue and lymph, along with fluid, fat and protein.)

Study #3: Li 2018

Sixty-four patients with stage 2 or 3 lymphedema with fibrotic tissue were recruited for this study. Eighteen had arm lymphedema, and forty-six had leg lymphedema. Their lymphedema was from a variety of causes, including breast cancer (25%), cervical cancer (19%), primary lymphedema (16%), ovarian cancer (13%), infection (9%), uterine cancer (6%), venous insufficiency (3%), Hodgkin's lymphoma (3%), trauma (3%) and other (3%).

They completed two-hour sessions of far-infrared therapy, five days a week, over four weeks. After treatment, their skin elasticity had improved significantly and fibrous banding, as viewed via ultrasound, was substantially reduced. Inflammation levels in lymphedema fluid had also decreased—specifically, levels of IL-18 and TGF-β. TGF-β is a cytokine (an inflammatory messenger) that is influential in fibrosis development. It is present in higher numbers in people with chronic lymphedema and fibrosis. There was no change in blood cytokine concentrations.

> **Anecdotal Report**
> "I've had patients use vibration plates and infrared saunas and swear by them, but do I not have the equipment to try in my clinic."
>
> —Ryan Schumacher, PT, CLT, Froedtert Health, Milwaukee, Wisconsin

Study #4: Xia 2022

Seventy-four women with lymphedema following surgery to remove gynecological tumors, and who had been cancer-free for at least five years, were split into two groups: The control group received compression bandaging, and the treatment group received bandaging + far-infrared therapy. One year after treatment, the treatment group's limb circumference and tissue fluid were significantly reduced compared with the control group. There was no increase in CA 125 (a tumor marker that indicates the presence of cancer cells), no recurrence of cancer and no adverse reactions. The authors concluded that "FIR is an oncologically safe treatment for lymphedema in gynecological tumor patients."

Side Effects/Risks

No side effects or adverse reactions were reported in these studies. The current position paper on risk reduction from the National Lymphedema Network says to "Avoid exposure to extreme heat and cold" (NLN 2012), but the organization has plans to update all of its position papers. In these studies, the impact of the heat may have been lessened because only the lymphedema limb was inside the far-infrared device.

> **User Experience**
> "I did ten sessions of far-infrared sauna at a gym-spa location several years ago; it seemed effective. I would like to do it again and more regularly."
>
> —**Meg, New York (lymphedema in both legs and abdomen post–ovarian cancer surgery)**

Bottom Line on Far-Infrared Sauna

The human body has a high water content—about 55% to 60% for adults. As far-infrared rays come in contact with the body's water, it heats up, increasing tissue temperature. In addition, far-infrared light produces radiation and resonance. The body's response to the heat, radiation and resonance is to dilate the blood and lymph vessels, which increases the circulation of blood and lymph and stimulates immune system activation, ultimately reducing pressure. The radiation also softens fibrotic tissue, and the resonance breaks down large protein molecules in the lymph.

The authors of the Chinese studies point out that, as helpful as the far-infrared treatments were, patients who don't follow them up with compression therapy could have their fibrosis return. Also, the treatments were time-intensive—two hours per day, five days a week, for four weeks. Could fewer and/or shorter treatments still offer benefits? We don't yet know the answer, but hopefully the positive results will provide impetus for the research to continue.

Although the researchers used a custom device made specifically for their studies, we may see a product like it in the future if they decide to make it commercially available and seek government approvals. There are currently no lymphedema studies I could find on the effects of the full-body far-infrared saunas found at health clubs and spas.

References for Far-Infrared Sauna

Li K, Xu H, Liu NF, et al. 2017. Far-Infrared Ray for Treating Chronic Lower Extremity Lymphedema with Dermatolymphangioadenitis: A Postoperative Complication of Gynecological Tumor Resection. *Arch Gynecol Obstet* 295 (6): 1441–50.

Li K, Zhang Z, Liu NF, et al. 2017. Efficacy and Safety of Far Infrared Radiation in Lymphedema Treatment: Clinical Evaluation and Laboratory Analysis. *Lasers Med Sci* 32 (3): 485–94.

Li K, Zhang Z, Liu NF, et al. 2018. Far-Infrared Radiation Thermotherapy Improves Tissue Fibrosis in Chronic Extremity Lymphedema. *Lymphat Res Biol* 16 (3): 248–57.

NLN Medical Advisory Committee. 2012. "Lymphedema Risk Reduction Practices." Position Statement of the National Lymphedema Network. Accessed April 22, 2025. https://lymphnet.org/page/risk-reduction/.

Xia L, Cui C, Nicoli F, et al. 2022. Far Infrared Radiation Therapy for Gynecological Cancer-Related Lymphedema Is an Effective and Oncologically Safe Treatment: A Randomized-Controlled Trial. *Lymphat Res Biol* 20 (2): 164–74.

Faradic Currents

What Are They?

Faradic currents are a type of electrical stimulation that uses short bursts of current to make muscles contract. They are typically given at a frequency of 50 to 100 hertz, with a pulse duration of 0.1 to 2 milliseconds (Physiopedia, n.d.). They are usually used to treat muscles with intact nerves, which is different from high-voltage electrical stimulation (see page 228).

Lymphedema-Specific Research

An Iranian clinical trial set out to be the first to study the effectiveness of combining complete decongestive therapy with either faradic currents or ultrasound (page 265) to treat individuals with breast cancer–related lymphedema (Hemmati 2022). It was a double-blind randomized controlled trial with thirty-nine women divided into three parallel groups. They all received CDT: five sessions per week with a physiotherapist, including manual lymphatic drainage; compression with short stretch bandages; skin care; and exercises for one hour a day. In addition, one group was treated with ultrasound (the Novin 215X) and another group was treated with faradic currents.

The faradic currents were administered to the muscles of the forearm using the Novin 710L, made in Iran, at a frequency of 30 hertz and a pulse duration of 300 microseconds, for an interval of two seconds on and five seconds off for ten minutes on each muscle. The electrodes were held in place with elastic bandages wrapped from the hand to the shoulder (from distal to proximal).

All of the treatment groups saw a significant reduction in circumference measurements at the middle of the forearm, elbow and mid upper arm. In addition, the faradic group had a significant reduction at the wrist and the area above the midway point of the upper arm.

Arm volume was also significantly reduced in all three groups. There was a nonsignificant difference between the faradic and control groups, but a significant difference between the ultrasound and control groups (but not the ultrasound and faradic groups). In other words, CDT + ultrasound was the most effective treatment for reducing volume. Pain and functional disability reduced significantly in all three groups, but significantly more in the faradic and ultrasound groups than in the control group.

To explain the results in the faradic group, the authors suggested that faradic currents trigger muscle contractions, increasing blood and lymph flow. Muscle contractions also stimulate the removal of intercellular proteins, which contributes to reduced edema.

Side Effects/Risks

None noted.

Bottom Line on Faradic Currents

Faradic currents are short bursts of electrical current used to stimulate muscle contractions, thereby improving intercellular protein removal and blood and lymph flow. The Hemmati study is an excellent example of how complementary therapies can enhance the effects of CDT to achieve even greater results. We can look forward to more studies to confirm the efficacy of faradic currents as a complementary therapy for lymphedema.

References for Faradic Currents

Hemmati M, Rojhani-Shirazi Z, Zakeri ZS, et al. 2022. The Effect of the Combined Use of Complex Decongestive Therapy with Electrotherapy Modalities for the Treatment of Breast Cancer-Related Lymphedema: A Randomized Clinical Trial. *BMC Musculoskelet Disord* 23 (1): 837.

Physiopedia. n.d. "Faradic Stimulation." Accessed July 17, 2025. https://www.physio-pedia.com/Faradic_Stimulation.

Fizyoflug

What Is It?

The Fizyoflug is a device that provides fluidotherapy, also known as dry heat therapy. Made by the Turkish company Fizyomed, it delivers convection heat by passing hot air through a special thermostat-controlled container filled with cellulose particles (Çakit 2024). The heated air moves the solid particles, separates them and creates a liquid-like medium. The temperature varies from 41°C to 48.9°C (105.8°F to 120°F). The temperature and particle movement settings are controlled by a clinician. The Fizyoflug has been used to treat pain, muscle spasms and edema in patients with post-stroke complex regional pain syndrome (Çakit 2024).

Lymphedema-Specific Research

Forty women with lymphedema in one arm following breast cancer treatment were randomly assigned to receive either standard CDT (MLD, short stretch multilayer bandaging, skin care and exercises) or CDT + fluidotherapy with the Fizyoflug (Çakit 2024). The final analysis included seventeen patients who received CDT alone and fifteen who received CDT + Fizyoflug (eight women had dropped out of the study). They all received treatment five days a week for three weeks. For the fluidotherapy group, it included twenty minutes of continuous mode therapy at 42°C (107.6°F), which resulted in greater pain reduction and volume reduction than was seen in the control group.

Side Effects/Risks

There were no side effects reported in the Çakit study. Of the original forty participants, three patients developed infection and dropped out, but the authors did not specify which group they belonged to or whether the infection was related to the treatment.

Bottom Line on Fizyoflug

The Fizyoflug joins the group of complementary therapies that appear promising but require additional larger trials. Despite positive findings in the one existing study, it's going to take more evidence to help the lymphedema community overcome the fear that heat boosts blood flow, increasing lymphatic load and worsening lymphedema. However, good science is willing to test even the most widely held and long-standing beliefs.

References for Fizyoflug

Çakit BD, Vural SP. 2024. Short-Term Effects of Dry Heat Treatment (Fluidotherapy) in the Management of Breast Cancer Related Lymphedema: A Randomized Controlled Study. *Clin Breast Cancer* 24 (5): 439–46.

Flowave

What Is It?

The Flowave was a product that worked using sound waves. Formerly made by the Italian manufacturer Talamonti, It has since evolved into the Manutech BH (see page 249). I'm including it in the event you run across this research and wonder why it wasn't included.

Lymphedema-Specific Research

Thirty women with breast cancer–related lymphedema were randomly assigned to receive either ten sessions of manual lymphatic drainage followed by ten sessions of Flowave, or Flowave first followed by MLD (Belmonte 2012). They received treatment once a weekday for two weeks. After the first ten sessions, the women received no treatment for a month (known as the washout period), then switched treatments.

The physicians who examined them pre- and post-treatment did not know which treatment they received first (a protocol known as single blinding). Comparing lymphedema volume before and after treatment with the Flowave, there was a nonsignificant reduction of 20 milliliters (0.7 ounces). Pain, heaviness and tightness also reduced. There was no significant difference between Flowave and MLD treatment, with neither leading to more than a 5% volume reduction. The authors attributed these results to the fact that the participants were all in the maintenance phase of treatment, and 87% regularly wore compression garments.

Side Effects/Risks

In the Belmonte trial, there was one episode of erysipelas (skin infection) on the fourth day of treatment with the Flowave, which resolved on its own. One patient reported skin irritation at an electrode point, but it resolved when the intensity was reduced.

Bottom Line on Flowave

The Flowave technology has been used to develop the Manutech BH (page 249). The Flowave itself is no longer available.

References for Flowave

Belmonte R, Tejero M, Ferrer M, et al. 2012. Efficacy of Low-Frequency Low-Intensity Electrotherapy in the Treatment of Breast Cancer-Related Lymphoedema: A Cross-Over Randomized Trial. *Clin Rehabil* 26 (7): 607–18.

Grounding Mats

What Are They?

Grounding, or earthing, has been defined as "reconnecting the conductive human body to the earth's natural and subtle surface electric charge . . . to influence the basic bioelectrical function of the body" (Menigoz 2020). Simply put, you make direct contact with the earth by walking barefoot, sitting on the ground or coming in direct contact with the earth (grass, soil, gravel, stone or sand) in some way. Grounding has been credited with reducing inflammation, pain and stress, and improving blood flow, energy, sleep and well-being (Menigoz 2020). It is also sometimes called "electromagnetic nutrition" and "vitamin G" (Sinatra 2023).

Grounding mats, pillows, bedsheets, body bands and patches allow for grounding to be done indoors. These devices contain a conductive material, such as silver threads. A cord plugs into the mat and then into the grounding port—the large round hole—in an electrical outlet. There are multiple manufacturers of grounding products.

Lymphedema-Specific Research

Although social media sites contain many anecdotal reports on the benefits of grounding, finding lymphedema-specific scientific research proved challenging.

Related Research

In an American study from the University of California at Irvine, forty middle-aged volunteers were randomly allocated to receive either indoor grounding or sham grounding (Chevalier 2015). They were to sit in a recliner for one hour with a grounding mat, a grounding pillow and four grounding patches placed on their palms and soles, all plugged into a connection box that was plugged into a power outlet. The control group used the same set-up, but the wires had been modified to disable grounding. The purpose of the study was to determine whether grounding promotes blood flow to the face, which would be an indication of an increase in blood-borne nutrients traveling to the face via the microcirculation of the skin.

Thermal imaging of the face, neck and torso was done before and after grounding to measure skin temperature at 5 millimeters (0.2 inches) deep, with the technicians blinded to which group the patients were in. The authors provided a detailed description of the results for three representative subjects from the treatment and control groups. Face temperature decreased after grounding in both groups, but significantly more in the control group. The researchers also measured temperature symmetry between the right and left sides of the face, which improved in the treatment group and got worse (more asymmetric) in the control group.

Most relevant to lymphedema was the temperature of the torso, which again showed an increase in symmetry. The treatment group experienced a statistically significant reduction in the temperature difference between hot and cold spots on the torso, while the control group had a non-significant increase in the difference between hot and cold. In the abdomen, the treatment group experienced a nonsignificant increase in temperature, while the control group had a significant decrease in temperature. The authors interpreted these findings in the treatment group as an increase in fluid return to the heart by the lymphatic and blood vessels. One patient in the treatment group reported less pain in areas where they experienced chronic pain, and two reported that their pain had disappeared.

The authors noted that temperature pattern changes generally take weeks to months, but with grounding they were seen within minutes, while there was no change in the control group other than what can be expected from relaxation. They credit a "surge in vascularity" brought about by grounding. In their discussion, they mention many times that venous-lymphatic return was improved, based on comparing thermal heat patterns before and after grounding. Extrapolating from these findings, patients with lymphedema may be good candidates for ongoing research of grounding devices.

In their conclusion, the authors observed: "The Earth possesses a form of easily accessible beneficial natural energy that has been demonstrated previously to positively influence human health." As a disclaimer, they acknowledged that the study was funded by Earth FX and the products used had been donated by earthing.com.

Side Effects/Risks

There were none noted in the Chevalier study, but a potential risk would be electrocution from faulty equipment or home wiring.

Bottom Line on Grounding Mats

Grounding products are very popular right now, which may make skeptics highly suspicious, as products that burst onto the scene often merit adjectives like "fad," "fringe" or "pseudoscience." The study I uncovered uses thermal imaging, which even the authors admit "has been widely misunderstood and criticized." Using a fringe device to prove the validity of another fringe device may not instill confidence in evidence-based stalwarts, but this trial did show that there were temperature changes in the patients who received grounding and none in the patients who received the sham treatment. Questions remain: Are these changes due to an increase in blood and lymph fluid return to the heart? If so, could grounding devices be a cost-effective and safe complementary therapy for lymphedema? Perhaps future studies will use outcomes like changes in limb volume, lymph flow rate (via lymphoscintigraphy) and extracellular fluid volume (via bioimpedance) that have an established record of use in lymphedema research.

If the low risk and relatively low cost of grounding products lead you to try one, be sure to observe—or better yet, measure—your lymphedema before and after use to assess the impact.

References for Grounding Mats

Chevalier G, Melvin G, Barsotti T. 2015. One-Hour Contact with the Earth's Surface (Grounding) Improves Inflammation and Blood Flow— A Randomized, Double-Blind, Pilot Study. *Health* 7 (8): 1022–59.

Menigoz W, Latz TT, Ely RA, et al. 2020. Integrative and Lifestyle Medicine Strategies Should Include Earthing (Grounding): Review of Research Evidence and Clinical Observations. *Explore* (New York) 16 (3): 152–60.

Sinatra ST, Sinatra DS, Sinatra SW, Chevalier G. 2023. Grounding—The Universal Anti-Inflammatory Remedy. *Biomed J* 46 (1): 11–16.

High-Voltage Electrical Stimulation

What Is It?

High-voltage electrical stimulation (HVES) is used in physical therapy to treat acute and chronic pain. Although HVES and faradic current treatments (see page 222) both use electrotherapy for rehabilitation, HVES uses high-voltage pulsed currents, while faradic currents are low-voltage alternating currents with interrupted pulses.

One hypothesis about why HVES might be effective for treating lymphedema is that the currents create an electrical field that can induce the lymphatic system to absorb excess fluid. HVES increases the speed of tissue regeneration, reconnects neural muscular partnerships and increases venous blood flow, all of which allow for absorption of edema. In addition, it activates muscle contractions, which also help the edema to be absorbed (Leal 2009).

> **Technical Breakdown**
> Did you know you can search for clinical trials on medical conditions? A searchable database at clinicaltrials.gov provides a catalogue of research that is currently recruiting, underway or completed. For example, when I type "lymphedema" into the "Condition/Disease" field, there are currently 628 trials listed. If you ever feel discouraged about the progress of research for lymphedema, you can look at the ongoing work that will help progress our understanding of how to prevent or treat it. You may even find you qualify for a study that is recruiting in your area and can reach out to the principle investigator to inquire.

Lymphedema-Specific Research

A review article on complementary therapies including pneumatic compression (page 256), laser therapy (page 241) and HVES summarized the results of three Brazilian studies published between 2005 and 2007 that examined the use of HVES for lymphedema (Leal 2009):

- **Garcia 2005a:** Twenty patients who received either HVES or MLD + compression sleeve experienced about the same improvement in lymphedema circumferences, but the HVES group achieved greater volume reductions.
- **Garcia 2005b:** For fifteen women with arm lymphedema following breast cancer treatment, HVES effectively reduced the volume and severity of the lymphedema.
- **Garcia 2007:** In this case study, three participants with bilateral lymphedema achieved a clinically important reduction after treatment with HVES.

Lymphedema Research in Animals

An animal study on rats with lymphedema experimented with HVES administered at a voltage below the threshold of a visible muscle contraction (Cook 1994). The blue dye injected into the animals to make lymph movement visible was immediately taken up by the animals that received electrical stimulation, while the control animals needed four hours to move the dye. But neither group had a significant reduction in lymphedema limb volume. The authors concluded that HVES "has the potential to reduce edema by increasing lymphatic uptake of proteins."

Side Effects/Risks

None noted.

Bottom Line on High-Voltage Electrical Stimulation

High-voltage electrical stimulation is a common tool of physical therapists who work with rehabilitation and pain. The only human trials that used HVES for lymphedema were published in Portuguese two decades ago, so it may be challenging to find a local practitioner who uses HVES for lymphedema. New research on whether HVES has value as a complementary therapy for lymphedema would be welcome.

References for High-Voltage Electrical Stimulation

Cook HA, Morales M, La Rosa EM, et al. 1994. Effects of Electrical Stimulation on Lymphatic Flow and Limb Volume in the Rat. *Phys Ther* 74 (11): 1040–46.

Garcia LB, Guirro ECO, Montebello MIL. 2005a. Availability of Different Physiotherapeutic Resources Does Not Control Post-Mastectomy Lymphedema. [In Portuguese.] *Rev Bras Mastol* 15 (2): 64–70.

Garcia LB, Guirro ECO, Montebello MIL. 2005b. Effects of High-Voltage Stimulation in Post-Mastectomy Lymphedema. [In Portuguese.] *Rev Bras Fisioter* 9 (2): 243–48.

Garcia LB, Guirro ECO, Montebello MIL. 2007. Effects of High-Voltage Electrical Stimulation in Postmastectomy Bilateral Lymphedema: Case Report. [In Portuguese.] *Fisioter Pesqui* 14 (1): 67–71.

Leal NF, Carrara HH, Vieira KF, Ferreira CH. 2009. Physiotherapy Treatments for Breast Cancer-Related Lymphedema: A Literature Review. *Rev Lat Am Enfermagem* 17 (5): 730–36.

Hivamat

What Is It?

Hivamat (also spelled HIVAMAT) is an acronym for "histologically variable manual technique." It is described on the US distributor's website as "a unique, patented, proven, non-invasive therapy method that creates biological oscillations using electrostatic attraction and friction" (KHG 2023). The device produces vibrations that penetrate 8 centimeters (3.1 inches) below the skin's surface, creating oscillations that have a gentle and deep-acting effect on all tissues. According to the German manufacturer, PhysioMed, the deep oscillation causes blood capillaries to constrict, reducing the loss of blood fluid to extracellular space. It can also dissolve hardened areas of edema and break down collagen fiber structures, providing an antifibrotic effect.

The Hivamat can be administered by a therapist, or you can purchase a personal device and provide your own treatment. The personal device consists of a controller—about the size of a small book—with a screen and a dial, connected by a cord to a handheld wand with a round treatment head. The treatment heads come in three sizes: 1.5 centimeters (0.6 inch), 5 centimeters (2 inches) and 9.5 centimeters (3.7 inches). The clinic version of the controller is a larger desktop unit, and the therapist can administer treatment either with a treatment head or by connecting themselves directly to the controller with an electrode and using their hands while wearing vinyl gloves.

> **Anecdotal Report**
> "I like the Hivamat—seems patients respond well to it and feel more lymph movement with that versus traditional MLD."
>
> —**Anonymous, Lymphedema therapist, Arizona**

Lymphedema-Specific Research

There have been three studies on using Hivamat to treat lymphedema, which I'll summarize in chronological order.

Study #1: Gasbarro 2006

Twenty patients with leg lymphedema had treatments with the Hivamat 200 twice a week for eight weeks. The device was applied for thirty minutes in a pattern that matches manual lymphatic drainage. Each treatment was divided into two phases: medium-high frequency (80 to 200 hertz) to soften the tissue and stimulate fluid transport; and low frequency (25 to 80 hertz) to stimulate a strong pumping effect. Following treatment, a compression garment was applied.

After eight weeks of treatment, ankle circumference had reduced by an average of 1 centimeter (0.4 inch), the upper third of the calf by 1 centimeter (0.4 inch) and the upper third of the thigh by 1.6 centimeters (0.6 inch). Skin thickness decreased by 0.15 centimeter (0.06 inch) for the ankle, 0.1 centimeter (0.04 inch) for the upper third of the calf and 0.19 centimeter (0.08 inch) for the upper third of the thigh. The authors concluded that the optimum treatment is two to three weeks of complete decongestive therapy + deep oscillation.

STUDY #2: JAHR 2008

Twenty-one patients with breast lymphedema were randomly assigned to one of two groups. The treatment group received fifteen minutes of manual lymphatic drainage plus forty-five minutes of deep oscillation in three sessions per week for four weeks ("the therapy"), then eight weeks of MLD on its own ("the treatment"). The control group received thirty to forty-five minutes of MLD of the breast, chest wall and arm, once or twice per week for twelve weeks (treatment only, no therapy).

The evaluation included subjective pain, swelling, range of motion and three-dimensional breast volume. Selected results are summarized in the table below.

Outcome Measure	MLD for 12 Weeks (Control Group)	MLD + Deep Oscillation for 4 Weeks + MLD Alone for 8 Weeks
Pain	No change	Significant reduction vs. pre-treatment and significant reduction vs. control at end of therapy (first four weeks)
Swelling (patient's subjective assessment)	Significant reduction after twelve weeks	Significant reduction after four weeks of therapy
Shoulder mobility	Significant reduction	No change
Cervical spine forward flexion	Worse	Slightly improved
Breast volume	Increased an average of 13 milliliters (0.4 ounces), with a range of −4 to +26 milliliters (−0.1 to +0.9 ounces)	Reduced an average of 16 milliliters (0.5 ounces), with a range of −35 to −6 milliliters (−1.2 to −0.2 ounces) after therapy
Satisfaction	Not reported	Highly satisfied

MLD = manual lymphatic drainage

The authors concluded that MLD + deep oscillation substantially improved outcomes of pain, mobility and lymphedema volume compared with MLD alone. I will point out, though, that the study was not a head-to-head comparison between MLD and deep oscillation, but rather a test of whether the addition of a four-week intensive therapy was superior to standard MLD treatment. The treatment group received more treatment sessions (three times per week for the first four weeks) than the control group (once or twice a week for the duration).

STUDY #3: TEO 2016

Three female patients with lipedema and two male patients with lymphedema had their larger leg treated with the Hivamat 200 and MLD, while the opposite limb was treated with MLD only. The thirty-minute treatments were two times per week for three weeks. After each treatment, the participants donned class 2 or 3 compression garments. The results were as follows:

Subject	Age	Gender	Diagnosis	Hivamat + MLD	MLD Only
1	57	M	Secondary lymphedema	−212 ml (−7.2 oz)	−1,440 ml (−48.7 oz)
2	56	F	Lipedema	−508 ml (−17.2 oz)	−13 ml (−0.4 oz)
3	52	M	Primary lymphedema	−1,723 ml (−58.3 oz)	−827 ml (−28.0 oz)
4	47	F	Lipedema	−920 ml (−31.1 oz)	−105 ml (−3.6 oz)
5	43	F	Lipedema	−1,573 ml (−53.2 oz)	−1,150 ml (−38.9 oz)

The average reduction in the Hivamat + MLD leg was 902 milliliters (30.5 ounces), versus 707 milliliters (24 ounces) in the MLD-only leg, a difference of 195 milliliters (6.6 ounces), which is considered nonsignificant. The authors concluded that while treating only the larger leg with deep oscillation could introduce some bias (the smaller leg has less fluid to move), the results of their pilot study were encouraging.

Side Effects/Risks

No side effects were observed in any of the studies. Contraindications for the Hivamat include acute infections, untreated malignant cancer, cardiac pacemakers and pregnancy (speak to your therapist for a full list). The contraindications apply to both the patient and the therapist if the therapist will be treating the patient with their hands. Hivamat is safe over pins, plates, prostheses, wounds and scars. It is recommended to be well hydrated for best results, and if your therapist is using their hands, they also need to be well hydrated (PhysioPod, n.d.).

Bottom Line on Hivamat

The Hivamat creates deep-acting electrostatic oscillations in tissues including skin, subcutaneous fat, muscle, and blood and lymph vessels. Treatment can be performed by a professional or self-administered, and benefits for lymphedema have been shown in three small studies, including one of breast lymphedema, which is often not included in research. This therapy seems promising, but more randomized controlled trials would be welcome to confirm efficacy and help determine the best timing, intensity and duration for best results.

References for Hivamat

Gasbarro V, Bartoletti R, Tsolaki E, et al. 2006. Role of HIVAMAT® (Deep Oscillation) in the Treatment for the Lymphedema of the Limbs. *Eur J Lymphology Relat Probl* 16 (48): 13–15.

Jahr S, Schoppe B, Reisshauer A. 2008. Effect of Treatment with Low-Intensity and Extremely Low-Frequency Electrostatic Fields (Deep Oscillation) on Breast Tissue and Pain in Patients with Secondary Breast Lymphoedema. *J Rehabil Med* 40 (8): 645–50.

Kismet Holdings Group (KHG). 2023. "The Authentic Hivamat® Deep Oscillation." Accessed July 4, 2025. https://www.hivamatus.com/.

PhysioPod UK Ltd. n.d. "FAQ Deep Oscillation Therapy for Practitioners and Patients." Accessed July 20, 2025. https://www.physiopod.co.uk/assets/pdfs/Physiopod-FAQbook2017.pdf.

Teo I, Coulborn A, Munnock DA. 2016. Use of the HIVAMAT 200 with Manual Lymphatic Drainage in the Management of Lower Limb Lymphoedema and Lipoedema. *J Lymphoedema* 11 (1): 49–53.

Hyperbaric Oxygen

What Is It?

Hyperbaric oxygen is oxygen delivered under pressure. You enter a hyperbaric oxygen chamber, which resembles a jet cockpit. The air pressure is increased, then 100% oxygen is pumped into the chamber, providing oxygen at 221% above what you would normally breathe. Under these conditions, the lungs can gather more oxygen, which the blood then carries throughout the body to promote healing. The results include vasoconstriction (narrowed blood vessels), reduced edema, increased dissolved oxygen in the plasma and increased oxygen attached to red blood cells (Claus 2017). Supplying oxygen to damaged tissues improves blood flow and generates new blood vessels, which promotes wound healing and reduces fibrosis (Koo 2020).

Hyperbaric oxygen is used to treat several conditions, including carbon monoxide poisoning, decompression illness, bone injury, diabetic wounds, air bubbles in blood (air embolism) and delayed radiation injury (Koo 2020).

How does hyperbaric oxygen therapy work? Air pressure is measured in atmospheres (ATM). Air pressure at sea level is 1 ATM. When you dive 12 meters (40 feet) below sea level, it is 2.21 ATM, and at 18 meters (60 feet) below it is 3 ATM. Inside a hyperbaric chamber, the air pressure is usually increased to 2 ATM (10 meters/33 feet below sea level). The normal composition of the air we breathe is 78% nitrogen and 21% oxygen. In the chamber, 100% oxygen is delivered.

Technical Breakdown
Did you know that hyperbaric medicine is a subspeciality of emergency medicine? Hyperbaric medicine specialists determine the best hyperbaric oxygen prescription to treat scuba divers and patients with slow-healing wounds and carbon monoxide poisoning, among other conditions.

Lymphedema-Specific Research

One case report and five studies have been published on using hyperbaric oxygen to treat lymphedema.

CASE REPORT: TEAS 2004

Within a pilot study (discussed below), the authors described an unpublished case study of a forty-one-year-old premenopausal women with arm lymphedema following mastectomy and chemotherapy (but no radiation). After twenty hyperbaric oxygen treatments, she experienced a 90% reduction in swelling. She gradually reduced the use of her compression garment during the treatment period until week three, after which she no longer wore it except for air travel. She also noted the resolution of her "chemo brain." Her results continued for three years post-treatment.

STUDY #1: TEAS 2004

In the same publication, the authors detailed a small pilot trial with ten healthy women who had developed arm lymphedema following breast cancer treatment that included surgery, axillary dissection and radiation. On average, they had had lymphedema for nine years. The hyperbaric oxygen treatments consisted of 100% oxygen for ninety minutes at 2.0 ATM, five times a week for four weeks. Lymphedema was measured by circumference and water displacement immediately before and after the sessions.

The results were inconsistent. Some women lost volume, some gained it, and some lost or gained it in different locations on the arm across fourteen to sixteen measurements. On average, there was a volume increase of 5 milliliters (0.2 ounces) after the final treatment, an increase of 42 milliliters (1.4 ounces) one month later and a loss of 75 milliliters (2.5 ounces) at the final measurement, seven to twenty months after the sessions ended (but this final follow-up included only seven of the original ten participants). Overall, the best results were in the hand.

In terms of individual responses, the greatest benefit was seen by subject #3, who had lost 291 milliliters (9.8 ounces) by the end of the treatment period and maintained a loss of 210 milliliters (7.1 ounces) months later. Some participants reported improvement in numbness, tightness or softness, but one women said her arm felt "lumpier."

In the end, no clinically or statistically significant changes in lymphedema were seen. But interestingly, the three women with the best outcomes did not wear a compression garment prior to or during the study, leading the researchers to speculate that active compression might inhibit the healing process offered by hyperbaric oxygen therapy.

Study #2: Gothard 2004

Twenty-one people with arm lymphedema following radiation therapy (and, for the majority, axillary surgery) received 100% oxygen at 2.4 ATM for 100 minutes, in thirty sessions over six weeks. Twelve months after the treatment period, three participants had experienced a 20% or greater reduction in lymphedema, and six participants had a 25% or greater improvement in lymph clearance, as seen in a lymphoscintigraphy. On average, there was a 7.5% reduction in lymphedema volume, which the authors described as clinically modest but statistically significant. More than half of the participants reported that their arms felt softer, and six reported improvements in shoulder mobility. Although there was no control group for comparison, the authors concluded that "there is sufficient evidence to justify a double-blind randomised controlled trial of hyperbaric oxygen."

Study #3: Gothard 2010

This randomized study focused on fifty-eight women with arm lymphedema following radiation treatment for breast cancer (fifty-six) or Hodgkin's lymphoma (two); the majority had also had surgery. Thirty-eight of the women received hyperbaric oxygen therapy, while twenty served as the control group. The treatment group received 100% oxygen at 2.4 ATM for 100 minutes, five days a week for six weeks.

After the final treatment, 30% of the women had an 8% or greater reduction in their lymphedema arm, compared to 19% of the control group; while positive, this difference is not statistically significant. Lymphatic clearance rates, as measured by lymphoscintigraphy, were not significantly improved in either the treatment or the control group. However, the treatment group had a greater improvement in extracellular fluid volume in the upper arm, detected using a dielectric moisture meter.

Study #4: Koo 2020

In this study, five patients with breast cancer–related lymphedema received CDT only, while another five received CDT + hyperbaric oxygen in five treatments per week for two weeks. During treatment, they breathed 100% oxygen at 2.4 ATM for 100 minutes, with two five-minute air breaks. At the end of the treatment period, bioimpedance showed more significant improvements in lymphedema for CDT + hyperbaric oxygen than for CDT alone.

Study #5: Ammitzbøll 2023

In this Danish study, nineteen women with breast cancer–related lymphedema completed forty hyperbaric oxygen therapy sessions every weekday for eight weeks and returned for follow-up after six months. Although there was no improvement in their lymphedema (as measured by arm mass, volume or lymphatic drainage), the women reported improved quality of life, physical functioning, insomnia and breast and arm symptoms. The authors recommended more research on hyperbaric oxygen therapy to explore treatment of soft tissue radiation injury.

Related Research

In addition to the lymphedema-specific research discussed above, there are two studies on the use of hyperbaric oxygen for cancer survivors.

Study #1: Teguh 2016

Fifty-seven cancer survivors with late radiation toxicity received forty-seven sessions of 100% oxygen at 2.4 ATM for eighty minutes. After the treatment period, when the participants were asked to rate their symptoms, 26% reported an improvement in hand and arm swelling, and 58% reported an improvement in breast swelling. The therapy was well tolerated, with minimal and reversible side effects.

Study #2: Batenburg 2021

This study included over 1,000 breast cancer survivors. Compared to the control group, those who were treated with hyperbaric oxygen reported reduced pain, breast and arm symptoms and improved quality of life. Interestingly, non-smokers and former smokers had better outcomes than current smokers. Also, participants who didn't respond to the therapy tended to be older. Based on these results, the authors are proceeding with a randomized controlled trial to further test the efficacy of hyperbaric oxygen in this population.

Side Effects/Risks

One study reported a single patient whose arm felt "lumpier" (Teas 2004). Risks include temporary and reversible tiredness, nearsightedness (myopia) and mild baro-trauma—damage, often of the inner ear, caused by pressure differences between gases within the body and those surrounding the body. Some moderate or severe non-reversible side effects reported in the Batenburg study were oxygen toxicity, sinus squeeze and cataracts.

Contraindications include claustrophobia, inability to clear the ears when pressure changes, sinus or ear surgery or infections, emphysema/chronic lung disease, hypo-glycemia or uncontrolled diabetes, uncontrolled fever, active cancer, HIV, eye conditions such as optic neuritis, and blood abnormalities such as sickle cell disease.

Bottom Line on Hyperbaric Oxygen

Based on the evidence to date, hyperbaric oxygen therapy definitely falls into the "results may vary" category. It has promise, but the trick seems to be figuring out who benefits from it. At this time, there isn't enough evidence to make broad recommendations on using it for lymphedema. If you are receiving hyperbaric oxygen for another condition, such as wound healing, speak to your specialist about whether you should wear a compression garment during treatment; based on the limited data, you may get more lymphedema benefit if you don't. The data also suggests that younger people and non-smokers benefit more. There is conflicting information on how soon after radiation this therapy should be done.

References for Hyperbaric Oxygen

Ammitzbøll G, Hyldegaard O, Forchhammer M, et al. 2023. Effects of an Early Intervention with Hyperbaric Oxygen Treatment on Arm Lymphedema and Quality of Life After Breast Cancer—An Explorative Clinical Trial. *Support Care Cancer* 31 (5): 313.

Batenburg MCT, Maarse W, van der Leij F, et al. 2021. The Impact of Hyperbaric Oxygen Therapy on Late Radiation Toxicity and Quality of Life in Breast Cancer Patients. *Breast Cancer Res Treat* 189 (2): 425–33.

Claus P, host. 2017. "Hyperbaric Oxygen Therapy." *Mayo Clinic Radio* (podcast), December 2. Accessed June 15, 2022. https://www.youtube.com/watch?v=QfdwLtPj5EY.

Gothard L, Haviland J, Bryson P, et al. 2010. Randomised Phase II Trial of Hyperbaric Oxygen Therapy in Patients with Chronic Arm Lymphoedema After Radiotherapy for Cancer. *Radiother Oncol* 97 (1): 101–7.

Gothard L, Stanton A, MacLaren J, et al. 2004. Non-randomised Phase II Trial of Hyperbaric Oxygen Therapy in Patients with Chronic Arm Lymphoedema and Tissue Fibrosis After Radiotherapy for Early Breast Cancer. *Radiother Oncol* 2004 70 (3): 217–24.

Koo JH, Song SH, Oh HS, Oh SH. 2020. Comparison of the Short-Term Effects of Hyperbaric Oxygen Therapy and Complex Decongestive Therapy on Breast Cancer-Related Lymphedema: A Pilot Study. *Medicine* (Baltimore) 99 (11): e19564.

Teas J, Cunningham JE, Cone L, et al. 2004. Can Hyperbaric Oxygen Therapy Reduce Breast Cancer Treatment-Related Lymphedema? A Pilot Study. *J Womens Health* (Larchmont) 13 (9): 1008–18.

Teguh DN, Bol Raap R, Struikmans H, et al. 2016. Hyperbaric Oxygen Therapy for Late Radiation-Induced Tissue Toxicity: Prospectively Patient-Reported Outcome Measures in Breast Cancer Patients. *Radiat Oncol* 11 (1): 130.

Kinetec Centura Lite

What Is It?

The Kinetec Centura Lite is a rehabilitation device that, according to the manufacturer's website, is designed to provide continuous passive motion (CPM) therapy at home (Kinetec 2025). Picture a chair with a small motor in the back, an armrest on one side and a metal frame with Velcro straps on the other side. When you sit in the chair, the therapist adjusts it to the proper height, then you place your affected arm in the metal frame and secure it with the straps. Your therapist adjusts the settings and turns on the device, which gently and repeatedly moves your arm in either flexion/extension or abduction/adduction motions. Rather than exercising, you are letting the machine do the work for you. The RAGodoy (see page 261) is another example of a passive motion device.

> **Technical Breakdown**
> Flexion/extension of the shoulder is when you move your arm forward, in front of your body, then return it to hang naturally beside your body, similar to swinging your arm as you walk or march. Abduction/adduction is the movement of raising your arm to the side and then lowering it, as you would when doing a jumping jack or making a snow angel.

Lymphedema-Specific Research

In a randomized controlled trial that included thirty women with breast cancer–related lymphedema, sixteen patients received complete decongestive therapy alone, while fourteen received CDT + continuous passive shoulder flexion (raising and lowering the arm in front of the body) using the Kinetec Centura Lite (Kizil 2018). The CPM exercises lasted for twenty minutes for the first five sessions, then thirty minutes for the next ten sessions. Arm volume was measured throughout the study. In addition, participants completed two questionnaires, one on their shoulder and arm disability, and the other evaluating their quality of life.

After the treatment period, all of the participants had reduced arm volume, with larger but not statistically significant reductions in the CPM group. Shoulder range of motion also improved for all participants, though surprisingly, it was not significantly greater in the treatment group. However, a statistically significant higher number of patients in the CPM group reported improved quality of life, which the authors postulated might be due to improved pain and patient satisfaction, two measures that were not included in their analysis.

Side Effects/Risks

None noted.

Bottom Line on Kinetec Centura Lite

To date, there is only one study on the use of the Kinetec Centura Lite to treat arm lymphedema with continuous passive shoulder movement. While all of the participants improved, the only statistically significant improvement between the treatment group and the control group was in quality of life. Future research could examine the treatment for patients with newly diagnosed lymphedema (the Kizil study used participants who'd had lymphedema for two years), the effects of passive shoulder abduction (the Kizil study used flexion only), changes in pain and patient satisfaction (which were not measured in the Kizil study) and longer-term follow-up. Despite lackluster initial outcomes, we may not have heard the last of the Kinetec Centura Lite for managing arm lymphedema.

References for Kinetec Centura Lite

Kinetec. 2025. "Centura Lite—Single Motor." Accessed July 20, 2025. https://www.kinetecusa.com/shop/cpm-active/shoulder-cpms/kinetec-centura-lite-single-motor/.

Kizil R, Dilek B, Şahin E, et al. 2018. Is Continuous Passive Motion Effective in Patients with Lymphedema? A Randomized Controlled Trial. *Lymphat Res Biol* 16 (3): 263–69.

Linforoll

What Is It?

Although the Linforoll (also spelled LINFORoll) looks like a small paint roller attached to an angled handle with push buttons, it is a sophisticated medical device made by Cizeta Medicali in Italy. The roller piece contains pressure sensors that transmit data wirelessly to a computer, where it is displayed on a screen. According to the company's website, the device shows the therapist objective data such as the force applied during lymphatic drainage, the number of passes to make in a particular area, whether they are achieving the proper speed of 3 centimeters (1.2 inches) per second, and the energy transferred to the patient. The Linforoll can be used for lymphedema, venous edema, post-traumatic edema and lipedema (Cizeta Medicali, n.d.).

Lymphedema-Specific Research

In a study of twenty individuals with lymphedema (fifteen leg and five arm), the affected limb was divided into sections. Each section was treated with twenty-five rolls at a speed of six rolls per minute and 15 centimeters (6 inches) per ten seconds, using a pressure between 80 and 120 mmHg for the leg and between 60 and 100 mmHg for the arm (Olszewski 2016). If the roller encountered hard tissue, more pressure would be applied, but if it exceeded 150 mmHg, a red light would indicate it should be eased. Any painful areas detected during rolling would be avoided in future passes. The treatments lasted an hour and were provided for fourteen days.

One of the benefits of Linforoll treatment is the ability to view the movement of fluid and continuously monitor and adjust the pressure. The patients experienced an increase in tissue elasticity, especially on the calf and forearm, which they felt was the most important outcome. Other results included decreased limb volume. There was no control group for comparison.

Additional research using this device is cited on the Italian Lymphoedema Framework's website (ILF 2022).

Technical Breakdown

The terms "objective" and "subjective" are very common in medical practice. In fact, there is a charting style called SOAP, which stands for "subjective, objective, assessment, plan." Subjective data includes a patient's complaints and how they present; for example: "A fifty-six-year-old woman post–breast cancer treatment complains of swelling and heaviness in her left arm. She reports she can no longer wear rings and her watch leaves an indentation in her wrist." Objective data would be measurements of, for example, the patient's height, current weight, usual weight and percentage of weight change. A lymphedema therapist would also include circumference measurements and arm volume calculations in their objective data. Medical professionals use subjective and objective data along with their critical thinking skills and experience to assess and make a treatment plan.

Side Effects/Risks

No side effects were noted, but the manufacturer's website notes several contraindications: tissue inflammation, venous thrombosis, post-traumatic tissue changes and pain during rolling (Cizeta Medicali, n.d.).

Bottom Line on Linforoll

The Linforoll quite literally takes manual lymphatic drainage out of therapists' hands and replaces them with a sophisticated medical device that provides objective data points. The Italian Lymphoedema Framework's website sums it up succinctly: "LIN-FORoll is a medical device that aims to make the Drainage of Edema 'OBJECTIVE and REPEATABLE'" (ILF 2022). The objectivity of the Linforoll replaces the subjectivity, experience and sensitivity of the therapist. I imagine this device will garner some pretty strong opinions from therapists. Those who have spent their careers feeling their way through MLD and developing a very sensitive touch may be resistant. Others may embrace the data-driven and purely objective feedback, particularly for treatment-resistant patients, where they may need some support.

The Linforoll may be most practical in remote or underserviced areas where highly trained, touch-sensitive practitioners are not available. At this point, a trained practitioner is still required to administer the device, which may increase its cost and decrease its accessibility in the short term. More research on the Linforoll would be welcome, but I admire the out-of-the-box thinking and medical engineering that led to its creation.

References for Linforoll

Cizeta Medicali. n.d. "LINFORoll®. Accessed July 6, 2025. https://www.cizetamedicali.com/en/product/linforoll-2/.

Italian Lymphoedema Framework (ILF). 2022. "LINFORoll®." Accessed June 29, 2025. https://www.italf.org/en/linforoll/.

Olszewski WL, Zaleska M, Michelin S. 2016. A New Method for Treatment of Lymphedema of Limbs: Standardized Manual Massage with a New Device Linforoll in Conservative and Surgical Therapy Protocols. *Lymphat Res Biol* 14 (4): 226–32.

Low-Level Laser

What Is It?

The word "laser" is an acronym for "light amplification by stimulated emission of radiation." Low-level laser therapy (LLLT) is also called light therapy, low-intensity laser therapy, cold laser therapy, laser phototherapy, photobiomodulation (PBM), and photobiomodulation therapy (PBMT). It uses visible red and near-infrared portions of the electromagnetic spectrum, which are highly absorbed by the body. It's a noninvasive form of phototherapy that uses wavelengths of light between 650 and 1,000 nanometers to deliver low-irradiance doses to the target tissue.

Laser is low energy density, but high enough to stimulate the membrane or organelles of cells. The chromophores in cells absorb photons. When stimulated by laser energy, they promote cell proliferation, resulting in changes to tissue properties such as structure, water content, thermal conductivity, heat capacity, density and the ability to absorb, scatter or reflect emitted energy (Arjmand 2021).

The RianCorp LTU-904, manufactured in Australia, is a low-level laser device that is FDA-approved for the treatment of lymphedema (FDA 2025) but has not yet been submitted for approval in Canada. It operates at 904 nanometers. A certification course is not required to use the device; in fact, it can be self-administered at home.

User Experience
"My current lymphedema therapist has a handheld low-level laser that really makes my ankle feel better. I have a compression pump that I use every day—if I have done any foam rolling or the vibration plate before using the pump, I notice more fluid movement out of my leg."

—Anonymous, Colorado (secondary lymphedema of the leg, abdomen and genitals)

Lymphedema-Specific Research

There is a lot of research on laser for lymphedema, with reviews and even a review of reviews.

OVERVIEW OF SYSTEMATIC REVIEWS: WANG 2022

Seven reviews were included in this overview of systematic reviews of low-level laser therapy in breast cancer patients with lymphedema. Although most studies have demonstrated efficacy in the management of breast cancer lymphedema, not all reviews have yielded positive outcomes. Some things to keep in mind:

- Energy density is important: If it's too low, there is no significant effect; if it's too high, unwanted inhibitory effects occur.
- The ideal energy density appears to be 1.5 to 2.4 joules per square centimeter.
- The sessions analyzed in the reviews lasted from seventeen to thirty-four minutes.
- Session frequency varied from daily for ten days to three times per week for twelve weeks.

For positive results, a well-conceived therapy schedule and an adequate laser configuration are necessary. Because the overview was not conclusive, the overview authors did their own review of individual studies. They concluded that:

- Low-level laser therapy leads to greater improvements than compression therapy, placebo laser or no treatment.
- There is no statistically significant difference in results between low-level laser therapy and complete decongestive therapy, manual lymphatic drainage or conventional therapy.
- Low-level laser therapy appears to be relatively safe.

So that clinical practice guidelines can be created, the overview authors advocated for more high-quality randomized controlled trials with large sample sizes and long-term follow-up.

Technical Breakdown
The energy density of a laser is measured in joules per square centimeter (J/cm^2): the total energy delivered by the laser, divided by the area of the beam. The total energy in joules is calculated by multiplying the laser's power in watts by the exposure time in seconds.

CLINICAL PRACTICE GUIDELINES: DAVIES 2020

The Academy of Oncologic Physical Therapy, an academy of the American Physical Therapy Association (APTA) has issued the following practice guidelines on low-level laser therapy for arm lymphedema: "Low-level laser therapy may be considered either in combination with compression or CDT in patients with established lymphedema of the upper extremity."

REVIEW #1: MAHMOOD 2022

This review, which was not included in the Wang overview, analyzed eight clinical trials on breast cancer–related lymphedema and found that low-level laser therapy led to a considerable reduction in arm circumference and volume that continued during long-term follow-up, but no significant improvement in pain or shoulder mobility.

> **User Experience**
> "I swear by my laser. I have patterns for the arms and legs. Both include the core, plus I have patterns for my head."
>
> **—Willa, British Columbia (full-body primary lymphedema tarda)**

REVIEW #2: WAHID 2024

This recent review looked at the efficacy of low-level laser, Endermologie (see page 212) and Kinesio taping (page 108) for lymphedema. It included nine studies on low-level laser therapy published between 2003 and 2020. The review authors concluded that there was a significant reduction in lymphedema volume when patients were treated with laser, that breast cancer survivors had better outcomes with laser than with conventional therapy, and that low-level laser provided more significant reduction in arm volume than Endermologie.

LASER VERSUS ENDERMOLOGIE: ZIETHAR 2021

In contrast to the Wahid review, this study, which compared Endermologie and low-level laser for lymphedema, found that Endermologie was more effective at reducing arm circumference and lymphedema fluid volume. See Endermologie (page 212) for more details on this study.

Related Research

A review of studies on low-level laser in oncology (Bensadoun 2020) observed the following therapeutic outcomes: tissue regeneration, wound healing, reduced inflammation and pain, immunomodulation, prevention of oral mucositis in head and neck cancer patients, and management of soft tissue necrosis and bone necrosis in cancer patients.

Side Effects/Risks

A 2020 systematic review warned that low-level laser therapy "should be used with caution in cancer patients until more studies are performed" (da Silva 2020). An earlier publication echoed this warning, saying: "Although evidence suggests that PBM using LLLT is safe in [head and neck cancer] patients, more research is imperative and vigilance remains warranted to detect any potential adverse effects of PBM on cancer treatment outcomes and survival" (Zecha 2016).

The Bensadoun review, which included sixty-seven studies (forty-three in vitro, fifteen in vivo and nine clinical trials), found conflicting data on the safety and efficacy of low-level laser therapy in oncology (Bensadoun 2020). It seems probable that different tumors react differently to the range of activity associated with low-level laser therapy.

Bottom Line on Low-Level Laser

Low-level laser appears to be a credible complementary therapy for lymphedema. The results of multiple studies and reviews have been positive for reductions in volume and circumference of the lymphedema limb, but less convincing for pain and range of motion. It is included in the clinical practice guidelines as a therapy worthy of consideration for physical therapists when treating lymphedema. One device approved by the FDA specifically for lymphedema (but not yet submitted for approval in Canada) is the RianCorp LTU-904 (Australia). Readers who are interested in low-level laser therapy should look for a therapist who has experience with this device where it is available. Caution is recommended for individuals with cancer.

References for Low-Level Laser

Arjmand B, Khodadost M, Jahani Sherafat S, et al. 2021. Low-Level Laser Therapy: Potential and Complications. *J Lasers Med Sci* 12 (August): e42.

Bensadoun RJ, Epstein JB, Nair RG, et al.; World Association for Laser Therapy (WALT). 2020. Safety and Efficacy of Photobiomodulation Therapy in Oncology: A Systematic Review. *Cancer Med* 9 (22): 8279–300.

da Silva JL, Silva-de-Oliveira AFS, Andraus RAC, Maia LP. 2020. Effects of Low Level Laser Therapy in Cancer Cells—A Systematic Review of the Literature. *Lasers Med Sci* 35 (3): 523–29.

Davies C, Levenhagen K, Ryans K, et al. 2020. Interventions for Breast Cancer-Related Lymphedema: Clinical Practice Guideline from the Academy of Oncologic Physical Therapy of APTA. *Phys Ther* 100 (7): 1163–79.

Food & Drug Administration (FDA). 2025. "LTU-904 Portable Laser Therapy Unit." Accessed July 20, 2025. https://www.accessdata.fda.gov/scripts/cdrh/devicesatfda/index.cfm?db=pmn&id=K030295.

Mahmood D, Ahmad A, Sharif F, Arslan SA. 2022. Clinical Application of Low-Level Laser Therapy (Photo-Biomodulation Therapy) in the Management of Breast Cancer-Related Lymphedema: A Systematic Review. *BMC Cancer* 22 (1): 937.

Wahid DI, Wahyono RA, Setiaji K, et al. 2024. The Effication of Low-Level Laser Therapy, Kinesio Taping, and Endermology on Post-Mastectomy Lymphedema: A Systematic Review and Meta-Analysis. *Asian Pac J Cancer Prev* 25 (11): 3771–79.

Wang Y, Ge Y, Xing W, et al. 2022. The Effectiveness and Safety of Low-Level Laser Therapy on Breast Cancer-Related Lymphedema: An Overview and Update of Systematic Reviews. *Lasers Med Sci* 37 (3): 1389–413.

Zecha JA, Raber-Durlacher JE, Nair RG, et al. 2016. Low Level Laser Therapy/Photobiomodulation in the Management of Side Effects of Chemoradiation Therapy in Head and Neck Cancer: Part 1: Mechanisms of Action, Dosimetric, and Safety Considerations. *Support Care Cancer* 24 (6): 2781–92.

Ziethar MMA, Waked IS, Toson RA, Sherif RRA. 2021. Endermologie Versus Low Level Laser Therapy on Post Mastectomy Lymphedema. *Med J Cairo Univ* 89 (4): 1359–66.

LymphaTouch

What Is It?

The LymphaTouch is a handheld mechanical device that delivers negative pressure—the same action as cupping (page 35), but with more precise mechanical controls. It is one of two negative pressure high-tech devices currently available; the other is the Vacumed (page 269). The LymphaTouch is approved as a medical device in the European Union (CE marking) and the United States (FDA approval).

Created in Finland in 2005 by LymphaTouch Oy, the LymphaTouch is designed to help people with lymphatic and circulatory issues. According to the manufacturer's website, "The patented technology of LymphaTouch combines negative pressure and mechanical high-frequency vibration, which activates the lymphatic circulation and soft tissues in the treated area" (LymphaTouch 2025). It delivers between 80 and 250 mmHg of suction pressure, which pulls your tissue into the suction cup (Ersoy 2023). It can be used for pain management, soft tissue mobilization, scar therapy and edema management.

Anecdotal Report

"In my experience, the LymphaTouch works well for fibrosis."

—Anonymous, lymphedema therapist, Arizona

Lymphedema-Specific Research

Two recent clinical trials and one narrative review that includes another five studies have looked specifically at using the LymphaTouch to treat lymphedema.

STUDY #1: LAMPINEN 2021

Twenty-eight breast cancer survivors with arm lymphedema living around San Franciso were randomly assigned to either MLD or negative pressure treatment with LymphaTouch. The treatment group received two or three one-hour LymphaTouch sessions per week for four to six weeks, for a total of twelve sessions. The control group received twelve one-hour sessions of MLD. The pressure used by the therapists for either treatment was based on their clinical judgment, taking into consideration patient comfort, tissue induration and amount of swelling. Compression sleeves were donned after each treatment and kept on for a minimum of two hours. Patients were assessed for circumference and bioelectrical impedance (a measure of extracellular fluid volume), and answered questions about their arm function on the DASH (Disabilities of the Arm, Shoulder and Hand) questionnaire. The assessor was blinded on the treatment received.

The limb volume of all participants improved, with significantly greater reductions in the women who received LymphaTouch treatments. Only the LymphaTouch patients saw improved bioimpedance scores, a result that was significantly greater than for the

MLD group. There were no differences in DASH scores when comparing pre- and post-treatment.

The authors concluded that the LymphaTouch may be more effective than MLD alone in reducing lymphedema severity, based on significant improvements in bioimpedance scores and changes in arm volume. These results were achieved even though the group randomly assigned to receive LymphaTouch treatment turned out to include more women who had had lymphedema for more than five years. This led the authors to suggest that LymphaTouch may be the superior treatment for chronic lymphedema. They hypothesized that the significant results may be due to the stimulation of lymphatic flow by stretching the skin and subcutaneous fascia, and that this may be beneficial when fibrosis is present. They speculated that the lack of improvement in the DASH survey could be because the women in this study had low functional impairments when they began the study.

Study #2: Ersoy 2023

This clinical trial enrolled thirty women who had developed lymphedema of the leg secondary to cancer treatment and had been in stage 1 or 2 for an average for five years. The participants were divided into two treatment groups for fifteen sessions, lasting forty-five minutes, of either MLD or negative pressure massage therapy with the LymphaTouch. In addition, they donned compression garments after their sessions and were taught and encouraged to do self-MLD.

All of the women experienced statistically significant improvements, but those receiving LymphaTouch treatment had better results for all six circumference measures. In their abstract, the authors stated that the LymphaTouch also reduced pain and discomfort significantly more than MLD, but a table in the full article seems to contradict that. I've reproduced the mean data from that table below so you can see the numbers for yourself. The numbers represent the difference between the pre-treatment and post-treatment results, so a larger number means a greater improvement.

	Difference Between Before and After Negative Pressure Massage Therapy	Difference Between Before and After Manual Lymphatic Drainage
10-Point Visual Analog Scales		
Pain	1.85 points	1.97 points
Discomfort	3.21 points	3.91 points
Circumference Measurements		
Metatarsophalangeal	1.2 cm	1.0 cm
Ankle	1.2 cm	1.0 cm
10 cm to ankle	3.4 cm	2.5 cm
20 cm to ankle	3.3 cm	2.1 cm
30 cm to ankle	2.2 cm	1.4 cm
40 cm to ankle	1.8 cm	1.0 cm

Narrative Review: Kimball 2018

This literature review included five small studies and an interview with a lymphedema therapist who had been using the LymphaTouch in their practice for several years. After reviewing the five articles, the author concluded that the Lympha-Touch reduces tissue stiffness, limb volume, inflammation, adipose tissue and fibrosis (Vuorinen 2013), and has potential to be used to screen for changes in soft tissue (Iivarinen 2013) and to reduce pain and lymphedema without discomfort for the patient (Airaksinen 2011). One of the studies suggested that continuous suction moves fluid more effectively than cyclical suction (Iivarinen 2016).

Related Research

Various studies have examined using the LymphaTouch to treat chemotherapy-induced peripheral neuropathy, radiation-induced fibrosis, low back pain, general post-operative swelling, sclerosis treatment and soft tissue issues. If any of these topics are of interest to you, you can read the results of the studies by following the links at https://lymphatouch.com/references/.

Side Effects/Risks

None noted.

Bottom Line on LymphaTouch

To date, results from studies of the LymphaTouch appear positive, and there are no noted side effects. Some lymphedema therapists are already using this device, and I suspect you will be hearing more about it. It seems to be worth exploring as a complementary therapy for lymph volume reduction, limb stiffness and pain, especially when used on the continuous setting or where lymphedema has been present for more than five years. There may even be a role for the LymphaTouch in diagnosing lymphedema. If your lymphedema therapist has one of these devices, it might be a good addition to your routine. Of course, more and larger studies would be welcome, to help strengthen recommendations for this therapy.

References for LymphaTouch

Airaksinen O, Vuorinen V-P, Raittila S. 2011. "Influence of LymphaTouch® Treatment Method for Pain and Edema in Context of Active Physiotherapy." LymphaTouch Internal Research Report.

Ersoy S, Kesiktaş N, Şirin B, et al. 2023. Comparison of Manual Lymphatic Drainage Massage and Negative Pressure Massage Therapy Efficacy in Lymphedema Patients: A Randomized Controlled Study. *Eur Res J* 9 (6): 1474–82.

Iivarinen JT, Korhonen RK, Julkunen P, Jurvelin JS. 2013. Experimental and Computational Analysis of Soft Tissue Mechanical Response Under Negative Pressure in Forearm. *Skin Res Technol* 19 (1): e356–65.

Iivarinen JT, Korhonen RK, Jurvelin JS. 2016. Modeling of Interstitial Fluid Movement in Soft Tissue Under Negative Pressure—Relevance to Treatment of Tissue Swelling. *Comput Methods Biomech Biomed Engin* 19 (10): 1089–98.

Kimball KD. 2018. "LymphaTouch as a Tool for Manual Lymph Drainage: A Therapist's Perspective." *Occupational Therapy: Student Scholarship and Creative Works* 3. Accessed February 4, 2024. https://core.ac.uk/reader/268401089.

Lampinen R, Lee JQ, Leano J, et al. 2021. Treatment of Breast Cancer-Related Lymphedema Using Negative Pressure Massage: A Pilot Randomized Controlled Trial. *Arch Phys Med Rehabil* 102 (8): 1465–72.e2.

LymphaTouch. 2025. "Operating Principle." Accessed July 8, 2025. https://lymphatouch.com/.

Vuorinen VP, Iivarinen J, Jurvelin J, Airaksinen O. 2013. "Lymphatic Therapy Using Negative Pressure: A Clinical Study with the Lympha-Touch® Device." Finnish Funding Agency for Technology and Innovation (5320003), 221.

Manutech BH

What Is It?

Through conductive gloves worn by the therapist, the Manutech BH measures impedance in body tissue as the therapist performs therapeutic movements and then delivers microcurrents with intensity and frequency patterns that are adjusted in real time by the device's artificial intelligence. Magnesium gel applied to the patient's skin optimizes the transmission of the electrical signals.

Developed by the Italian manufacturer Talamonti, the Manutech BH can be used to treat many different conditions, including lymphedema and lipedema (Talamonti Group 2022). It evolved from two of their previous products, the Flowave and the Transponder, which both demonstrated potential in small studies on their efficacy for lymphedema (see pages 224 and 264).

Lymphedema-Specific Research

The Manutech BH was the device used in the Cavezzi study discussed under "Integrative Therapy" (page 7) in "Complementary, Alternative and Integrative Care." To recap, forty-one patients with stage 2 or 3 leg lymphedema completed an intensive six-day program of MLD, lymphatic drainage with the Manutech BH, multilayer short stretch bandaging, a low-carbohydrate diet, anti-inflammatory supplements and exercise. After seeing progressive improvement in limb volume and reduced extracellular fluids over the treatment period, the authors concluded that their protocol was beneficial in the short term (Cavezzi 2020).

This was the only English-language study I could find that included the Manutech BH in its protocol. Obviously, further research is needed to isolate the effects of the device and determine its role as a complementary therapy for lymphedema.

Side Effects/Risks
None noted.

Bottom Line on Manutech BH
This device sounds exciting, but we need to see studies evaluating the Manutech BH on its own, not only as part of a holistic protocol. By refining its previous products, the Flowave and Transponder, and learning from their successes and weakness, Talamonti has presumably improved the technology and will continue to do so. The Manutech BH is definitely one to watch, and hopefully research will confirm its efficacy for treating lymphedema.

References for Manutech BH

Cavezzi A, Urso SU, Paccasassi S, et al. 2020. Bioimpedance Spectroscopy and Volumetry in the Immediate/Short-Term Monitoring of Intensive Complex Decongestive Treatment of Lymphedema. *Phlebology* 35 (9): 715–23.

Talamonti Group. 2022. "Manutech BH." Accessed July 9, 2025. https://www.talamontigroup.solutions/manutechbh/.

Microcurrent Therapy

What Is It?
Microcurrent therapy uses low electrical currents, applied to the skin, to stimulate healing. The intensity of the currents is less than 1 milliampere, below the threshold that would activate muscle contraction. Microcurrent therapy is thought to work at a cellular level, and is used to reduce musculoskeletal pain, treat wounds, reduce fibrosis, decrease inflammation and promote the creation of new blood vessels (Cho 2023).

Lymphedema-Specific Research
I was unable to locate any human studies using microcurrent therapy to treat lymphedema.

Lymphedema Research in Animals
Twelve rats had forelimb lymphedema induced by axillary (armpit) lymph node dissection (Cho 2023). After a two-week recovery, half of the rats received microcurrent therapy using a device made in South Korea, while the others received a sham therapy. The microcurrent treatment intensity was 25 microamperes at a frequency of 8 hertz, applied for one hour per day for two weeks.

Circumference measurements at the carpal joint (wrist) and 2.5 centimeters (1 inch) above the carpal joint were made three days after surgery, before treatment began, weekly during treatment and at a two-week follow-up after the treatment period ended. After treatment, the rats in the treatment group had significantly less swollen wrists and a greater number of blood vessels in the forelimb than the rats in the control group. The area above the wrist was reduced in both groups, with no significant difference between them.

The level of vascular endothelial growth factor C (VEGF-C), a protein important for blood and lymph vessel growth and maintenance, was also higher in the treatment group. In addition, the microcurrent therapy significantly reduced fibrosis.

The authors concluded that microcurrent therapy promotes angiogenesis (the formation and growth of blood vessels) and improves fibrosis in secondary lymphedema. But they conceded that their research was limited by a small sample size and a short treatment period, and recommended that future studies evaluate different intensities, frequencies and durations.

Side Effects/Risks
None noted.

Bottom Line on Microcurrent Therapy
A relatively recent animal study using microcurrent therapy to treat secondary lymphedema found that it improved swelling, fibrosis and VEGF-C levels. While the Cho study used the device on newly induced lymphedema, the fact that microcurrent therapy can treat scar tissue and fibrosis may make it effective for long-standing fibrotic lymphedema. But before it can be recommended as a complementary therapy, more research, including lymphedema-specific human studies, is needed to determine the ideal protocol.

References for Microcurrent Therapy

Cho SC, Sung WJ, Lee YJ, Cho HK. 2023. Therapeutic Effect of Microcurrent Therapy in a Rat Model of Secondary Lymphedema. *Ann Palliat Med* 12 (4): 729–37.

Microwave Therapy
What Is It?
Microwave therapy uses electromagnetic waves to heat tissue. The word "microwave" makes me think of a microwave oven, and from a description of the device used in a 1996 study, it even sounds a bit like one: a chamber lined with lead, with three radiation antennae attached to the inner wall generating 120 watts of energy (Gan 1996). The cylindrical chamber has an opening at one end, with shielding cloth to mini-

mize microwave leakage, and the lymphedema limb is placed on a splint inside and its skin temperature maintained at 39°C to 41°C (102°F to 106°F).

Lymphedema-Specific Research

At least eight studies of microwave treatment for lymphedema were conducted between 1984 and 1996, and the five most recent ones (Chang 1992, Chang 1996, Gan 1996, Liu 1993 and Zhang 1986) were included in a review of heat and cold therapies for lymphedema (Hill 2024). The review authors made the following observations:

- One randomized controlled trial (Chang 1996) found that significantly more patients in the treatment group reported an improvement in swelling and restricted mobility than in the placebo group. For feelings of burning pain or heaviness, there was no significant difference between the groups in the proportion of patients who reported improvements.
- In a non-randomized trial (Liu 1993), microwave therapy improved circumference more than hot water therapy, but hot water therapy more effectively reduced limb volume.
- All five studies demonstrated improvements in circumference and limb volume from baseline to end of study. Three found the circumference improvement to be significant, and four found the volume improvement to be significant.
- Two of the studies (Gan 1996 and Zhang 1986) found a significant improvement in the number of skin infections with microwave treatment.

Side Effects/Risks

The Hill review concluded that there was no evidence that heat therapy was unsafe for people with lymphedema. It did, however, point out that the studies were done in a controlled laboratory setting—in other words, "Don't try this at home."

> **Between Professionals**
> When a research trail goes cold, I wonder why. Microwave therapy had multiple studies with positive results, yet research on it stopped after 1996. It could be that the researchers who were championing this therapy retired or lost funding, or that new treatments were developed that worked better, or that there were safety or regulatory concerns. Without details, it's hard to know why a therapy loses popularity, or if there might someday be a revival of interest.

Bottom Line on Microwave Therapy

Despite positive results in eight studies, there has been no new research on microwave therapy in almost thirty years, and no one has offered a potential mechanism of action to explain the findings. If it is to be revived as a complementary therapy, new research with current equipment will need to be conducted.

References for Microwave Therapy

Chang TS, Gan JL, Fu KD, Huang WY. 1996. The Use of 5,6 Benzo-[Alpha]-Pyrone (Coumarin) and Heating by Microwaves in the Treatment of Chronic Lymphedema of the Legs. *Lymphology* 29 (3): 106–111.

Chang TS, Gan JL, Huang WY, et al. 1992. A Modified Microwave Oven in the Treatment of Chronic Lymphedema of the Extremities. *Eur J Plast Surg* 15 (5): 242–46.

Gan JL, Li SL, Cai RX, Chang TS. 1996. Microwave Heating in the Management of Postmastectomy Upper Limb Lymphedema. *Ann Plast Surg* 36 (6): 576–80; discussion 580–81.

Hill JE, Whitaker JC, Sharafi N, et al. 2024. The Effectiveness and Safety of Heat/Cold Therapy in Adults with Lymphoedema: Systematic Review. *Disabil Rehabil* 46 (11): 2184–95.

Liu NF, Olszewski W. 1993. The Influence of Local Hyperthermia on Lymphedema and Lymphedematous Skin of the Human Leg. *Lymphology* 26 (1): 28–37.

Zhang DS, Han LY, Gan JL, Huang WY. 1986. Micro-wave: An Alternative to Electric Heating in the Treatment of Chronic Lymphedema of Extremities. *Chin Med J* 99 (11): 866–870.

Music Medicine

What Is It?

Music medicine, also known as physioacoustic or vibroacoustic therapy, uses electronic devices to convert sound (music and/or low-frequency sound waves) into vibrations via specialized speakers called transducers. This therapy uses vibration at 40 hertz (40 clicks per second, close to low E on a piano). The goal is to stimulate blood circulation, leading to an endothelial cell response that results in the release of nitric oxide and a change in blood flow, among other physiological reactions (Bartel 2021). Some music medicine devices are chairs or loungers with built-in speakers in which the user both hears and feels the vibration. It is different from music therapy (page 91).

Lymphedema-Specific Research

I was unable to find research specifically on music medicine for lymphedema.

Related Research

In a review and meta-analysis of vibroacoustic therapy for pain, most of the studies included music along with a sound vibration device (Kantor 2022). Some of the devices used were the Next Wave Physioacoustic Chair, Sound Oasis VTS-1000, Music Vibration Table (MVT), Taikofon FeelSound Player, Multivib 10 mattress, Somatron recliner and SL5 Nexneuro.

The results showed a nonsignificant reduction in pain. The review authors recommended using 40 hertz for at least twenty minutes, with more frequent (daily) sessions when treating acute pain, and using music along with the sound vibration for added psychological impact. They suggested that future research should include detailed reporting of the frequency, amplitude, pulsation and loudness of the sound therapy.

Potential improvements in pain would be important to some individuals with lymphedema, but the nonsignificant results and lack of specific recommendations available so far mean this therapy needs more research. Outside of pain management, it's unknown what effect music or vibroacoustic therapy devices might have on lymphedema. But vibration is being explored as a therapy for lymphedema, delivered via other high-tech modalities such as vibration plates (page 270), ultrasound (page 265) and deep oscillation (see Hivamat, page 230).

Side Effects/Risks

None noted.

Bottom Line on Music Medicine

Music medicine is unexplored for lymphedema. Although sound vibration stimulates blood circulation and endothelial cells, it is unclear what effect this has on the lymphatic system or lymphedema. Until more research is done, continue to enjoy your favorite music, sing, dance or play an instrument with a joyful and curious mind. As you do, you can observe whether sound vibration has any benefit for your lymphedema.

References for Music Medicine

Bartel L, Mosabbir A. 2021. Possible Mechanisms for the Effects of Sound Vibration on Human Health. *Healthcare* (Basel) 9 (5): 597.

Kantor J, Campbell EA, Kantorová L, et al. 2022. Exploring Vibroacoustic Therapy in Adults Experiencing Pain: A Scoping Review. *BMJ Open* 12 (4): e046591.

Neuroglide

What Is It?

The Neuroglide is a back and neck pad that looks like a narrow mattress. According to the website of its manufacturer, Eva Medtec, it inhibits the transmission of pain signals to the brain and restores the body's natural ability to heal. It also mimics manual lymphatic drainage using a patented Stretch n' Release technology with sixteen air bladder chambers that inflate and deflate sequentially to help move the lymph (Eva Medtec 2023). The principle is similar to a pneumatic compression pump (see page 256), but you lie on top of a mat instead of donning a garment with inflatable chambers.

Lymphedema-Specific Research

A 100-person study has been submitted for publication but was not yet available at the time of writing. In the meantime, we have one case study of four individuals: a patient with complex regional pain syndrome and lymphedema; a healthy patient; a breast cancer survivor with chronic pain; and a patient with a history of abdominal surgery (Aldrich 2024). Although case studies are near the bottom of the hierarchy of evidence (see page 4), they are a good way for new technologies to establish proof of concept.

The patients were injected with indocyanine green and a baseline recording was made of their lymphatics. They then had one hour of treatment on the Neuroglide, during which lymph imaging continued. An image analyzer added up the number of pulses observed and the pulse frequency per minute. Both increased and decreased lymphatic pulse frequencies were observed, even within different limbs of the same patient. After treatment, the three patients with pain reported improvement in their pain level.

The authors, two of whom are the inventors and patent holders of the device, concluded that Neuroglide may improve lymphatic contractility.

Between Professionals

I have a client who I think could benefit from the Neuroglide. He is confined to his bed and needs assistance to get into and out of the inflatable garments for pneumatic compression pump therapy. When the pump is running, he experiences pain in his knees due to arthritis. Because of these issues, his use of the pump is limited. If the Neuroglide is proven effective, he and others with similar challenges would likely use the treatment more consistently.

Side Effects/Risks

None noted, but the manufacturer's website does list several contraindications, including pregnancy, heart problems, vascular problems, deep vein thrombosis and back injury, as well as a general warning that it is "not to be used if you are under a physician's care" (Eva Medtec 2023).

Bottom Line on Neuroglide

The Neuroglide appears to be based on the principle of promoting pain management via proper drainage of inflammatory mediators from extracellular fluid compartments. It's exactly the kind of out-of-the-box thinking (or in this case, out-of-the-inflatable-pants thinking) that could be a game changer for many lymphedema patients. Now we just need clinical trials to demonstrate that it's effective for lymphedema.

References for Neuroglide

Aldrich MB, Rasmussen JC, Karni RJ, et al. 2024. Case Report: The Effect of Automated Manual Lymphatic Drainage Therapy on Lymphatic Contractility in 4 Distinct Cases. *Front Med Technol* 6 (July): 1397561.

Eva Medtec. 2023. "Neuroglide." Accessed July 9, 2025. https://www.neuroglide.com/.

Pneumatic Compression Pump

What Is It?

A pneumatic compression pump is a mechanical, prescription-only medical device that delivers intermittent pneumatic compression ("pneumatic" means air under pressure). They are also called compression pumps, lymphatic pumps, lymphedema pumps, arm pumps, leg pumps, lymphedema machines, compression machines, pneumatic compression machines, intermittent pneumatic compression (IPC) devices and sequential compression devices (SCDs). There are basic and advanced models. You can read more about different pumps and their features on the websites of these manufacturers:

- Airos Medical: airosmedical.com
- Bio Compression Systems: biocompression.com
- LymphaCare: lymphacare.com
- Lympha Press: lymphapress.com
- Tactile Medical: tactilemedical.com

To use a pump, you first put on the device, much like slipping into bulky pants or a bulky jacket. The legs or sleeves contain individual chambers that you connect via tubing into the pump. Once the pump is turned on, air-powered compression squeezes your limb from your fingers or toes toward the top of your arm or leg (from distal to proximal). In some devices, the garment portion includes the abdomen or chest, which gets the lymph closer to the subclavian veins—its ultimate destination. The compression pump directs the movement of lymph by using the highest compression in the distal area—the chamber farthest away from your trunk—and the lowest pressure in the proximal area, near the trunk of the body. The pressure difference tells the lymph fluid to go toward the subclavian area (the area behind your collarbones), also called the terminus. The pump cycles through inflation and deflation sequences with the amount of pressure that has been recommended and set by your therapist.

According to the Canadian Agency for Drugs and Technologies in Health, "Intermittent pneumatic compression (IPC) can be used in the treatment of lymphedema as an adjunct to CDT, particularly in patients with compromised mobility or physical exercise. Although lymphedema reduces after application, the use of IPC remains controversial due to its adverse effects, including the recurrence of edema due to residual proteins remaining in the interstitial space, and potential lymphatic structure damage due to high pressure application" (Tran 2017).

User Experience
"With my lymphedema, the pneumatic compression pump has been very helpful with moving the lymph fluid up my arm, around the underarm, with keeping the swelling down and helping with the arthritic pain in the left shoulder. I have used the arm/torso and leg pump for the last eight months."

—Robin, Washington (left arm, hand and underarm lymphedema)

Lymphedema-Specific Research

Unlike many other complementary therapies, there are several studies on compression pumps. I'll highlight some below.

STUDY #1: ZALESKA 2014

What happens when you use a pump for years? In this study, eighteen participants used a pneumatic compression pump for forty-five minutes a day for three years, wearing compression garments between sessions. The pump was an eight-chamber model by Bio Compression, with a sequential inflation of 100 to 120 mmHg for fifty seconds.

Participants were evaluated monthly, and initially saw decreased limb circumference, decreased tissue stiffness and increased tissue elasticity, followed by maintained circumference and tissue elasticity. Most importantly, they did not experience either genital lymphedema or a fibrotic ring at the top of the thigh, two issues that had been reported in previous studies.

STUDY #2: KARACA-MANDIC 2015

This study looked at the outcomes of over 700 health insurance customers with lymphedema who had received compression pumps in Minnesota, based on an analysis of private insurance and Medicare databases from 2007 to 2013. The patients' health care costs one year before and after receiving the pump—the Flexitouch system by Tactile Medical—were compared. After using the pump for a year, non-cancer patients had a 75% reduction in cellulitis episodes and 54% fewer inpatient hospitalizations, while cancer patients had a 79% reduction of cellulitis episodes and 22% fewer inpatient hospitalizations. As a result, costs went down for all patients. Cellulitis is expensive to treat, often requiring emergency room care and sometimes inpatient care, and patients also needed fewer outpatient sessions with a lymphedema therapist.

It seems like the pumps were being used—at least in part—to replace manual lymphatic drainage by a certified lymphedema therapist. It's also possible that the patients were not reliably doing self-MLD in the year before they received their pumps but were more compliant with the pumps. Less cellulitis is certainly a big win; however, this study does not report on other aspects of lymphedema management, such as limb volume reduction, pain and quality of life.

STUDY #3: ALDRICH 2017

In this small study, four lymphedema patients donned multi-chambered pants with clear windows. Their lymph fluid movement was scanned with near-infrared fluorescence lymphatic imaging during the treatment and for thirty minutes afterward. Comparing the results with previous scans, the authors concluded that the pneumatic compression pumps improved the movement of lymph.

STUDY #4: SORAN 2022

In this clinical trial, sixty-nine patients received "standard lymphedema care." In addition, fifty patients were given a pneumatic compression pump. For the pump users, infection rates reduced by 32%, hospitalization due to infection decreased by 14%, and the need for physical therapy reduced by 24%. Pump compliance was 84%, while compliance to manual lymphatic drainage was 53%. The authors concluded that pneumatic compression pumps are good value for the patient and the health care system, due to the reduced need for hospitalization and physiotherapy.

Side Effects/Risks

In general, the same contraindications apply to compression pumps as to MLD. Some examples include active infection, lymphangiosarcoma, active deep vein thrombosis, blood clots, congestive heart failure, inflammatory phlebitis or pulmonary embolism, untreated or infected wounds, gangrene, recent skin grafts and dermatitis.

Reported side effects include recurrence of edema due to residual proteins remaining in the interstitial space, and potential lymphatic structure damage due to high pressure application (Tran 2017). An older study noted lymphedema moving into the groin (Boris 1998), and it's unclear whether the technology has evolved enough that this is no longer a risk. Be vigilant about observing the changes you experience while using a pump.

Bottom Line on Pneumatic Compression Pumps

Your lymphedema therapist will advise you on whether you are a good candidate for a pneumatic compression pump and, if so, which device is most appropriate, what settings to use, how often you should use it and for how long. They may also help monitor your results and suggest changes to your treatment plan.

Given that recent studies show both benefits and cost-effectiveness, pumps may become more popular as a complementary therapy. If you live in the US, your insurance company may incentivize pump use due to studies showing a cost savings. Be sure to discuss the best options with your therapist. The inflation pattern, duration and pressure vary by pump and manufacturer, so it's best not to simply order a pump online and fiddle with the settings yourself. As the anecdotal report on page 259 noted, using a pneumatic compression pump along with self-MLD to clear the proximal lymphatics may provide better results; speak with your therapist.

References for Pneumatic Compression Pumps

Aldrich MB, Gross D, Morrow JR, et al. 2017. Effect of Pneumatic Compression Therapy on Lymph Movement in Lymphedema-Affected Extremities, as Assessed by Near-Infrared Fluorescence Lymphatic Imaging. *J Innov Opt Health Sci* 10 (2): 1650049.

Boris M, Weindorf S, Lasinski BB. 1998. The Risk of Genital Edema After External Pump Compression for Lower Limb Lymphedema. *Lymphology* 31 (1): 15–20.

Karaca-Mandic P, Hirsch AT, Rockson SG, Ridner SH. 2015. The Cutaneous, Net Clinical, and Health Economic Benefits of Advanced Pneumatic Compression Devices in Patients with Lymphedema. *JAMA Dermatol* 151 (11): 1187–93.

Soran A, Toktas O, Grassi A, Sezgin E. 2022. Adding Pneumatic Compression Therapy in Lower Extremity Lymphedema Increases Compliance of Treatment, While Decreasing the Infection Rate. *Lymphat Res Biol* 20 (3): 315–18.

Tran K, Argáez C. 2017. "Intermittent Pneumatic Compression Devices for the Management of Lymphedema: A Review of Clinical Effectiveness and Guidelines [Internet]." Canadian Agency for Drugs and Technologies in Health, May 12.

Zaleska M, Olszewski WL, Durlik M. 2014. The Effectiveness of Intermittent Pneumatic Compression in Long-Term Therapy of Lymphedema of Lower Limbs. *Lymphat Res Biol* 12 (2): 103–9.

RAGodoy

What Is It?

The RAGodoy is a mechanical lymphatic drainage device that works by performing passive flexion and extension exercises of the ankle or the elbow to stimulate lymphatic drainage. It is made by Dr. José Maria Pereira de Godoy and Dr. Maria de Fátima Guerreiro Godoy from the Godoy Clinic and the Godoy & Godoy International School of Lymphatic Therapy in Brazil. For leg lymphedema, the RAGodoy is used in the supine position (lying on your back), allowing gravity to assist. A foam wedge helps bear the weight of the lower legs. The arm apparatus is used in the seated position, without a wedge.

Between Professionals

This device makes me think of a client I had when I worked in home care. She had mobility issues and was confined to her bed for most of the day. One of the movements she could do, though, was point and flex her toes. While someone with similar challenges could do this on their own for a short period of time, the motion could be done passively by strapping their feet into the device. I would be curious to know if the RAGodoy has been used in this population.

Lymphedema-Specific Research

There are multiple studies on the RAGodoy's use for lymphedema, as well as a review article (Pereira de Godoy 2022). According to the review, the lower leg device has been tested in forty studies since 2004. In ten of the studies, it was the only therapy; in the rest, it was part of a multi-treatment protocol. The studies showed that the device leads to mobilization of macromolecules as visualized on lymphoscintigraphy, reduction of edema volume, stimulation of venous blood return and reduction of skin fibrosis. There was one finding of a massive (50%) volume reduction when the RAGodoy was used for a multi-hour session, combined with a compression machine, over a five-day treatment cycle.

Studies of the arm device began in 2009 and have also demonstrated volume reduction.

The review authors concluded that using the RAGodoy for mechanical lymphatic drainage assists considerably in treatment and in maintaining results. It is effective on its own, but results are superior when it is used in combination with compression.

Side Effects/Risks

None are noted, but I would think muscle cramping might be an issue. There may also be contraindications, but none were listed in the review paper.

Bottom Line on RAGodoy

The Godoys are innovators in the lymphedema community who have also developed their own MLD technique. The 2022 review says there are forty published studies of their device. I counted thirty-eight in the reference section, of which only three did not have one of the Godoys as an author. They have been prolific in publishing research on their device, but I'm confused by their disclosure that there are no financial conflicts of interest for the device they created—not that such a conflict would diminish the impressive results. Still, cautious investigators may want to run their own trials before adopting the RAGodoy into their practice.

I did a quick search of the FDA website and Health Canada's Medical Devices Active Licence Listing, and I don't see the RAGodoy listed. For now, it appears it is not approved in the US or Canada (or not under that name). But if the device becomes available where you live, you can be assured that it has a strong history of positive results. It may be especially useful for anyone who is bedridden.

References for RAGodoy

Pereira de Godoy JM, Guerreiro Godoy MF, Pereira de Godoy HJ. 2022. Mechanical Lymphatic Drainage (RAGodoy®): Literature Review. *Cureus* 14 (1): e21263

Transcutaneous Electrical Acupoint Stimulation

What Is It?

Transcutaneous electrical acupoint stimulation (TEAS) is a combination of two therapeutic approaches: traditional acupressure and electrical nerve stimulation (Zhou 2025). A practitioner programs the device with the electric current frequency, then places the electrodes strategically on acupoints on the skin while asking the patient for feedback about the intensity and adjusting accordingly. TEAS has been used to treat pain, improve gastrointestinal function, treat infertility, enhance cognitive function, promote recovery and reduce fatigue (Zhou 2025). It is ideal for a patient who wants to have acupuncture but is afraid of the needles or can't have needle insertion.

Lymphedema-Specific Research

I located two studies using TEAS for lymphedema prevention and treatment, described below in chronological order.

Study #1: He 2016

In this study, for which I could only access the abstract, 100 women who had had a radical mastectomy for breast cancer were assigned to either TEAS or a control group that received the usual postsurgical nursing care. Two weeks after the surgery and the postsurgical treatment, limb swelling was compared. Those that received TEAS had a 22% occurrence rate of abnormal upper limb sensations, compared to 84% of the control group. Incidence of swelling in the TEAS group was 4%, while the control group's was 24%. Both of these outcomes are statistically significant.

The authors concluded that TEAS can effectively prevent and release early-stage arm swelling after radical mastectomy.

Study #2: Lu 2023

This study included fifty-two patients with breast cancer–related lymphedema. Roughly half (twenty-seven) were assigned to the control group, who received complete decongestive therapy consisting of manual lymphatic drainage, compression bandaging, skin care and functional exercise. They were also taught to do self-MLD, which they were instructed to perform two to three times per day. The remaining twenty-five patients received TEAS combined with warm acupuncture. Specific acupoint sites were treated, as well as any areas of the limb with noticeable swelling or hard spots. The TEAS device used was the HANS-200A.

After four weeks of treatment, all participants experienced a reduction of lymphedema compared to pre-study levels. Likewise, they all reported a reduction in their sensation of swelling, with the TEAS group noting significantly greater perceived improvements. In a clinical assessment of lymphedema stage before and after treatment, all of the participants improved. In the TEAS group, thirteen had a markedly effective response, five effective and seven ineffective, for an overall response rate of 72%. In the CDT group, twelve experienced a markedly effective response, three effective and twelve ineffective, for an overall response rate of 56%.

Side Effects/Risks

No serious adverse events occurred in the Lu study. Small bruises at individual acupoints resolved on their own, and the authors attributed occasional aggravations of the edema to "improper self-management" or to radiation therapy or other cancer treatments that the patients were receiving simultaneously.

Bottom Line on TEAS

TEAS combines traditional Chinese medicine with modern electro-stimulation. Two studies have demonstrated its efficacy in preventing and treating lymphedema in the short term. Benefits in the Lu study included improvements in perceived swelling, circumference measurements and clinical effectiveness, with the TEAS group responding better than the CDT group. Because TEAS was combined with warm acupuncture in the Lu study, it's unclear what effect the TEAS had or whether it would be effective on its own. This therapy is appealing for patients who are drawn to acupuncture but concerned about needle punctures; however, larger, well-designed studies of longer duration are needed before TEAS can be recommended with confidence.

References for TEAS

He JG, Chen XJ, Wang YJ. 2016. Clinical Study on Transcutaneous Electric Acupoint Stimulation for Swelling Limb After Breast Cancer Operation. *Shanghai J Acupunct Moxibust* 12: 301–3.

Lu C, Li GL, Deng DH, et al. 2023. Transcutaneous Electrical Acupoint Stimulation Combined with Warm Acupuncture for Breast Cancer Related Upper Limb Lymphedema: A Retrospective Cohort Study. *Chin J Integr Med* 29 (6): 534–39.

Zhou W, Li J, Shen X, et al. 2025. Transcutaneous Electrical Acupoint Stimulation (TEAS): Applications and Challenges. *World J Acupunct - Moxibustion* 35 (1): 10–16.

Transponder

What Is It?

The Transponder was an "electro-sound wave and vacuum medical device" (Cavezzi 2013) developed by Talamonti. It is no longer in production.

Lymphedema-Specific Research

In the first of two studies, eight patients with leg lymphedema were given daily sessions with the Transponder for ten days (Cavezzi 2013). Total limb volume decreased by 5%, and lower leg volume reduced by 8%. In the second study, eight patients with lymphedema or lipedema had two Transponder sessions then self-administered the remaining treatments (Elio 2014). After six days of treatment, limb volume had decreased by an average of 154 milliliters (5.2 ounces), a 2% reduction. Heaviness had decreased by 47%, dysesthesias by 58% and pain by 64%.

Side Effects/Risks

None noted.

Bottom Line on Transponder

The Transponder is no longer available, but its manufacturer, Talamonti, currently makes the Manutech BH (see page 249).

References for Transponder

Cavezzi A, Paccasassi S, Elio C. 2013. Lymphedema Treatment by Means of an Electro-Medical Device Based on Bioresonance and Vacuum Technology: Clinical and Lymphoscintigraphic Assessment. *Int Angiol* 32 (4): 417–23.

Elio C, Guaitolini E, Paccasassi S, et al. 2014. Application of Microcurrents of Bioresonance and Transdermal Delivery of Active Principles in Lymphedema and Lipedema of the Lower Limbs: A Pilot Study. *G Ital Dermatol Venereol* 149 (6): 643–47.

Ultrasound

What Is It?

We know of ultrasound as a diagnostic tool, and every pregnant woman sees those grainy grey-and-white images of their baby. When used to create images, it is also called sonography or ultrasonography, and the image it creates is called a sonogram. But ultrasound is also a treatment tool (often called therapeutic ultrasound) used by physical therapists, as the sound wave vibration can loosen lesions by creating cell and tissue movement (Liu 2023). You can think of ultrasound as an internal massage that works through high-intensity sound waves. Ultrasound is safe, it does not produce radiation, and it is noninvasive. Ultrasound devices are made by multiple manufacturers.

Lymphedema-Specific Research

Most of the human research on ultrasound for lymphedema focuses on using it as a diagnostic tool or an assistive device during surgery. But I located two studies that used therapeutic ultrasound to treat lymphedema.

Study #1: Balzarini 1993

In this Italian study, fifty patients with postsurgical arm lymphedema received two cycles of ultrasound treatment, four months apart. Each cycle contained ten sessions lasting thirty minutes each. The researchers connected acupressure points along the arm with ten fixed sequenced transducers from the Liposonic10 ultrasound device. After treatment, half of the patients wore elastic compression, while the other half did not. They were then compared to 100 patients who had used a pneumatic compression pump (the Jobst Extremity Pump).

The ultrasound group lost more lymphedema volume in the first four months, but the reduction did not persist for the full year of follow-up. A year later, they did not show a significant difference in lymphedema volume, but they did have a softer arm, better pain relief and greater range of motion, and they required fewer anti-inflammatory and analgesic drugs.

The authors concluded that ultrasound is a useful therapeutic tool. Besides an overall shorter length of treatment, it offers advantages including softer tissue, pain relief and less joint stiffness, and it eliminates the need for a compression sleeve between treatments. They stated that the trial was ongoing and they would publish more, but I was unable to locate further results. A later study by the same lead author (Balzarini 2001) used ultrasound as a diagnostic tool, not a treatment tool.

Study #2: Hemmati 2022

This Iranian clinical trial (also discussed in the chapter on faradic currents) compared complete decongestive therapy on its own to CDT + faradic currents and to CDT + ultrasound to treat breast cancer–related lymphedema. It was a double-blind randomized controlled trial with thirty-nine women divided into three groups. They all received CDT: five sessions per week with a physiotherapist, including manual lymphatic drainage; compression with short stretch bandages; skin care and exercises for one hour a day. In addition, one group was treated with ultrasound (the Novin 215X) and another group was treated with faradic currents (the Novin 710L).

The thirteen women in the ultrasound group received three minutes of ultrasound (1 megahertz and 2 watts per square centimeter) for each section of the arm. Each treatment lasted about seventy-five minutes, and they received ten sessions in total.

All of the treatment groups saw a significant reduction in circumference measurements at the middle of the forearm, elbow and mid upper arm. Only the treatment groups (faradic current or ultrasound) saw a reduction at the wrist. Arm volume was also significantly reduced in all three groups. There was a nonsignificant difference between the faradic and control groups, but a significant difference between the ultrasound and control groups (but not the ultrasound and faradic groups). In other words, CDT + ultrasound was the most effective treatment for reducing volume. Pain and functional disability reduced significantly in all three groups, but significantly more in the faradic and ultrasound groups than in the control group.

To explain the results in the ultrasound group, the authors suggested that therapeutic ultrasound generates micromassage through sound waves, which modifies microcirculation and cell metabolism. It also produces stress on the cell membranes and increases cell permeability, which can result in improved lymph flow and reduced fibrosis. All of these actions, working together, lead to improved swelling, pain and hardness of the lymphedema limb.

Technical Breakdown
Sound waves are measured in hertz (Hz): how many times a sound wave is produced per second. The normal human sound range (what we are able to hear) is 15 to 20,000 hertz. Dogs can hear up to 45,000 hertz; dolphins, 150,000 hertz; and bats, 250,000 hertz. Far beyond this, at 1 million hertz (1 megahertz) is the frequency of sound waves used in medical ultrasound (Dolphin Communication Project, n.d.).

Lymphedema Research in Animals

The focus of an animal study on ultrasound as a potential treatment tool was to determine if low-intensity pulsed ultrasound, using the WED-100 ultrasonic therapy machine, could reduce lymphedema by enhancing anti-inflammatory macrophage circulation (Liu 2023). Lymphedema was induced in the rats' tails. Three days after the induction surgery, half of the rats received three minutes of pulsed ultrasound, while the other half served as the control group. The ultrasound therapy continued for twenty-eight days.

After treatment, tail circumference and skin thickness in the ultrasound group were reduced by 30%, there were fewer collagen fibers, and tail blood flow was better, with fewer macrophages and less inflammation. The authors concluded that ultrasound's influence on macrophages and microcirculation was responsible for improving the lymphedema.

Side Effects/Risks

None noted.

Bottom Line on Ultrasound

The 1993 trial using therapeutic ultrasound to treat lymphedema and the 2022 study comparing CDT on its own to CDT + ultrasound or faradic currents seem promising. In 2023, an animal study on pulsed ultrasound offered more encouraging results. It is early days yet, but if studies continue to provide good outcomes, then ultrasound may be validated as a complementary therapy for lymphedema. Future research can also provide details on the ideal duration, location and intensity of treatments. The good news about this modality is that therapeutic ultrasound machines are very popular and are already in many public and private clinics, so implementation may be easier than for emerging technologies.

References for Ultrasound

Balzarini A, Milella M, Civelli E, et al. 2001. Ultrasonography of Arm Edema After Axillary Dissection for Breast Cancer: A Preliminary Study. *Lymphology* 34 (4): 152–55.

Balzarini A, Pirovano C, Diazzi G, et al. 1993. Ultrasound Therapy of Chronic Arm Lymphedema After Surgical Treatment of Breast Cancer. *Lymphology* 26 (3): 128–34.

Dolphin Communication Project. n.d. "So High It Hertz." Accessed July 23, 2025. https://www.dolphincommunicationproject.org/the-dolphin-pod-36/.

Hemmati M, Rojhani-Shirazi Z, Zakeri ZS, et al. 2022. The Effect of the Combined Use of Complex Decongestive Therapy with Electrotherapy Modalities for the Treatment of Breast Cancer-Related Lymphedema: A Randomized Clinical Trial. *BMC Musculoskelet Disord* 23 (1): 837.

National Institutes of Health (NIH), National Institute of Biomedical Imaging and Bioengineering. 2023. "Ultrasound." Accessed July 23, 2025. https://www.nibib.nih.gov/science-education/science-topics/ultrasound.

Liu Z, Li J, Bian Y, et al. 2023. Low-Intensity Pulsed Ultrasound Reduces Lymphedema by Regulating Macrophage Polarization and Enhancing Microcirculation. *Front Bioeng Biotechnol* 11 (May): 1173169.

Vacumed

What Is It?

Like cupping (see page 35) and the LymphaTouch (see page 246), the Vacumed is a negative pressure device. It is a large cylindrical vacuum tube in which the body is enclosed from the feet to the top of the pelvis (the iliac crest). A seal is made with nylon cinched around the waist (much like a kayaker would use), sealing the lower body in the tube. The device alternates between low and normal pressure cycles, leading to an increase in blood flow.

The Vacumed has its origins in space medicine: According to the German manufacturer, Weyergens High Care Medical, it was developed in conjunction with the Institute of Aerospace Medicine of the German Aerospace Center "to prevent orthostatic complications during manned space missions in microgravity" (Weyergens 2025).

Lymphedema-Specific Research

Fifty patients with primary or secondary leg lymphedema underwent an integrated protocol that the authors called "Complete Lymphedema Functional Treatment" (Campisi 2015). It included lymphatic microsurgery, physical therapy, manual and pneumatic sequential compression pump treatment, lymphatic drainage, compression garments, exercise with an emphasis on swimming, and intermittent negative pressure using the Vacumed. The protocol had three phases: pre-surgery, post-surgery and long-term maintenance.

In the two weeks pre-surgery and two to three weeks post-surgery, patients completed twenty-minute sessions of negative pressure between −35 and −40 mmHg. Their results were compared to those of fifty previous patients, who had received the same treatment but without the Vacumed. The average post-treatment volume reduction for the Vacumed group was 83%, versus 76% for the earlier group, an improvement that the authors determined was clinically significant. In addition, all patients had low rates of infection, and they reported that the treatment was enjoyable.

Side Effects/Risks

None noted.

Bottom Line on Vacumed

Who wouldn't want to be treated in a giant, comfy vacuum designed for astronauts in space? That's one big pro for this technology: It's a great conversation starter. But access to the Vacumed is currently limited—unless you happen to be having microvascular surgery in Europe. I look forward to more research, which could look at using this device outside of a surgical protocol to see if it might be a good complement to CDT. I suspect we are a few years away from more widespread availability, as the Vacumed would have to receive government approvals, be adopted by hospital systems and be covered by insurance, but it's nice to know that promising new treatment options are in the pipeline.

References for Vacumed

Campisi CC, Ryn M, Campisi CS, et al. 2015. Intermittent Negative Pressure Therapy in the Combined Treatment of Peripheral Lymphedema. *Lymphology* 48 (4): 197–204.

Weyergens High Care Medical. 2025. "Welcome to Vacumed®." Accessed July 12, 2025. https://www.vacumed.de/en/vacumed-home.html.

Vibration Plate

What Is It?

A vibration plate is a sturdy platform you can stand or sit on that provides adjustable vibration. At the moment, these devices seem to be everywhere, having burst onto the scene from multiple manufacturers, and there are lots of social media testimonials about how beneficial they are for lymphedema and lipedema. But since they are marketed to the masses rather than the medical community, the research on vibration plates is limited.

Vibration plates are sometimes said to provide "whole-body vibration," but that description can also refer to other devices, so when you're reading research papers, make sure to note the exact device used. Even if you confirm that the study is discussing vibration plates, the results may not be transferable to the particular device you are considering, as different models deliver different frequencies and amplitudes of vibration. For example, in a study comparing the Galileo 900, Power Plate Pro5 and Juvent 1000 (Spain 2021), the examiners found that the Juvent 1000 did not deliver vibration above the knee, while the other two models delivered vibration to the femoral neck (at the top of the thigh) and lumbar spine (lower back).

> **Anecdotal Report**
> "In my experience, most patients like vibration plates."
>
> —Anonymous, lymphedema therapist, Arizona

Lymphedema-Specific Research

I found only a single case study of lymphedema treatment that included a vibration plate, which I described briefly in "Complementary, Alternative and Integrative Care" (page 8). A woman in her mid-fifties with primary lymphedema, obesity, severe neuropathy in her lower extremities and elevated stress levels was treated with a holistic treatment designed to address mind, body and spirit (Hamlett 2013). The four-month treatment protocol consisted of resistance and cardiovascular training, whole-body vibration with the I-Shape vibrating platform, daily meditation and reflection, chair yoga and healthy eating with the guidance of a registered dietitian, using the WeightWatchers Points program.

Vibration was included in the protocol because the researcher believed it would increase skin blood flow. Three minutes of whole-body vibration at 25 hertz was followed by ten minutes of cardio at 70% perceived exertion, then twenty-five minutes of resistance training for the whole body, then three minutes of vibration at 65 to 70 hertz.

With a multidisciplinary approach, it is difficult to tease out the effect of a single component, but in this case, whole-body vibration was part of a holistic protocol that produced successful results: The client lost 20 kilograms (45 pounds), her cholesterol was reduced, her legs had increased fluid movement and less swelling, and her overall health, stress, quality of life and general outlook on life greatly improved.

User Experience
"The vibration plate is new to me as of two months ago. I am easing into this slowly, but it seems to wake up my lymphatic and circulation systems. My legs feel like they have been on a walk without going anywhere. We'll see about this therapy."

—Robin, Washington (left arm, hand and underarm lymphedema)

Side Effects/Risks

I could not find any reported risks, but common sense says one might lose their balance and fall off a vibration plate; for this reason, a model with handles may be a safer choice. Read the fine print to learn whether there are any contraindications for the vibration plate you are considering, especially if you have a prosthetic device, a pacemaker or other such considerations.

Anecdotal Report
"I highly recommend vibration plates and use them regularly."

—Deanna, lymphedema therapist, Virginia

Bottom Line on Vibration Plates

Vibration plates are available in department stores and online shops, are relatively affordable and don't seem to require special training. But there is no published evidence that they benefit lymphedema, and no guidance on model, intensity, frequency or timing. If you plan to try a vibration plate, "start low and go slow," and, of course, seek input from your certified lymphedema therapist, who may have anecdotal experience with these devices.

References for Vibration Plates

Hamlett P. 2013. "A Holistic Approach to Lymphedema Treatment and Case Study." Accessed July 12, 2025. https://www.researchgate.net/publication/273772739_A_HOLISTIC_APPROACH_TO_LYMPHEDEMA_TREATMENT_1_A_Holistic_Approach_to_Lymphedema_Treatment.

Spain L, Yang L, Wilkinson JM, McCloskey E. 2021. Transmission of Whole Body Vibration—Comparison of Three Vibration Platforms in Healthy Subjects. *Bone* 144 (March): 115802

Wii Fit

What Is It?

The Wii is a virtual reality game console made by the Japanese company Nintendo. Released in 2006, it features a motion-detecting handheld wireless controller you can use to play various games, including sports. In 2008, the company added the Wii Fit (and in 2009, the Wii Fit Plus), which comes with a balance board that allows you to do a home workout and improve your balance through active gaming, as well as yoga, strength-building and aerobic exercises.

Lymphedema-Specific Research

A recent study set out to explore ways to address one aspect of life with unilateral lymphedema: balance dysfunction (Sayed 2022). Sixty women with stage 1 or 2 post-mastectomy lymphedema were divided into two groups. The first group did Wii Fit balance exercises, including ski slalom, advanced skiing, ski jumping and jump rope, three times a week for four weeks. The control group performed core stability exercises, including abdominal bracing, curls, bridges, planks and bird dogs, three times a week for four weeks.

Before and after the treatment period, a therapist tested the women's balance using two measures: an assessment with the Wii Fit balance board, which evaluates how much pressure each side of the body is placing on the board; and the timed up and go (TUG) test, which times how long it takes to get up from a chair, quickly walk 3 meters (9.8 feet), turn around and sit back down. The two groups had similar scores in both measures pre-treatment.

After treatment, the patients in both groups had a significant improvement in TUG test times compared to their baseline. The Wii Fit group's center of pressure, as assessed by the balance board, also significantly improved over baseline, while there was no significant difference for the participants in the control group. Comparing the two groups' post-treatment measures, the Wii Fit group had significantly better TUG values than the control group, and nonsignificantly better balance board scores.

The authors concluded that exercises using the Wii Fit balance board more effectively correct imbalance for patients with unilateral lymphedema than core stability exercises.

Between Professionals
One of my students in an online class confirmed that balance was an issue for her, along with proprioception—the body's ability to sense its position and movement in space, also known as kinesthesia. If you think your balance and/or proprioception are off, ask your physical therapist to assess them.

Side Effects/Risks
None noted.

Bottom Line on Wii Fit
Before reading the Sayed study, I hadn't given much thought to the balance issues people with lymphedema on only one side of the body might experience. But of course it makes sense, with one side being considerably heavier and larger than the other. Working out with the Wii Fit balance board seems like a low-risk, enjoyable practice that might encourage people to be consistent about doing corrective exercises to improve their balance.

References for Wii Fit

Sayed S, Baky A, Waked I, Mohamed A. 2022. Virtual Reality Balance Training Versus Core Stability Exercises on Balance in Patients with Unilateral Lymphedema. *Int J Health Sci* 6 (S2): 5151–60.

High-Tech Devices Summary

The therapies in this category use every conceivable means to try to move lymph, including light, sound, heat, compressed air, electrical stimulation, hyperbaric oxygen, passive movement, vibration and electrostatic fields. High-tech devices are often more costly than other therapies, but they do tend to have lymphedema-specific research (electric blankets, grounding mats, vibration plates, and the Wii Fit are the exceptions, as they are not medical devices and are much more affordable). Be sure to consult the individual chapters and the references included there for more details. As a reminder, speak to your health care professional before trying these therapies, and follow the directions for safe use.

Device	What It Is	Claims	Lymphedema Research	Results	Side Effects/ Risks
BEMER	Pulsed electromagnetic field therapy	Dilates lymphatic capillaries to increase flow	One study of 10 patients undergoing supermicro-surgery	No change in lymph fluid movement	None noted
Chi Machine	A device that provides passive ankle motion and elevation	Improves circulation of blood and lymph	One study of 30 patients with leg lymphedema	Reduced volume, extracellular fluid and body weight	Easily resolved knee pain, dizziness, neck pain and ankle discomfort
Chinese heat therapy	A homemade device using light bulbs as a heat source	Heat is beneficial for lymphedema	One case series + one study of patients with filarial lymphedema	Reduced volume, softened skin	Potential risk of burns
CO_2 laser	A laser used to remove damaged outer layers of skin	Addresses advanced, treatment-resistant lymphedema	Three case studies of five patients	Softened scar, reduced leg circumference, improved appearance, reduced skin lesions and lymphorrhea	None noted
CVAC therapy	A device that simulates rapid altitude changes	Offers similar benefits to exercise, without exertion	One study of 10 patients with adiposis dolorosa	Significantly reduced pain, improved mental functioning, increased fat mass and reduced non-fat mass	Difficulty equalizing ear pressure
Dayspring	A portable non-pneumatic compression pump	Reduces lymphedema	Three studies with a total of 121 parti-cipants	Better volume reduction, response rate, QoL and adherence than pneumatic pump	No serious side effects noted
Dolphin Neurostim	A handheld device that provides DC microcurrents	Manages pain and improves scars	None	Reduced pain in a study of pain management and scar therapy	None noted
Electric blanket	A blanket with internal heating coils	Heat is beneficial on its own or in combination	One study on an electric blanket + RAGodoy with 7 participants	No benefit from electric blanket versus room temperature	Risk of burns
Electronic moxibustion	The heating of acupressure points with an electronic device	Improves circulation of qi and blood	One study of 10 breast cancer patients	Temporarily improved circumference but not bioimpedance	Skin burns

Device	What It Is	Claims	Lymphedema Research	Results	Side Effects/ Risks
Endermologie	A device with two motorized cylinders that lift and roll the skin	Massages skin and sculpts the body	Six studies with a total of 194 participants + one review	Improved pain, circumference, volume, fibrosis, skin thickness, dermal backflow, RoM, heaviness, tightness and hardness	Increased thirst and urination
Extracorporeal shock wave therapy	High-energy sound waves	Regenerates tissue, regulates inflammation, relieves pain, prevents fibrosis	One systematic review and meta-analysis of studies with a total of 193 participants	Improved volume, skin thickness and RoM better than CDT alone	None noted; contraindicated with metastatic disease, vascular disease, infection and blood thinners
Far-infrared sauna	Heat from infrared light	Infrared rays penetrate the skin and resonate with body water	Three studies with a total of 160 participants	Improved pain, infection rates, uncomfortable limb sensations, circumference, skin thickness and elasticity, and QoL	None noted
Faradic currents	Electrical stimulation with short bursts of current	Increases blood and lymph flow, reduces edema	One study of 39 patients post–breast cancer	Reduced pain better than CDT alone	None noted
Fizyoflug	A device that provides dry heat by convection	Treats pain, muscle spasms and edema	One study of 40 women post–breast cancer	Reduced pain and volume better than CDT alone	None noted, but possibly infection
Flowave	A discontinued device that delivered sound waves	Increases lymph flow	One study of 30 women post–breast cancer	Nonsignificant reduction in volume, reduced pain, heaviness and tightness	Skin irritation; product replaced by the Manutech BH
Grounding mats	Mats and other devices with conductive material that connect to the grounding port of an outlet	Improves inflammation, pain, stress, blood flow, energy, sleep and well-being	None	n/a	Electrocution if home wiring or device is faulty
High-voltage electrical stimulation	Electrical stimulation	Improves edema absorption	Three studies with a total of 38 participants + one animal study	Reduced volume better than MLD + compression, and reduced circumference	None noted

n/a = not applicable; CDT = complete decongestive therapy; RoM = range of motion; MLD = manual lymphatic drainage

Device	What It Is	Claims	Lymphedema Research	Results	Side Effects/ Risks
Hivamat	A device that produces deep-acting oscillation	Constricts blood capillaries, antifibrotic	Three studies with a total of 46 participants	Reduced circumference, volume, skin thickness, pain and swelling	None noted; contraindicated with acute infections, malignant cancers and pregnancy
Hyperbaric oxygen	100% oxygen delivered under pressure	Promotes wound healing and reduces fibrosis	One case report + four studies with a total of 99 participants	Improved volume, lymph clearance, tissue softness and mobility, but with inconsistent results	Barotrauma, myopia, tiredness, oxygen toxicity, sinus squeeze, cataracts; multiple contraindications
Kinetec Centura Lite	A device that provides continuous passive motion of the shoulder	Exercise without exertion	One study of 30 women post–breast cancer	Improved RoM, nonsignificant improvement in arm volume and significant improvement in QoL versus CDT alone	Note noted
Linforoll	A roller device that assists with lymphatic drainage	Replaces MLD with objective and repeatable data and results	One study with 20 participants	Improved tissue elasticity and lymphedema volume	None noted; contraindicated with tissue inflammation, venous thrombosis, post-traumatic tissue changes and pain during rolling
Low-level laser	Phototherapy using red and near-infrared light	Stimulates cells	Multiple studies and reviews	Reduced volume and circumference; mixed results for pain and RoM	Limited, but use caution when cancer is present
LymphaTouch	A negative pressure device	Lifts the skin and improves lymph flow	Two studies with a total of 58 participants + one narrative review that cites five small studies	Reduced circumference (but not pain or discomfort) more than MLD; reduced volume, inflammation, adipose tissue and fibrosis; improved bioimpedance	None noted
Manutech BH	A device that delivers microcurrents based on real-time feedback from sensors	Stimulates lymphatic drainage	One study using a holistic protocol with 41 participants	Holistic protocol improved lymphedema	None noted
Microcurrent therapy	Low electrical currents	Reduces pain, fibrosis and inflammation, promotes angiogenesis	One animal study	Reduced fibrosis and swelling, increased VEGF-C levels	None noted

RoM = range of motion; QoL = quality of life, CDT = complete decongestive therapy; MLD = manual lymphatic drainage; VEGF-C = vascular endothelial growth factor-C

Device	What It Is	Claims	Lymphedema Research	Results	Side Effects/ Risks
Microwave therapy	A heating chamber	Heat may be safe for lymphedema	Eight studies + one review	Improved volume, circumference, skin infections and mobility	None noted
Music medicine	Sound vibration	Stimulates blood flow and nitric oxide release	None	n/a	None noted
Neuroglide	An air mattress with stretch and release inflatable bladders	Mimics MLD, promotes healing	Case studies of 4 patients	Improved pain; both increased and decreased lymphatic pulse frequencies	None noted; contraindicated with heart and vascular issues, deep vein thrombosis, back injury and pregnancy
Pneumatic compression pumps	A wearable device that delivers air under pressure in a sequence designed to move lymph	Provides an automated version of MLD	Multiple studies	Improved lymph movement, limb circumference, stiffness and elasticity, reduced cellulitis incidence and hospitalization	Recurrence of edema, potential lymphatic structural damage; similar contraindications as MLD
RAGodoy	A device that performs passive flexion and extension of the ankle or elbow	Stimulates lymphatic drainage	Forty studies + one review	Improved volume, venous blood return and fibrosis	None noted
Transcutaneous electrical acupoint stimulation (TEAS)	A combination of electrical nerve simulation and acupressure	Stimulates acupoints to harmonize qi without needles	Two studies with a total of 152 partici- pants	Reduced swelling post- mastectomy; TEAS + warm acupuncture reduced swelling and lymphedema stage better than CDT	None noted

MLD = manual lymphatic drainage; CDT = complete decongestive therapy

Device	What is it	Claims	Lymphedema Research	Results	Side Effects/ Risks
Transponder	A discontinued device that delivered electro-sound waves	Improves lymph flow	Two studies with a total of 16 participants	Reduced volume, heaviness, pain and dysesthesias	None noted; product replaced by the Manutech BH
Ultrasound	High-intensity sound waves	Creates cell and tissue movement	Two studies with a total of 89 participants + one animal study	Improved volume, pain, softness, RoM and inflammation	None noted
Vacumed	A vacuum tube that alternates low and normal pressure cycles	Increases blood flow	One study of 50 patients with leg lymphedema	Improved volume reduction after microsurgery	None noted
Vibration plate	A platform that provides adjustable vibration	Increases blood flow	One case study of a holistic protocol	Holistic protocol improved swelling, overall health, stress, QoL and general outlook	None noted
Wii Fit	A virtual reality game console with a balance board	Improves balance	One study of 60 women post–breast cancer	Significantly improved balance	None noted

RoM = range of motion; QoL = quality of life

Part Five
Final Thoughts

Final Thoughts

You've got options. That's the message I want you to take away from this book if you're unhappy with the state of your lymphedema or, if you're a therapist, the results you're achieving with your clients. There is a huge range of complementary therapies, and you'll know which ones you're drawn to, whether they're natural remedies or the latest technologies. I also want to point out that you don't have to use any of them. After reading this book, if you are unimpressed with the state of the evidence or simply aren't drawn to any complementary therapies, that's okay too. But now you know what's out there.

If you do want to try a complementary therapy, you need to decide which one. To do so, consider the specific issue you are trying to solve. Some treatments work better for certain complaints, such as recurrent cellulitis, fibrotic tissue, pain, swelling or thickened skin. The tables on pages 284 and 285 may help you determine where to begin your exploration. They are based only on the lymphedema-specific human research reviewed in this book and do not include the anecdotal reports from the survey respondents or any therapies that were tested only as part of a holistic protocol. Some of the therapies in this book did not make it into the tables because they lacked human trials on lymphedema or failed to show efficacy.

Not every study measures every outcome; for example, if researchers don't measure pain reduction, their reporting won't note improvements in pain, even if they occurred. Also, these tables don't distinguish between short-term and long-term benefits. Therefore, be careful to think of them only as a general guide to help you decide which therapies to look into more closely, through the chapters in this book and your own independent research.

It's important to point out that the majority of the research cited in this book was done on women with breast cancer–related lymphedema. It's not clear how applicable this research is to other types of lymphedema. But for now, this information forms the basis of our understanding of complementary therapies for lymphedema.

	Cellulitis/Infection	Edema*	Fibrotic Tissue	Pain	Thickened Skin	Other Improvements
Traditional Therapies						
Acupressure		X				Inflammation
Acupuncture		X		X		
Ayurveda		X				
Cupping		X		X	X	
Moxibustion		X		X		Fatigue, WBC, GI toxicity
Qigong		X				Blood flow
Traditional Chinese medicine				X		RoM, muscle strength, ADL
Tuina		X				
Wenyang Huoxue compress						ADL
Yoga				X		QoL, RoM, insomnia, fatigue
Body Work						
Ai chi		X				
Aqua therapy		X				
Art therapy						Group support, empowerment, courage, confusion loneliness, reframing negative experiences
Circle of Healing						Weight loss, RoM, QoL, mood, bioimpedance, general health
Deep breathing		X				Heaviness, tightness, pins and needles
Dry needling				X		
Lidong needling therapy		X				
Pilates		X		X		RoM, QoL, grip strength, social anxiety
Progressive muscle relaxation						Anxiety, depression
Reflexology		X		X		Body image, stress, self-confidence, mobility, well-being
Stress reduction						Weight loss, chronic stress, distance walked
Taping		X				Interstitial microcirculation
Natural Health Products						
Astragalus + peony		X*				Heaviness
Coumarin	X	X		X		Skin softness, temperature, hardness, heaviness, mobility
Cyclo 3 Fort		X				
Daflon 500		X				Heaviness, lymphatic migration speed
Ginkor Fort						Lymphatic migration speed, heaviness, tightness, lymph drainage, lymph stasis
Goreisan		X				Weight loss, extracellular water
Hwanggigyejiomul-tang		X				RoM
Hydroxytyrosol						Itchy skin
Linfadren		X				Functional abilities
Meliven 3					X	Functional abilities
Robuvit	X	X			X	Proteins in interstitial fluid
Selenium	X	X			X	Weight loss, nighttime urination, vision, dry skin, mood, heat sensitivity, antioxidant levels, need for tracheostomies
Synbiotics		X				Inflammation, antioxidants
Unguentum Lymphaticum						Skin softness, pitting refill
Wobenzym N		X		X	X	

	Cellulitis/ Infection	Edema*	Fibrotic Tissue	Pain	Thickened Skin	Other Improvements
High-Tech Devices						
Chi Machine		X		X		Body weight, body fat, tightness, heaviness, dryness, extracellular water, perceived leg size
Chinese heat therapy		X				Skin softness
CO_2 laser		X	X		X	Skin appearance, lymphorrhea, softening of scar tissue
CVAC therapy				X		Mental functioning
Dayspring		X				QoL
Electronic moxibustion		X				
Endermologie		X	X	X	X	Dermal backflow, heaviness, tightness, hardness, RoM
Extracorporeal shock wave therapy		X			X	RoM
Far-infrared sauna	X	X		X	X	Tightness, heaviness, hardness, fullness, tingling, numbness, skin elasticity, QoL, inflammation
Faradic currents		X		X		Functional disability
Fizyoflug		X		X		
High-voltage electrical stimulation		X				
Hivamat		X		X	X	
Hyperbaric oxygen		X*				Lymph clearance, tissue softness, mobility, numbness, tightness, softness, RoM, QoL, insomnia
Kinetic Centura Lite		X				QoL
Linforoll		X				Tissue elasticity
Low-level laser		X		X*		RoM (mixed results)
LymphaTouch		X	X			Inflammation, stiffness, inflammation
Microwave therapy	X	X				Mobility
Neuroglide				X		Changes in lymphatic pulse frequencies
Pneumatic compression pump	X	X				Stiffness, lymph movement, elasticity, hospitalizations
RAGodoy		X	X			Venous blood return
Transcutaneous electrical acupoint stimulation		X*				Post-mastectomy swelling, abnormal upper limb sensations
Ultrasound		X		X		Softness, RoM, inflammation, joint stiffness, functional disability
Vacumed						Volume after microsurgery
Wii Fit						Balance

RoM = range of motion; QoL = quality of life; ADL = activities of daily living; WBC = white blood cells; GI = gastrointestinal;
* Edema includes reduction in limb size by either circumference or volume measurements; X* = mixed results

Don't throw the kitchen sink at your lymphedema. Instead, try new complementary therapies in a methodical way, one at a time, so you can be sure which treatments are working and which are not. I've developed a tool to make this process easier: the Lymphedema Journal, a convenient way to track your self-care, lymphedema and complementary therapies. It is available in different formats—for men or women, and daily or weekly—on Amazon; search for "Lymphedema Journals by Jean LaMantia."

Although I didn't discuss nutrition in this book, I am a big believer that your diet is a key complementary therapy, and I have lots of nutrition resources to help you, including:

- One-on-one virtual nutrition counseling
- Free and low-cost webinars
- Lymphedema Nutrition School Live program
- Lymphedema Nutrition School Self-Study program
- Lymphedema Nutrition for Health Professionals Self-Study Program
- CEUs for Professionals through PESI.com
- Lymphedema Teaching Tool Templates for Professionals
- *The Complete Lymphedema Management and Nutrition Guide*, 2nd edition

You can learn more about all of these options at my website: www.jeanlamantia.com.

Therapy Commonalities

As I was writing this book, I was thinking about what the complementary therapies have in common. In some cases, I've pointed similarities out in the write-ups. In terms of mechanism of action, most of the therapies seem to rely on one of twelve broad categories. If you are drawn to one therapy but feel you need to substitute another because of cost, accessibility or other reasons, the tables that follow may help you find an alternative that works with a similar mechanism of action. You may also want to design a plan that incorporates different mechanisms of action, and these tables can help you with that. I've included all the therapies except the ones that are no longer available and the Wii Fit, which stands alone as a balance device. Be sure to consult the chapter on each therapy for more details. There are several that would fit into more than one grouping, and you might choose to categorize them differently.

Aligning Qi	Anti-Inflammatory	Compression	Electrical Conductivity
Acupressure	Apple cider vinegar	Aqua therapy	BEMER
Acupuncture	Astragalus + peony	CVAC therapy	Dolphin Neurostim
Ai chi	Cabbage leaves	Dayspring	Faradic currents
Ayurveda	Castor oil	Hyperbaric oxygen	Grounding mats
Cupping	Escin	Neuroglide	High-voltage electrical stimulation
Electronic moxibustion	Ginger	Pneumatic compression pumps	Manutech BH
Lidong needle therapy	Hydroxytyrosol		Microcurrent therapy
Moxibustion	Linba Fang		Transcutaneous electrical acupoint stimulation
Qigong	Omega-3 fatty acids		
Tai chi	Procurcuma		
Traditional Chinese medicine	Robuvit		
Transcutaneous electrical acupoint stimulation	Selenium		
Tuina	Serrapeptase		
	Sulfuretin		
	Synbiotics		
	Vitamin D		
	Wobenzym N		

Heat	Mechanical Action	Mind-Body Connection	Negative Pressure
Balneotherapy	Dry brushing	Art therapy	Cupping
Chinese heat therapy	Dry needling	Circle of Healing	LymphaTouch
CO_2 laser	Endermologie	Deep breathing	Taping
Electric blanket	Foam roller	Essential oils	Vacumed
Far-infrared sauna	Linforoll	Homeopathy	
Fizyoflug	Pilates	Hypnosis	
Low-level laser	Pyro-drive jet injector	Meditation	
Microwave therapy	Rebounding	Music therapy	
Wenyang Huoxue compress	Reflexology	Progressive muscle relaxation	
	Scar therapy	Qigong	
		Stress reduction	
		Tai chi	
		Visualization	
		Yoga	

Passive Movement	Reduced Vessel Permeability	Sound Waves	Vibration
Chi Machine	Benzopyrones	Extracorporeal shock wave therapy	Far-infrared sauna
Kinetec Centura Lite	Coumarin	Ultrasound	Hivamat
RAGodoy	Cyclo 3 Fort		Music medicine
	Daflon 500		Singing bowls
	Garlive		Tuning fork
	Ginkor Fort		Ultrasound
	Goreisan		Vibration plate
	Linfadren		
	Meliven 3		
	Pycnogenol		
	Unguentum Lymphaticum		

Identifying Credible Sources

There are a lot of myths and misinformation about complementary therapies on the web and social media. Be sure you are getting credible information from credible practitioners. Here are some ways you can tell when a source is not credible:

- People misrepresent their credentials—for example, calling themselves "Doctor," with the implication that they are a medical doctor, when they are doctors of something other than medicine, such as chiropractors or PhDs. Trustworthy professionals will be transparent about their credentials.
- A certain protocol—a specific supplement or therapy—claims to be right for anyone with lymphedema. In my experience, the protocol should fit one's individual issues, goals and lifestyle.
- Statements such as "studies show" or "clinically proven" are not backed up by specific study citations (you can see that I was careful to cite every study in this book).
- Cited research is from animal studies, but that fact is not explicitly stated— for example, saying "studies show that this supplement reduced lymphedema volume" without specifying that the studies were done on animals, not humans.
- Research backing up a recommendation is from a completely different human population, but that fact is not explicitly stated—for example, the study was on people with edema due to liver disease, not lymphedema.

Listen to your "spidey sense": If something doesn't feel right and has you questioning it, then it's probably not credible. I know it can be confusing, especially when you hear the same information from multiple sources, but maintain a healthy dose of skepticism— if something sounds too good to be true, keep investigating.

Bottom Line on Complementary Therapies for Lymphedema

Continue with complete decongestive therapy and a healthy diet, and if you are using or planning to try a complementary therapy, communicate openly about it with your lymphedema therapist and health care team. You may also want to ask others with lymphedema and the professionals you work with for their anecdotal experiences with various therapies.

I researched therapies for this book month after month, study after study, in the hope that lymphedema patients and therapists will find value here, that my book will increase awareness of lymphedema and complementary therapies, and that researchers will be inspired to conduct more studies. By recommending this book to others, writing reviews and sharing your thoughts on social media, you can help me to spread the word to the lymphedema community about complementary therapy options, and I appreciate you very much for helping me with this goal. Thank you!

Glossary

Adjunctive, which means "added to something else as a supplement rather than an essential part," is another word for "complementary" that is often used in scientific literature.

Allopathic means modern evidence-based medical practice, also called standard, conventional, Western, mainstream or biomedicine.

Alternative therapy is done in place of, or as an alternative to, the standard therapy. It is not the same as complementary therapy, but people often use the terms interchangeably.

Blinding means a study participant or researcher does not know whether the patient is receiving the treatment or the placebo. It is done to prevent bias. *See also* Double blinding.

CAM, which stands for "complementary and alternative medicine," is a popular term in oncology. CAM therapy includes unconventional treatments done either in addition to or instead of standard care.

Complete decongestive therapy (CDT) is the gold standard of treatment for lymphedema—the allopathic therapy. It consists of four parts: compression, manual lymphatic drainage, skin care and exercise.

Contraindications are conditions that make a therapy inappropriate. For example, using a pneumatic pump is contraindicated (not recommended) when you have an active infection.

Control group is the set of participants in a study that don't receive the treatment. Their results are compared against the treatment group's results at the end of the study.

Controlled trial is a type of scientific study that compares the effects of different treatments on groups of people to determine whether a treatment is safe and effective.

Complementary therapy is done in addition to, or as a complement to, standard therapy.

Conservative treatment means the focus is on preventing a condition from getting worse. In lymphedema research, the term is often used to mean complete decongestive therapy.

Distal means farther from the center of the body; it is used as a comparative in conjunction with "proximal." If a therapy is applied on a limb "from distal to proximal," it means from the fingers to the shoulder or from the toes to the hip.

Double blinding means neither the evaluator/researcher nor the study participant knows whether they are getting the treatment or the control or placebo. It is done to reduce bias.

Dysesthesias is a sensory experience in which the skin feels painful or unusual.

Erysipelas is a bacterial skin infection usually caused by group A streptococcus bacteria. It affects the dermis (middle) layer of skin and may also extend to the superficial lymphatics.

Holistic is a form of healing that considers the whole person—body, mind, spirit and emotions—in the quest for optimal health and wellness.

Integrative health aims to bring conventional and alternative therapies together by using a well-coordinated multidisciplinary team to treat the patient. Usually, the professionals practice within the same institution to make sharing information easier.

Integrative therapies is another term for "holistic therapies"—those that consider the whole person and often combine conventional and complementary approaches.

Lymphangitis, a contraction of "lymph," "angio" and "itis," means inflammation of the lymphatic vessels.

Lymphoscintigraphy is a procedure that provides images of the lymphatic system. It begins with the injection of the radioactive isotope Technetium-99m, then special gamma cameras are used to show the movement of the lymphatic fluid. The rate of movement can be measured and expressed as the flow rate.

Manual lymphatic drainage (MLD) is a hands-on gentle skin stretching technique done by a certified lymphedema therapist to move lymphatic fluid. When you perform MLD on your own body, it is called self-MLD.

Meta-analysis is a type of research that involves gathering all of the studies on a specific treatment, then analyzing the data to determine the overall effect of the treatment. It can be considered a "study of studies."

Nonsignificant means that the difference in outcome between the treatment and control groups is not statistically significant, and the results could have occurred by chance rather than due to the efficacy of the treatment.

Phlebolymphedema is lymphedema that develops as a result of venous insufficiency. It is the most common cause of leg lymphedema.

Pilot study is usually the first study of a particular therapy. Pilot studies are often small and lack blinding. They are done to test whether it is worthwhile to move forward with larger, more well-designed studies.

Placebo is a substitute that looks just like the real treatment but has no medical effect. In the case of a supplement, the placebo might be a look-alike sugar pill.

Placebo-controlled means a study uses a placebo for the control group. If everyone in the study receives the test treatment, it is more difficult to gauge what the treatment's true effects are.

Proximal means closer to the center of the body; it is used as a comparative in conjunction with "distal."

Pruritus means itchiness. For example, Olivamine-based skin care products were tested to see if they could help with pruritus secondary to lymphedema.

Random, or randomly assigned, means neither the researchers nor the participants choose who receives the treatment and who doesn't. It is done to reduce bias.

Self-MLD. *See* Manual lymphatic drainage (MLD).

Significant, or statistically significant, means that the difference in outcome between the treatment and control groups is sizable enough that it cannot be due to chance, and the treatment demonstrates efficacy. Statistical significance is dependent on a large enough sample size.

Stemmer sign is a simple, validated test to help diagnose lymphedema. It is done by using your thumb and index finger to try to pinch and tent the skin at the base of the second toe or finger. The inability to do so is a positive Stemmer sign that indicates lymphedema may be present.

Systematic review is a research process in which the researcher defines their search engines, search terms and criteria, then carefully selects all the published research that meet the criteria so that results can be examined from a broad view. A systematic review can be followed by a meta-analysis.

Tissue induration means hardening or thickening of the skin. If a study reports improvements in tissue induration, that means the treatment softened the skin.

Traditional medicine, also called traditional and complementary medicine, is an approach to health and healing based on indigenous cultural models, such as traditional Chinese medicine or Ayurveda, that predate contemporary biomedicine.

Whole person health means helping individuals, families, communities and populations to improve and restore their health in multiple interconnected domains—biological, behavioral, social and environmental—rather than just treating a disease.

Acknowledgments

First, I want to thank the researchers and all those who volunteer to be part of research protocols. Without you, this book would be nothing. Collectively, we are moving forward to a better quality of life for people with lymphedema.

I started researching complementary therapies as one of the modules for a program I created called Lymphedema Nutrition for Health Professionals. That expanded to a three-part course on twenty complementary therapies. From there, I thought I would write a book about those twenty therapies. But when I pored through the research to make sure I had covered all the options, what I found surprised me: There is so much out there! And the more I uncovered, the more convinced I became that there is still even more to discover.

Thank you to my good friend Linda Kelemen, DrPH. I'm so glad we met early in our careers as dietitians. I'm grateful for your support over the years, and I'm so impressed with your academic excellence.

Thank you to Kerry Upson, an excellent proofreader and sounding board, who told me readers would find value in this book and encouraged me to keep going!

Thank you to my students at Lymphedema Nutrition School who are willing to test the crazy ideas I present to them and report back to me with their findings. Together we've found some real winners, and your feedback enables me to guide the students and clients who come after you.

To my survey respondents, thanks for taking the time out of your day to complete my survey and share your experiences with the different therapies. Your lived experience is very valuable to my readers.

To Nesreen Hajjar, who created a beautiful book cover that I am very proud of. Your design skills have no limits!

Thanks to Sue Sumeraj, my go-to editor since my first book. Your eagle eye and attention to the most minute details give me confidence that this book is a professional work.

To my kids, who are used to me being on my laptop all evening and weekend and don't complain. I hope your mom makes you proud.

This is my first venture in self-publishing a book, having previously worked with publishers. It's a real leap of faith to believe in oneself this way, and I'm grateful to my family for giving me the courage to do it.

To all my readers, I hope this book provides inspiration, sparks ideas and may even encourage you to either conduct or participate in new research that will help us find safe, cost-effective and helpful complementary therapies for lymphedema.

Index

negative pressure therapies, 287. *See also specific therapies*
Neuroglide, 255–56, 278, 285, 287
nutrition, ix–x, 286

O

olive pomace. *See* hydroxytyrosol
omega-3 fatty acids, 154–56, 189, 287
onion extract, 104
osteoarthritis, 28–29, 169, 183–85, 244
oxygen (hyperbaric), 233–37, 277, 285, 287

P

pain reduction, 17, 284–85
passive movement therapies, 287. *See also specific therapies*
peony, 121–22, 187, 284, 287
phlebolymphedema, 136, 142, 259
Pilates, 93–94, 113, 284, 287
placebo effect, 146
pneumatic compression pumps, 256–61, 278, 285, 287
prebiotics/probiotics. *See* synbiotics
Procurcuma, 157–58, 189, 287
progressive muscle relaxation, 95–96, 113, 284, 287
Pycnogenol, 158–60, 189, 287
pyro-drive jet injectors, 96–98, 113, 287

Q

qi alignment therapies, 287. *See also specific therapies*
qigong, 48–49, 68, 284, 287

R

RAGodoy, 209–210, 261–62, 278, 285, 287
rebounding, 85, 95, 98–100, 113, 287
reduced vessel permeability therapies, 287. *See also specific therapies*
reflexology, 100–102, 113, 284, 287
relaxation techniques, 95–96, 113, 284, 287
Robuvit, 160–62, 189, 284, 287

S

sauna, far-infrared (FIR), 218–22, 276, 285, 287
scar therapy, 33, 102–106, 113, 100, 287
selenium, 162–68, 189, 284, 287
serrapeptase (serratiopeptidase), 132, 169–72, 189, 287
silicone gel, 102–105
singing bowls, 51–51, 68, 254, 287

skin conditions, 21–22
sound-wave therapies, 287. *See also specific therapies*
stress reduction, 95–96, 106–1, 113, 284, 287 *See also specific methods*
sulfuretin, 172–73, 189, 287
supplements. *See* natural health products
synbiotics, 174–78, 189, 284, 287

T

tai chi, 52–53, 69, 287
tape
    athletic (Kinesio), 108-10, 113, 284, 287
    microporous (paper), 104
traditional Chinese medicine (TCM), 54–55, 69, 284. *See also specific remedies*
traditional therapies, 13–69. *See also specific therapies*
    summary, 66–69
trampolines. *See* rebounding
transcutaneous electrical acupoint stimulation (TEAS), 262–64, 278, 285, 287
Transponder, 254–65, 279
trolamine, 104
tuina, 56–57, 69, 284
tuning forks, 110–11, 113, 287
turmeric, 134, 149. *See also* Procurcuma

U

ultrasound, 265–68, 279, 285, 287
Unguentum Lymphaticum, 178–80, 190, 284, 287

V

Vacumed, 269–70, 279, 285, 287
vibration plates, 260, 270–72, 279, 287
vibration therapies, 287. *See also specific therapies*
visualization, 57–59, 69, 287
vitamin D, 180–83, 190, 287

W

weight loss, 20
Wenyang Huoxue (WYHX) compress, 59–61, 69, 284, 287
Wii Fit, 272–73, 279, 285
Wobenzym N, 183–85, 190, 284, 287
wound healing, 33. *See also* scars

Y

yoga, 39, 61–66, 69, 284

www.ingramcontent.com/pod-product-compliance
Lightning Source LLC
Chambersburg PA
CBHW081804200326
41597CB00023B/4145